THE HISTORY OF SURGERY
IN THE UNITED STATES
1775–1900

VOLUME 1

Textbooks, Monographs,

and Treatises

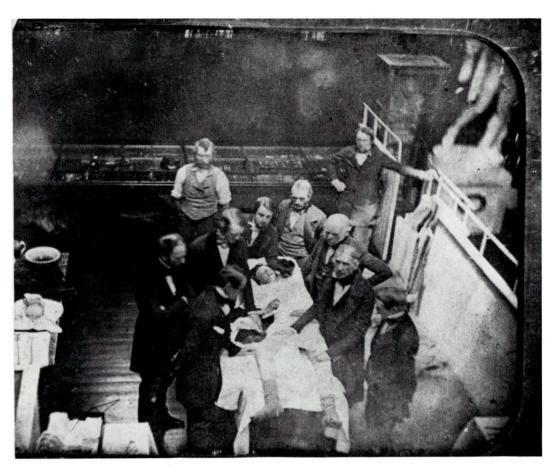

The first operation using ether as an anesthetic, at Massachusetts General Hospital on October 16, 1846. Facing the camera on the right is John Collins Warren, who performed the surgery. In the foreground on the left is Henry Jacob Bigelow who announced the discovery to the world in his scientific paper "Insensibility during surgical operations produced by inhalation" (*Boston medical & surgical journal* XXXV, {1846–47} 309– 17, 379–82).

The reproduction is from an early twentieth-century copy print of an original daguerreotype by Southworth and Hawes. Actually the photograph was posed sometime after the original operation because photographer Josiah H. Hawes was so unnerved at the sight of blood during the first operation on October 16 that he left the scene before taking any photographs. By the time this photograph was taken the team was administering ether with a sponge rather than with the glass flask originally used. (Courtesy of Stanley B. Burns, M.D. and the Burns Archive.)

THE HISTORY OF SURGERY
IN THE UNITED STATES
1775–1900

VOLUME 1

Textbooks, Monographs,

and Treatises

by

IRA M. RUTKOW, M.D.

Norman Publishing

San Francisco

1988

Copyright © 1988 by Ira M. Rutkow

Published by Norman Publishing
Division of Jeremy Norman & Co., Inc.
442 Post Street
San Francisco, California 94102–1579

Library of Congress Cataloging-in-Publication Data

Rutkow, Ira M.

The history of surgery in the United States, 1775–1900.

(Norman bibliography series ; no. 2) (Norman surgery series ; no. 2)
Includes index.
Contents: v. 1. Textbooks, monographs, and treatises.
1. Surgery—United States—History—Bibliography.
I. Title. II. Series: Norman bibliography series ; 2. III. Series: Norman surgery series ;
no. 2. [DNLM:1. Surgery—history—United States. WO 11 AA1 R9h] Z6666.R87 1988
016.617′0973   87-62662

[RD27.3.U]

ISBN 0–930405–02–1 (v.1)

Ira M. Rutkow, 1948–

The photographs in this book come from the collection of the author with the following exceptions: The frontispiece and jacket photograph is reprinted courtesy of Stanley B. Burns, M.D. and the Burns Archive. Figs. 85–86 come from the collection of Jeremy Norman & Co., Inc. Figs. 20–27, 52, 54, 55, 61, 64, 70, 77, and 121 have been reproduced courtesy of the Historical Collections of the Library, College of Physicians of Philadelphia.

Norman Bibliography Series, No. 2

Norman Surgery Series, No. 2

This book is printed on acid-free paper, and its binding materials have been chosen for strength and durability.

Manufactured in the United States of America.

Contents

Illustrations

Foreword

Only the man who is familiar with the art and science of the past is competent to aid in its progress in the future.

— THEODOR BILLROTH

In this admirable treatise Ira Rutkow has assembled an astonishing collection of surgical literature and biographical data. In a prodigious and extremely important study, he has compiled for the first time a list of every book, monograph, or treatise written by an American surgeon from the Revolution to the beginning of the twentieth century. This work provides an unexcelled source of information about American surgical literature of the eighteenth and nineteenth centuries. More than one hundred illustrations, each carefully selected and remarkably well reproduced, are included in the work. The author has identified 552 individual works from this formative era of American surgery. Of the total, 197 are in the field of general surgery, 86 in ophthalmology, 75 in otorhinolaryngology, 61 in orthopedics, 58 in gynecology, 47 in genitourinary surgery, 22 in colon and rectal surgery, and 6 were devoted to neurological surgery. The annotated bibliography is in itself quite praiseworthy, presenting as it does a brief summary of each work and a biographical sketch of its author.

The initial entry describes the text of John Jones (1729–91), the first surgical work written by an American and printed in North America. Jones was a respected surgeon reputed to have been among the first American lithotomists, and his book became the accepted guide to surgical practice during the Revolutionary War. Jones later became professor of surgery at the newly created Medical School of King's College, now Columbia University. He was also known for his role as the founder of the New York Hospital and later the College of Physicians in Philadelphia. The author provides a detailed description of this special work and its impact on surgical practice in the latter part of the eighteenth century.

The contributions of John Syng Dorsey (1783–1818) also receive special attention. Syng's *Elements of surgery: for the use of students* was the first systematic treatise on surgery authored by an American. The book appeared in 1813 and was followed by a second edition in 1818. Dorsey was the nephew of Philip Syng Physick (1768–1837), who held the chair in surgery at the University of Pennsylvania. Since Physick was not a good writer, he asked his nephew to organize his teachings in the form of a surgical handbook. The result was a 72-chapter text entitled *Elements of surgery*. Dorsey held the chair of materia medica (1816) and of anatomy (1818) at the University of Pennsylvania. He also performed the first successful ligation of the external iliac artery in America; an excellent illustration of this procedure is reproduced in the text.

Quite appropriately, the classic work *Experiments and observations on the gastric juice and physiology of digestion* by William Beaumont (1785–1853) is reviewed with a concise description of this historic contribution, including the experiments performed on Alexis St. Martin, the French Canadian hunter who had sustained a shotgun wound of the upper abdomen and developed a chronic gastric fistula which opened widely onto the abdominal wall. A wood engraving from Beaumont's work showing the prolapsed gastric mucosa of this fistula is reproduced in the text. This work is one of the best-known of all the early American surgical classics and was internationally recognized. A German edition was published in 1834 and a British edition in 1838.

Rutkow describes in detail the surgical master John Collins Warren (1778–1856) and his *Surgical observations on tumours, with cases and operations*. This text is one of the great classics of American medicine and is considered to be Warren's best. An important figure in early American surgery, Warren was professor of anatomy and surgery at Harvard and a surgeon at Massachusetts General Hospital. This text contains sixteen hand-colored plates by David Claypoole Johnston and is divided into fourteen sections describing the characteristics of a variety of tumors.

Rutkow gives considerable attention to Samuel David Gross (1805–84) and his important text *Elements of pathological anatomy*. The founder of both the American Medical Association and the American Surgical Association, Gross was an extraordinary figure, widely known and respected. Gross's work is divided into two parts, one devoted to general principles of pathological anatomy and the other a special pathological anatomy section of twenty-seven chapters on specific organs. This admirable work contains ninety-seven wood engravings and five color plates. Gross later described this work and its background in his autobiography:

> It was from dissections, from an elaborate course of reading, and from numerous visits to pork and slaughter houses of Cincinnati that I derived the knowledge upon which I founded my work on Pathological Anatomy, issued in 1839, in two octavo volumes of more than five hundred pages each. The work was illustrated by numerous wood-cuts and several colored engravings . . . . As far as I know mine was the first attempt ever made in this country, or indeed, in the English language, to systematize the subject and to place it in a connected form before the profession.

Rutkow reviews several other key contributors to surgical science in the latter half of the nineteenth century, including Keen, Nancrede, Deaver, Crile, DaCosta, Cheever, Senn, Park, and Lewis Atterbury Stimson, the noted professor of surgery at Columbia University. Attention is also given to Pilcher, the first editor of the *Annals of surgery*, who held this post for fifty years.

The history of surgery in the United States, 1775–1900 is a masterwork that is splendidly written and illustrated. It undoubtedly will become one of the most frequently cited texts in future references to this period of American surgery. Moreover, those familiar with the publisher will recognize the high quality of production in this special work, including a striking excellence in reproduction of the classic illustrations from the original texts. Ira Rutkow's work will be sought and read by surgical academicians and by thoughtful surgeons at large who seek a complete and meaningful description of the development of American surgery from the Revolution to the beginning of the twentieth century.

David C. Sabiston, Jr., M.D.
James B. Duke Professor of Surgery
and Chairman of the Department
Duke University Medical Center
February 1988

Introduction

The history of surgery in the United States, 1775–1900, Volume 1: textbooks, monographs, and treatises is intended to be a comprehensive record of all books relating to the early clinical development of surgery in the United States. It may be looked on as a close relative of Francisco Guerra's *American medical bibliography, 1639–1783,* Robert B. Austin's *Early American medical imprints: a guide to works printed in the United States, 1668–1820,* and Francesco Cordasco's *American medical imprints, 1820–1910.* However, unlike these volumes, the present one is limited to works written by surgeons living in the United States.

The genesis of this project lies in the problems I encountered in attempting to study the history of American surgery. To trace the evolution of what I do as a surgeon and to understand it from a historical perspective has long been one of my intellectual goals. As a medical student in St. Louis and a surgical resident in Boston, Baltimore, and Newark, I was intrigued to learn about surgical history. I have always been fascinated by the stories my fellow surgeons tell about their predecessors and their discussions of events in the history of surgery. However, it seemed odd that few of these vignettes were ever about eighteenth- or nineteenth-century American surgeons. Was it that my mentors and colleagues ignored their surgical ancestors in the United States or simply that they knew little about them?

As my historical interests focused on American surgery I began to do research on the subject and to collect original editions of American surgical works. I became acquainted with a body of literature which was surprising in its originality and sometimes possessed of a crude eloquence. However, my initial research was frustrated by the lack of histories of American surgery. It was evident that the general history of surgery in our country had been poorly served by historians. For various reasons, neither surgeons nor historians have done much research on the development of surgery in America. As a result, most articles on American surgical history in clinical journals represent little more than a regurgitation of previous papers. Certainly, the few books written about surgery in the United States have been half-hearted and mediocre endeavors to understand a rather broad subject.

I was disappointed in my attempts to learn about the social, economic, and political forces which contributed to the evolution of American surgery, but my greatest frustration came in attempting to collect American surgical textbooks, monographs, and treatises published before World War I. I often found it impossible to obtain information on many of the items I acquired. More important, I was unable to find a definitive source of information to guide me in building such a collection.

As I became familiar with the existing books and papers on surgical history, I realized that the ingenuity and boldness with which early American surgeons approached seemingly unsolvable surgical problems was a stirring but largely unrecognized chapter in medical history. It was obvious to me that a definitive history of American surgery needed to be written.

I believe that to truly understand a country's surgical past, a researcher must first be familiar with three specific areas. These are (1) primary textbooks, monographs, and treatises relating to the surgical sciences; (2) articles written by surgeons for medical periodicals, including separately printed pamphlets; and (3) biographical information about the numerous individuals who wrote works on surgery. With this core of knowledge, it is possible to write a narrative history of American surgery.

Unfortunately, none of these areas has ever been adequately researched. Thus, the study of our country's surgical past is an especially difficult—and important—task. Before the present work there were no bibliographies of eighteenth- and nineteenth-century American surgical texts. In addition, before the beginning of the twentieth century, almost every major American city had its own medical journal. Most of these journals are no longer in existence, and copies of some cannot be found.

To understand a surgeon's role in advancing the art of surgery, it is often necessary to know the story of his life's work. But the task of writing a history of American surgery is made even more difficult by the fact that as late as 1876 there was considerable confusion in determining who was and who was not a surgeon. Samuel David Gross (1805–84) in his memorable article on the history of American surgery (*American journal of the medical sciences* 71:431–84, 1876) pointed out this problem at the time:

> There are, strange to say, as a separate and distinct class of surgeons, no such persons among us. It is safe to affirm that there is not a medical man on this continent who devotes himself exclusively to the practice of surgery.

To make matters worse, it is extremely difficult to find biographical data on many of the lesser known eighteenth- and nineteenth-century American physicians.

The confusion and lack of concise information about our country's surgical past ultimately presented a challenge I could not resist. W. B. Saunders Company asked me to serve as editor for the seventy-fifth anniversary issue of the *Surgical clinics of North America* (published in December 1987). While establishing the parameters for this volume, I decided to prepare a chronological short-title list of American textbooks, monographs, and treatises relating to the surgical sciences for the years 1775 to 1900.

My research began in the spring of 1986. By January 1987 I had found 540 individual works to be listed. Most of the titles were obtained from three sources: previously written bibliographies; the Index Catalogue of the Library of the Surgeon-General's Office; and the Historical Collections of the Library of the College of Physicians of Philadelphia. I also contacted the National Library of Medicine, the New York Academy of Medicine, and the Countway Library. Finally, rare book dealers were helpful in providing information about obscure titles.

After preparing the text I wrote a short note to Jeremy Norman seeking his expertise and advice regarding my research. He wrote back (January 9, 1987):

> What a treat to receive your bibliographical essay on reference books concerning the history of American surgery together with the chronological bibliography! . . . If you would consider writing a sentence or two annotating each entry I would be interested in publishing the bibliography as a monograph. This could be an intermediate step on the way to writing your definitive history. The bibliography could also be enhanced with illustrations and attractively printed . . . . The notes could be as long or short as you would be interested in writing. Such a bibliography would appeal to a wide audience of book collectors, librarians, surgeons, and historians . . . . Let me know your thoughts.

Jeremy Norman's letter was all the coaxing I needed to write the book you have before you. I began the project in February and completed the entire manuscript a few days before Thanksgiving 1987.

This volume is planned as the first of four volumes which will record the history of surgery in the United States from 1775 to 1900. Volume II will encompass all articles in periodicals as well as separately published pamphlets from 1797 to 1900. In-depth biographies of all the authors covered in the first two volumes will constitute Volume III. Volume IV will present a detailed narrative history of American surgery, describing not only the development of clinical medicine but also the social, political, and economic forces which helped mold this country's early practice of surgery. These volumes will be written and published consecutively.

Because the present volume is the first such compilation ever attempted, a few clarifications are in order. Before World War I, it was not uncommon for journal articles to be longer than 100 pages. In many instances, these articles were then separately paginated and published as monographs. Such articles, or in today's terms *offprints* or *reprints*, have generally been excluded from my bibliography. Accordingly, most items in the list are either first editions of a textbook or the initial printing of a treatise or monograph. In some instances, a collection of journal articles relating to a particular topic was published in book form, and these works have been included. I have included a few works that are under fifty pages long because of their importance to the development of surgery. Most published manuscripts (i.e., those not initially printed in a journal) less than fifty pages long have been excluded. These smaller works were usually case reports and tended not to have a major impact on the course of American surgery.

The most perplexing problem I had during the research was trying to determine if a particular surgeon was from the United States. Unfortunately, none of the previously written bibliographies on early American imprints make that distinction. I have not included books translated by an American surgeon from a foreign-language work or British texts edited and updated by Americans. In the entry for each work I have included a short biography of the author and a description of the his post-1900 surgical works. In addition, I have listed all non-surgical and other non-clinical texts (i.e., literary works, autobiographies, etc.).

I have made a conscious decision not to include information about the library location of individual books. My intent in compiling this bibliography is to create a work that hopefully will be useful indefinitely. Libraries frequently misplace or lose books, and there is no guarantee that the present library locations of books in this bibliography will be valid years from now. While doing the research for this volume I was often frustrated by the inaccuracy of information about book locations in previous bibliographies.

In addition, it proved an arduous task to find certain birth and death dates. Some of the authors are unknown, and in these cases I have noted the lack of information with question marks. In a number of the specialties, there was particular difficulty in determining which works should be listed. Within general surgery, I have included anatomy texts and works on anesthesia written by surgeons. Ophthalmology has been construed to include works by both ophthalmologists and opticians, mainly because prior to the twentieth century there was considerable confusion in the public mind regarding the difference between the two types of practice. For otorhinolaryngology, I have included items which do not necessarily deal with surgical problems (i.e., auralists, laryngologists, etc.) but which illustrate the growth of the specialty. The section on urology includes works on venereal diseases by surgeons. Finally, the most difficult decisions concerned gynecology. I excluded general obstetrical works and those on midwifery but included those on uterine surgery. However, some textbooks tended to combine information about obstetrical and gynecological problems. These have been included, as were volumes which dealt strictly with medical gynecology. Because little is known about them, I have given special attention to the listing of texts written by homeopathic and eclectic surgeons.

I have personally examined all of the texts except three. They are OT10 (Knapp), OT18 (Bosworth), and OP59 (Buffum). After extensive searching I have been unable to locate them. However, they are known to have once existed, since all are listed in the Index Catalogue of the Library of the Surgeon-General's Office or in other publications.

Many of the illustrations are from books in my own collection. I have chosen them as representative of the various types of illustration found in eighteenth- and nineteenth-century American medical publications. Some are literally works of art by distinguished artists. Others are nothing more than crude engravings or woodcuts.

This annotated bibliography is intended to be as comprehensive as possible; however its true completeness will only be judged over the course of time. I look forward to receiving corrections, additions, or other information. This volume represents the better part of my waking existence for the past two years. It is my hope that along with the future volumes of the *History of surgery in the United States* it will stimulate the study of the history of American surgery.

Ira M. Rutkow, M.D., M.P.H., Dr.P.H.
Marlboro, New Jersey

February 1988

Acknowledgments

This work could not have been accomplished without the support of my family. They have tolerated a rather desultory writing schedule, made especially difficult by my clinical surgical practice. To my wife, Beth, and our children, Lainie and Eric, I dedicate this project. You provide all that a husband and father could possibly ask. Your love, patience, and encouragement were vital to the entire enterprise. Nor can I forget my parents, Bea and Al Rutkow. You taught me how important an education is.

I owe special debts of gratitude to many people. Jill Rotenberg, Manager of Norman Publishing, deserves commendation for her editorial guidance. Thomas Horrocks and his staff at the Historical Collections of the Library of the College of Physicians of Philadelphia gave valuable assistance in gathering the research material. To Robin Siegel, librarian at the Freehold Area Hospital, goes a special thank you for helping to locate many of the rare volumes.

I am indebted to Drs. David Sabiston, Jr. and Gert Brieger, for graciously preparing a foreword and a preface, respectively, to this work. Their perspectives, from both a surgeon's and historian's viewpoint, are very important. Finally, I must publicly acknowledge the vital role that Jeremy Norman played in stimulating me to actually undertake this endeavor. Without his persuasion and patronage it is unlikely that it would ever have been completed.

Ira M. Rutkow, M.D.

Preface

The study of the history of surgery in America, as is true for the history of medicine in general, is slowly but surely growing in size and scope as well as in sophistication. We are beginning to approach a better understanding of the culture of surgery and of surgeons in the varying periods of our past. It is no longer sufficient to describe simply who did what first. We are beginning to ask better questions, questions that range from the economic circumstances of the practitioners and their patients to the nature of the creation of new surgical knowledge and its acceptance and use.

Our research must continue to dig deeply in many sources, manuscripts as well as printed ones. All of us who wish to write about surgical history depend on access to these sources. One form of access continues to be bibliographic compilations such as this array of books in general surgery and the surgical specialties published by American authors between 1775 and 1900. It is safe to say that no existing biographical dictionary, and certainly no history of surgery, contains as much information about these books and their authors as Dr. Rutkow has managed to pull together in one convenient volume.

As recently as 1954, Dr. Estelle Brodman in her now classic history of medical bibliography could still write that her field was

> . . . groping in the dark for techniques which will allow it to do successfully what it has been so painfully and incompletely doing since its very beginning: namely to cover the entire medical literature, in whatever form, wherever published, and in whatever language, and to cover it accurately, promptly, and in easily usable form. Each time medical bibliography has reached the point where it seemed to have gained mastery over the literature, the literature has grown in size or changed in form . . . .

The purposes of bibliography are many, and in this day of ever more rapid growth in medical knowledge, the number of publications necessary to contain it has grown apace. Dr. Rutkow has provided in this volume a list of published works that anyone who wishes to study the history of surgery in this country must know about and use.

Gert H. Brieger, M.D.
William H. Welch Professor
of the History of Medicine
The Johns Hopkins University
School of Medicine
February 1988

I. GENERAL SURGERY

GS1. JOHN JONES (1729–91). *Plain concise practical remarks on the treatment of wounds and fractures; to which is added, a short appendix on camp and military hospitals; principally designed for the use of young military surgeons in North America.* 92pp. New York: John Holt, 1775. [G-M 2155]

The first surgical work written by an American and printed in North America, the *Remarks* was the accepted guide to surgical practice during the Revolutionary War. Jones was well known as a surgeon and is said to have been among the first American lithotomists. In 1767, he was named professor of surgery and obstetrics in the newly created medical school of King's College in New York. He was also a founder of the New York Hospital and later the College of Physicians of Philadelphia. The *Remarks* is exceptionally rare because few were printed and most copies were used as field manuals by the Continental Army. It provides little more than a condensation of the teachings of Percival Pott (1713–88), Henri-François LeDran (1685–1770), and other European surgeons, most of whom Jones had studied with in 1751. Jones writes in the preface:

> The present calamitous situation of this once happy country, in a peculiar manner, demands the aid and assistance of every virtuous citizen; and though few men are possessed of those superior talents, which are requisite, to heal such mighty evils as now threaten the whole body politic with ruin and desolation; yet, every man has it in his power to contribute something towards so desireable an end; and if he cannot cure the fatal diseases of this unfortunate country, it will, at least, afford him some consolation, to have poured a little balm into her bleeding wounds. Influenced by these motives, I have endeavoured to select the sentiments of the best modern surgeons upon the treatment of those accidents, which are most likely to attend our present unnatural contest . . . .

Within the text are two major notes of originality. On pages 59–60, Jones describes a successful case of trephining for delirium eighty days following a head injury. The second case (pages 68–69) involved a fourteen-year-old boy who sustained a fracture of the parietal bone. Following trephination, there were repeated problems with cerebral swelling which forced tissue through the wound. Three times the swelling was ligated at its base with eventual sloughing. The youngster died, and autopsy demonstrated destruction of the entire left lobe of the cerebellum and conversion of half the right lobe into pus. The first edition is dedicated to Thomas Cadwalader (1708–79) and consists of ten chapters: "Wounds in general"; "Inflammation"; "Division of wounds"; "Penetrating wounds of the thorax and abdomen"; "Simple fractures of the limbs"; "Compound fractures"; "Amputation"; "Blows on the head"; "Injuries arising from concussion or commotion"; "Injuries arising from a fracture of the skull"; and "Gunshot wounds." There are no figures or plates. The appendix, "Structure and oeconomy of hospitals," is drawn almost entirely from John Pringle's (1707–82) well-known work, *Observations on the diseases of the army*.

A second edition of the *Remarks* appeared in Philadelphia in 1776, soon followed by a slightly modified version in which the new publisher, Robert Bell, placed an additional page of medical book advertisements.

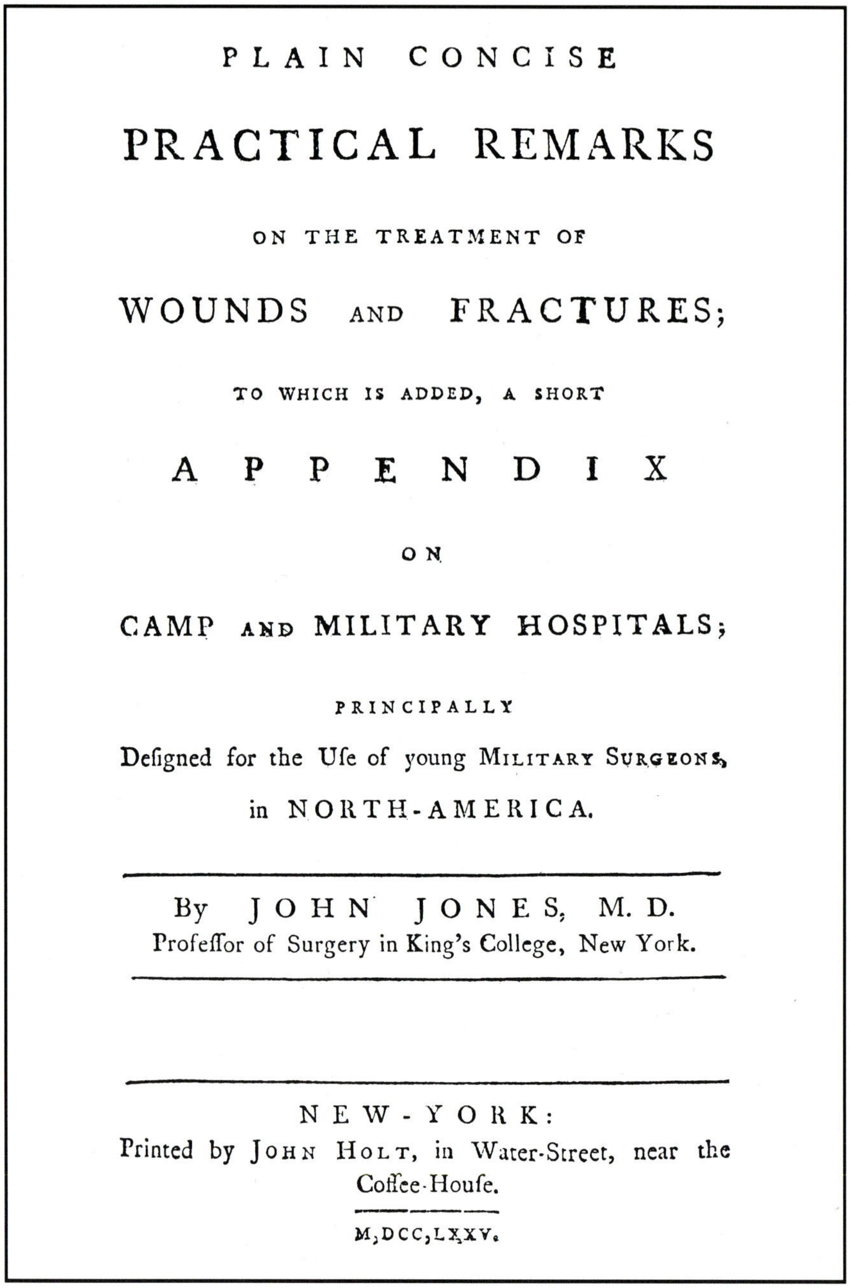

PLAIN CONCISE

PRACTICAL REMARKS

ON THE TREATMENT OF

WOUNDS AND FRACTURES;

TO WHICH IS ADDED, A SHORT

APPENDIX

ON

CAMP AND MILITARY HOSPITALS;

PRINCIPALLY

Defigned for the Ufe of young MILITARY SURGEONS, in NORTH-AMERICA.

By JOHN JONES, M. D.
Profeffor of Surgery in King's College, New York.

NEW-YORK:
Printed by JOHN HOLT, in Water-Street, near the Coffee-Houfe.

M,DCC,LXXV.

Fig. 1. (GS1) The title page from the first surgical treatise written by a surgeon in the United States. There are less than a dozen known copies of the 1775 first edition.

The second edition and its modification are notable in that they are usually found bound with Gerard van Swieten's (1700–72) *The diseases incident to armies*. This unusual binding arrangement must have occurred because Bell was the printer of both works and Jones was the translator of van Swieten's book. The third and final edition was printed in 1795 under the title *The surgical works of the late John Jones*, and included a short account of his life. Two minor works were also added: "Case of anthrax" (pages 173–77); and "Uncommon case of hydrocele" (pages 179–81). The original New York edition was reprinted in facsimile by the Society of the New York Hospital in 1871 in honor of its centennial celebration.

GS2. **VALENTINE SEAMAN** (1770–1817). *Pharmacoepia [sic] chirurgica in usum Nosocomii Novi Eboracencis. Being an account of the applications and formulae of the remedies employed in the clinical practice of the surgical department of the New-York Hospital.* 47pp. New York: Samuel Wood, 1811.

Interleaved with blank pages, this is the earliest known formulary for a civilian hospital in the United States. Seaman was on the medical staff of the New York Hospital at the time of its publication. He introduced vaccination for smallpox in New York City, but argued that yellow fever was not contagious. The *Pharmacoepia* has been described in *Drug intelligence and clinical pharmacy* 6:425–34, 1972. Seaman's other medical books consisted of *A dissertation on the mineral waters of Saratoga* (New York: Samuel Campbell, 1793); *An account of the epidemic of yellow fever, as it appeared in the city of New-York in the year 1795* (New York: Hopkins & Webb, 1796); the first American textbook on midwifery, *The midwives monitor, and mothers mirror: being three concluding lectures of a course of instruction on midwifery* (New York: Isaac Collins, 1800); and *A discourse upon vaccination, or kine-pock inoculation* (New York: Samuel Wood, 1816).

GS3. **JOHN SYNG DORSEY** (1783–1818). *Elements of surgery: for the use of students.* 2 vols., 407pp. and 308pp. Philadelphia: Edward Parker & Kimber & Conrad, 1813.

The first systematic treatise on surgery authored by an American. A second edition was printed in 1818 but was largely a reprint of the first edition with additional footnotes, case histories, a new section on harelip, and an additional plate. A third edition with twenty-eight plates was printed in 1823 and a fourth in 1831. Dorsey's *Elements* was unique in many respects, although little of its contents were original to Dorsey. Dorsey was the nephew of Philip Syng Physick (1768–1837), who occupied the chair of surgery at the University of Pennsylvania. Unfortunately, Physick never became a competent writer. Physick therefore asked his nephew to organize his teachings in the form of a surgical handbook. The *Elements* has seventy-two chapters. They range from general remarks on accidental injuries and their effects (chapter 1) to schirrus and cancer (chapter 72). The twenty-five plates are of interest in that Dorsey drew and engraved numbers 1, 5, 6, 12, 17, 22, 23, and

25 himself. In some instances they were hand-colored. Dorsey writes in the preface:

> Numerous circumstances combine to render necessary an American Epitome of Practical Surgery . . . . An American, although he must labour under many disadvantages in the production of an elementary treatise, is in one respect better qualified for it than an European surgeon. He is,—at least he ought to be,—strictly impartial, and therefore adopts from all nations their respective improvements. Great Britain and France have been foremost in the cultivation of modern surgery, but their deficiency in philosophick courtesy and candour has in some instances greatly retarded its progress . . . . As the present

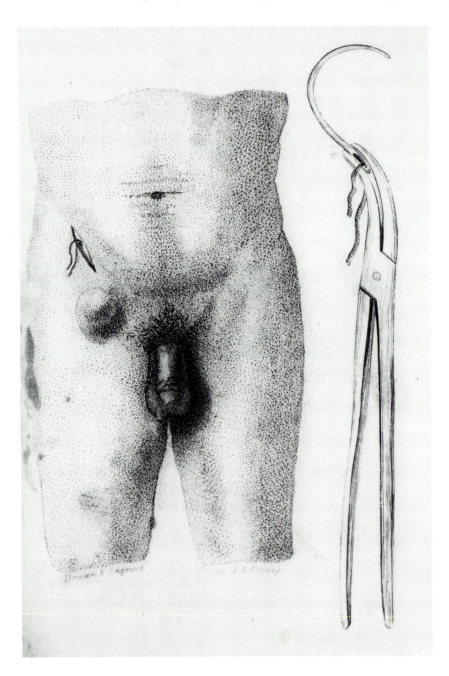

Fig. 2. (GS3) Dorsey performed the first successful ligation of the external iliac artery in America in 1811. This hand-colored plate, figure 23 on page 186 in volume 2, was drawn and engraved by Dorsey and depicts his patient and the instrument used to place the ligature.

work is intended chiefly for the use of students, it is to be considered in the light of a mere introduction to other surgical writers . . . .

Dorsey occupied the chairs of materia medica (1816) and anatomy (1818) at the University of Pennsylvania. He also performed the first successful ligation of the external iliac artery in America [G-M 2930].

GS4. **JAMES MANN** (1759–1832). *Medical sketches of the campaigns of 1812, 13, 14. To which are added, surgical cases, observations on military hospitals, and flying hospitals attached to a moving army.* 317pp. Dedham: H. Mann, 1816.

Mann was an army surgeon who served three years in the Revolution and another three years in the War of 1812. His chief writing was the *Sketches*, which gives probably the best and most vivid picture of early nineteenth-century American military life. The chapter on surgery (pages 206–33) is especially invaluable for its first-hand descriptions of the treatment of wounds. Interestingly, the initial five pages include Richard Willmott Hall's (1785–1847) translation of Dominique Jean Larrey's (1766–1842) *Memoirs of military surgery* (Baltimore: Joseph Cushing, 1814), specifically the section on amputations and gunshot wounds. Mann follows this translation with detailed discussions of amputations and treatment of their complications. Following the war, he became a consulting physician to the Massachusetts General Hospital, where he was among the first to successfully excise the elbow joint.

GS5. **WILLIAM ANDERSON** (?–?). *System of surgical anatomy. Part first; on the structure of the groin, pelvis, and perineum, as connected with inguinal and femoral hernia; tying the iliac arteries, and the operation of lithotomy.* 199pp. New York: J. V. Seaman, 1822.

Anderson was an English surgeon and anatomist who came to the United States in 1820. He settled in New York and lectured on surgical anatomy. The *Anatomy* is dedicated to Valentine Mott (1785–1865) and contains nine plates. The dedication reads:

> To Valentine Mott professor of surgery in the University of the State of New York, whose private life is to his credit as a man; whose liberal motives and honourable endeavors to improve his profession, are an example to his brethren, and whose acquirements in the several departments of scientific and practical surgery, are an honour to his country, this volume is presented in testimony of the esteem, respect, and friendship of the author.

Four of the nine plates were drawn by the celebrated engraver and landscape painter, Asher Brown Durand (1796–1866), and all were engraved by him. Four other plates were executed by Benjamin A. Vitry, who later studied medicine in Paris. It was Anderson's intention to complete a yearly series of works on surgical anatomy, but this plan was never carried out.

GS6. **JAMES THACHER** (1754–1844). *A military journal during the American Revolutionary War, from 1775 to 1783.* 603pp. Boston: Richardson & Lord, 1823.

Thacher was appointed surgeon's mate under John Warren (1753–1815) just after the Battle of Bunker Hill. He served through the war and was eventually promoted to the position of surgeon in the army. He obtained wide experience in medicine and military surgery and was present at many important events. Although the *Journal* does not have a specific section on surgery, it provides interesting anecdotes of a Revolutionary War surgeon. Included is the scalping and subsequent treatment of a wounded soldier and observations on a gunshot injury to the sole of the foot obtained while the wounded was fleeing from the enemy, an act which Thacher describes as "cowardice treason." A second edition was

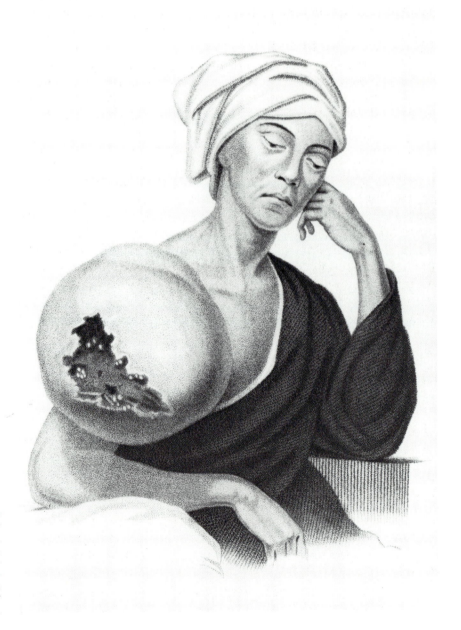

Fig. 3. (GS7) Drawn from nature by Gibson and engraved by C. Tiebout, this hand-colored plate, figure 7 on page 313 in volume 1, depicts a fungus hematodes of enormous proportions. This now obsolete term denotes a soft, fungating, easily bleeding, malignant neoplasm.

published in 1827. Thacher was a voluminous writer and is best remembered for his *American medical biography* (Boston: Richardson & Lord & Cottons & Barnard, 1828) [G-M 6710]. Among his other medical writings are *The American new dispensatory* (Boston: T. B. Wait, 1810), *Observations on hydrophobia* (Plymouth: Joseph Avery, 1812), and *American modern practice* (Boston: Ezra Read & C. Norris, 1817).

GS7. **WILLIAM GIBSON** (1788–1868). *The institutes and practice of surgery; being the outlines of a course of lectures.* 2 vols., 469pp. and 542pp. Philadelphia: Edward Parker, 1824.

The second systematic American textbook of surgery. It became one of the most popular medical texts of its day, passing through eight editions, in 1827, 1832, 1835, 1838, 1841, 1845, and 1850. Like Dorsey's *Elements* (GS3), much of its material was extracted from lectures by Philip Syng Physick (1768–1837), although Gibson also consulted foreign authors. Gibson writes in the preface:

> . . . the work must be considered a mere outline of the lectures, which will be filled up by numerous illustrations, derived chiefly from an extensive collection of models, morbid preparations, magnified drawings, and imitations of disease on the dead subject . . . . I do not presume to offer these Outlines to the experienced members of the profession. They are designed exclusively for those young friends in whose interest I take a lively concern . . . .

The eight chapters in the first volume include topics such as "Inflammation"; "Wounds"; "Abscesses"; "Ulcers"; and "Fractures." The sixteen chapters of the second volume discuss diseases of specific organs. Among the eighteen plates, numbers 4 through 7 are hand-colored, with 4, 6, and 7 being drawn by Gibson himself. In 1819, Gibson succeeded Physick in the chair of surgery at the Univef Pennsylvania. In 1812, Gibson performed one of the earliest ligations of a common iliac artery for traumatic aneurysm [G-M 2944]. His only other book is *Rambles in Europe in 1839 with sketches of prominent surgeons, physicians, medical schools, hospitals, literary personages, scenery, etc.* (Philadelphia: Lea & Blanchard, 1841).

GS8. **NATHAN RYNO SMITH** (1797–1877). *Surgical anatomy of the arteries.* 104pp. Baltimore: J. D. Troy & W. R. Lucas, 1830.

The son of Nathan Smith (1762–1829), Nathan Ryno was professor of surgery at the University of Maryland and one of the surgeons of the Baltimore Infirmary. The first edition of Smith's *Anatomy* was reprinted in 1832, and a second edition of 133 pages appeared in 1835. The eighteen hand-colored plates are copied from the *Anatomie de l'homme* of Jules Germain Cloquet (1790–1883) and are executed by the noted early American lithographer J. Swett. For this volume, the arterial diagrams are printed in red in the text, which is an unusual feature from the point of view of book production at that time. Smith writes in the preface:

> I have been induced to attempt a work on the Anatomy and Surgery of the Arteries, by the acknowledged fact, that on this subject we have no

American publication which perfectly meets the wants of the pupil, or
the practitioner . . . . The object is to convey to the eye, at a glance, an
idea of the absolute and relative length and diameter of each of the
more important arteries—also of the number of their branches, and the
order in which they are given off . . . .

Part 1 (pages 2–28) consists of general observations on the anatomy,
physiology, and pathology of the arteries. Part 2 (pages 29–104) comprises four sections that explain the arterial anatomy of particular organs. Throughout Part 2 are surgical observations listed for each artery
discussing arterial wounds and dissecting techniques to provide exposure during an operation. Among Smith's other medical books is *A
physiological essay on digestion* (New York: E. Bliss & E. White, 1825). (See
also OR19.)

GS9. **WILLIAM BEAUMONT** (1785–1853). *Experiments and observations
on the gastric juice, and the physiology of digestion.* 280pp. Plattsburgh, N.Y.: F. P. Allen, 1833. [G-M 989]

Beaumont, an army surgeon, was the first to study digestive physiology and the movements of the stomach in vivo. His investigations were
carried out on Alexis St. Martin, a French-Canadian hunter whom
Beaumont treated for a shotgun wound of the upper abdomen. The *Experiments* is one of the best known of all early American surgical classics.
It describes a series of four experiments and discusses such diverse topics
as "Hunger and thirst"; "Mastication"; "Deglutition"; and "Chylifi-
cation." A second edition was printed in Burlington, Vermont, in 1847.
This edition's preface notes that the first edition consisted of 3,000
copies. In 1834, copies of the Plattsburgh edition were also issued by
Lilly & Wait of Boston, with a cancel title page. The book received
worldwide attention, and in 1834 a German translation was published.
Another edition was printed in Edinburgh in 1838. A facsimile reprint
was published by the Harvard University Press in 1929.

GS10. **DUDLEY ATKINS** (1798–1845). *Medical and surgical cases and observations.* 127pp. New York: P. Hill, 1834.

Atkins held no academic posts and was a general practitioner in
New York. This book is dedicated to James Jackson (1777–1867) of Boston. Atkins writes in the preface:

The following collection of cases is thrown together without method,
for it was not easy to fix upon any principle of arrangement, when
scarcely two were alike. They are published from a variety of motives,
which it may not be amiss briefly to state. In the first place, I thought
some of them were worthy of record from their singularity . . . . In the
second place, I thought there were many of them which were of a
character very much to encourage the young physician, in his attempts
to relieve cases apparently desperate in their circumstances . . . . In the
third place, I recollected that most of them occurred in places remote
from my present residence, and that any reputation they might have
given me, whether deserved or not, could only be regained by their
publication here . . . .

Among the surgical cases are an undescribed affection of the eye, operation for the stone upon a child of three years, treatment of a case of paraplegia in a child, cases of compound fracture of the leg, bandage for transverse wounds of the extremities, and remarks upon hemorrhoidal tumors. There was only one edition. Atkins's other medical text is *Reports of hospital physicians, and other documents in relation to the epidemic cholera of 1832* (New York: G. & C. & H. Carvill, 1832).

GS11. HEBER CHASE (?–?). *A treatise on the radical cure of hernia by instruments; embracing an analysis of the mechanical properties of the various trusses now in use, a description of the new instruments invented by the author, and general directions to patients for the safe employment of these instruments, with hints to surgeons in their application, etc.* 195pp. Philadelphia: J. G. Auner, 1836.

This is the first American textbook dealing solely with the treatment of hernias. It consists of eleven chapters, six of which are devoted to the use of the truss. There are thirty-two figures but no plates. Numerous case studies are presented, including a "tabular statement" of 100 hernias (pages 180–84). Chase, although not known as a surgeon,

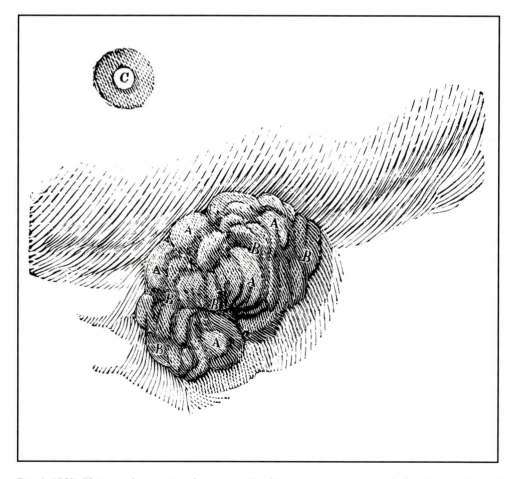

Fig. 4. (GS9) This wood engraving from page 29 of Beaumont's classic work depicts a portion of Alexis St. Martin's prolapsed gastric mucosa. His nipple is at C to provide orientation.

had an active interest in the treatment of surgical problems by nonsurgical or mechanical measures. Regarded as an outsider in the world of Philadelphia medicine, publication of this book provided him with a measure of respect from his fellow physicians. As Chase writes in the preface:

> It is hardly necessary to apologize to the public for the appearance of the following treatise . . . . Much of the business of treating hernia by trusses, has gradually passed from professional hands into those of the patients themselves, or has been consigned to others who pretend to medical skill without having employed the means, by which alone such skill can be acquired. Practitioners of the latter class have but too frequently no further purpose in view than the mere pecuniary result of the sale of their instruments; for they are not held in check by the necessity of maintaining unimpeached that most delicate of all possessions, a professional reputation; nor are they restrained like the patient, by the dread of personal suffering from their own ignorance or incompetency. It is chiefly with the view of shielding the patient at once from those evils so frequently resulting from illgrounded self-confidence on one hand, and from improper faith in the pretensions of empyrics and mere machinists on the other, that the following pages are offered to the world . . . .

(See also GS14.)

GS12. **AUGUSTUS SIDNEY DOANE** (1808–52). *Surgery illustrated, compiled from the works of Cutler, Hind, Velpeau and Blasius.* 200pp. New York: Harper Brothers, 1836.

Doane received his M.D. from Harvard in 1828. After studying for two years in Paris, he settled in New York, where he established a successful general practice. His *Surgery* was designed with no pretensions to originality. Doane felt that medicine benefited more from a compilation of facts than an original book of theory. His simple aim was to be useful. The book is divided into three major sections: "Bandages"; "Fractures of the extremities"; and "Surgical operations." The fifty-two plates are largely copies of European works, but Doane wrote the text himself. Of major interest is the fact that Nathaniel Currier (1813–88) was lithographer for plates 29, 30 (hand-colored), 31 (hand-colored), 35, 36, 39 (hand-colored), and 42. W. K. Hewitt, who drew Currier's first great success on stone, the Lexington boat fire of 1840, also executed some of the plates in this volume. Currier began business in 1834, and the records of his production before 1840 are incomplete. Medical subjects were rare in Currier's output in any period, and none of these plates are noted in books on Currier. Doane's other books are translations of foreign medical texts.

GS13. **JOSEPH PARRISH** (1779–1840). *Practical observations on strangulated hernia, and some of the diseases of the urinary organs.* 330pp. Philadelphia: Key & Biddle, 1836.

Incorporating seventy-five detailed case reports, this volume provides an excellent account of early nineteenth-century treatment of strangulated hernia and bladder and prostate problems. Parrish dedi-

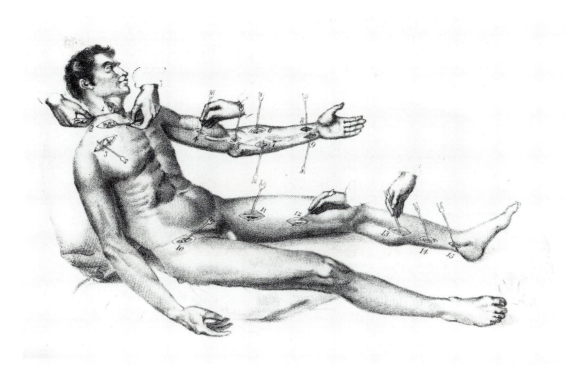

Fig. 5. (GS12) W. K. Hewitt drew on stone and Nathaniel Currier produced the lithograph for Doane's plate, figure 29 on page 126. It depicts various incisions and methods used to ligate blood vessels.

cated the book to Philip Syng Physick (1768–1837), whom he succeeded in 1816 as surgeon to the Pennsylvania Hospital. In the preface, Parrish provides an interesting thought regarding the disposition of books:

> Should this work meet a favourable reception, perhaps it may prove the prelude to a series of medical and surgical observations, to appear in due course. But if its value has been overrated, it may at least be permitted quietly to occupy some nook or corner of the storehouse already noticed, where it may repose in oblivion, along with its author.

GS14. **HEBER CHASE** (?–?). *The final report of the committee of the Philadelphia Medical Society on the construction of instruments, and their mode of action, in the radical cure of hernia . . . .* 243pp. Philadelphia: J. G. Auner, 1837.

In 1834, the Philadelphia Medical Society, of which Chase was an honorary member, formed a committee to investigate the use of trusses. Based on these efforts two short preliminary papers were published, and this volume was the committee's final report. The work contains a table discussing over 200 cases of hernias (pages 208–16). Most of the text is devoted to a detailed description of Chase's truss (deemed by the committee to be the most efficient) and its mode of operation. There are twenty-three figures. Another of Chase's books is *The medical student's guide; being a compendious view of the collegiate and clinical and medical schools, the courses of private lectures, the hospitals, and almshouses and others* (Philadelphia: J. G. Auner, 1842). (See also GS11.)

GS15. **JOHN COLLINS WARREN** (1778–1856). *Surgical observations on tumours, with cases and operations.* 607pp. Boston: Crocker & Brewster, 1837. [G-M 2611.1]

One of the great classics in American medicine and considered to be Warren's magnum opus. Warren was professor of anatomy and surgery at Harvard University and surgeon to the Massachusetts General Hospital at the time of its writing. The work was the first American treatise on tumors. It is divided into fourteen sections plus a glossary of distinguishing characteristics of tumors. Among the topics are "Epidermoid tumors"; "Dermoid tumors"; "Tumors of the cellular membrane"; "Muscular tumors"; "Periosteal tumors"; "Osseous tumors"; "Tumors of the glands"; "Tumors of the testis"; "Tumors of the secreting glands"; "Tumors of the mucous glands"; "Tumors of the vascular texture"; "Tumors of the membranous textures"; "Encysted tumors"; and "Abdominal tumors." It also contains sixteen hand-colored plates by the engraver, David Claypoole Johnston (1799–1865), who is best known for his caricatures. Although Warren wanted to publish an enlarged second edition, numerous other commitments and his advanced age of fifty-nine kept him from doing so. A two-volume biography of Warren, *The life of John Collins Warren,* appeared in 1860 (Boston: Ticknor & Fields), edited by his son Edward Warren (1804–78). According to this account (volume 1, pages 276–81):

> Before his departure for Europe in 1837, Dr. Warren published his work on tumours,—one of the largest surgical books which he ever found time to compile. There can be no doubt that it was his original intention to prepare a more elaborate treatise on this, and probably upon other subjects. The care with which he had preserved the records of his hospital practice (forming six large folio volumes), in addition to the records of private practice, seems to indicate such a design. They afforded an immense mass of facts and observations, and ample materials for treatises upon all subjects of operative surgery . . . . But he found, as he states in his preface, "practical men, called as they are to every kind of medical duty, possessing no time they can devote to study but what is robbed from hours which the wearied faculties require for repose, can estimate the obstacles to any literary labor among us. Compelled to accomplish this publication under an unusual pressure of affairs, or to defer it to an uncertain period, I thought it right to relinquish the attempt at an elaborate and finished production, to clothe the facts in the best dress that circumstances permitted me to give them, and to content myself with the expectation that the errors which may have escaped me now will be readily discovered hereafter, both by myself and others . . . .

Warren is also credited with having introduced the operation of staphylorrhaphy for the treatment of fissure of the soft palate [G-M 5742]. (See also GS26, GS27.1, and OR1.)

Fig. 6. (GS15) Warren had
David Claypoole Johnston
draw a massive lymphangioma
of the cheek in this hand-
colored plate, figure 9 on page
166.

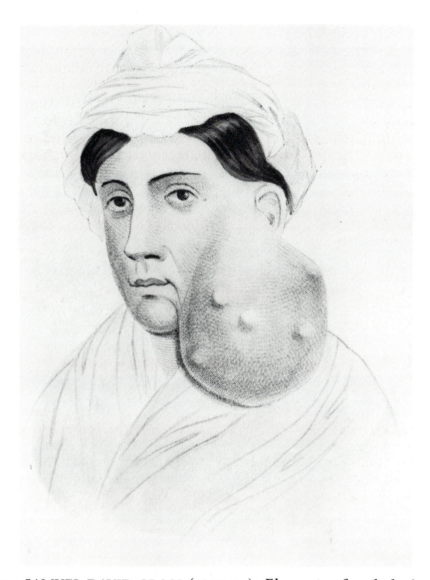

GS16. **SAMUEL DAVID GROSS** (1805–84). *Elements of pathological anatomy.* 2 vols., 518pp. and 510pp. Boston: Marsh, Capen, Lyon & Webb, and James B. Dow, 1839. [G-M 2292]

Gross was one of the most prominent American surgeons of the nineteenth century. His remarkable career included the founding of the American Medical Association and the American Surgical Association. The *Elements*, written when he was professor of general anatomy, physiology, and pathological anatomy in the medical department of the Cincinnati College is considered the first exhaustive study in English of the subject. Dedicated to Daniel Drake (1785–1852), the book consists of two parts: a general principles of pathological anatomy and a special pathological anatomy section of twenty-seven chapters on specific organs. The *Elements* has just ninety-seven wood-engraved figures and only five colored plates. Two later editions were published in 1845 and

1857. Gross writes in his *Autobiography* (Philadelphia: George Barrie, 1887; volume 1, pages 72–74):

It was from dissections, from an elaborate course of reading, and from numerous visits to the pork and slaughter houses of Cincinnati, that I derived the knowledge upon which I founded my work on Pathological Anatomy, issued in 1839, in two octavo volumes of more than five hundred pages each. The work was illustrated by numerous wood-cuts and several colored engravings . . . . As far as I know, mine was the first attempt ever made in this country, or, indeed, in the English language, to systematize the subject and to place it in a connected form before the profession. The book was well received. A second edition, greatly enlarged and thoroughly revised, much of it having been rewritten, was issued in 1845 by Barrington & Haswell, of Philadelphia, in one large octavo volume of eight hundred and twenty-two pages, illustrated by

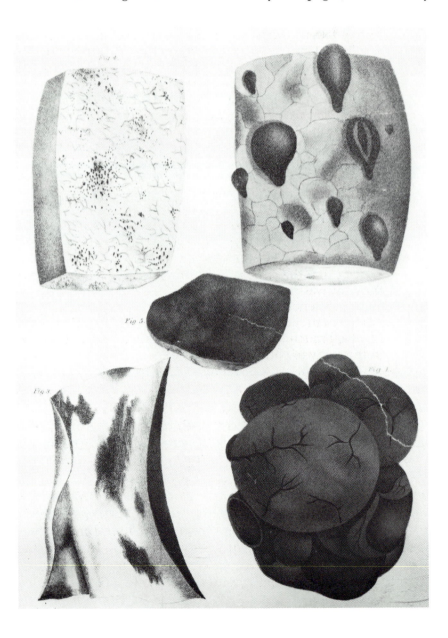

Fig. 7. (GS16) In this hand-colored fold-out plate, E. W. Bouve, the lithographer for Gross's work, has shown multiple forms of melanosis in varying human tissues (figure 2 on page 171 in volume 1).

colored engravings and two hundred and fifty wood-cuts. It was full of marginal references, which greatly enhanced its value. A third edition—the last one—modified and carefully revised, and illustrated by three hundred and forty-two engravings on wood, appeared in 1857 from the press of Blanchard & Lea. It formed an octavo volume of seven hundred and seventy-one pages. It was, in some degree, an abridgment of the second edition, and yet it comprised a very good outline of the existing state of the science. I was assisted in its preparation, especially the microscopical portion, by Dr. J. M. DaCosta, now my distinguished colleague, who was well informed on the subject. The labor of rewriting and dovetailing of course devolved upon me. I never liked this edition. It always seemed to me as if the work had been emasculated, inasmuch as I left out all marginal references and all that related to diagnoses. The work, in its original form, cost me much labor and anxiety. It was written when I was a young man, without any one to advise or guide me, in my leisure hours, often snatched from sleep, and under the exhaustion of fatigue, when one is ill-qualified for healthful mental exertion. A solitary lamp was generally my only companion, in a basement office, and it was often past the hour of midnight before my head pressed its pillow. Upwards of three years were spent upon its composition. When the manuscript was completed I offered it to different publishers in Philadelphia and New York, but no one was willing to undertake its publication, and it was only after a good deal of hard work that I finally succeeded in inducing Marsh, Capen, Lyon & Webb, of Boston, to bring it out. After much delay it at length appeared, under the title of *Elements of Pathological Anatomy*. For this edition I received no remuneration. The Boston house failed soon after its publication, and did not even pay the proof-reader, the late Dr. Jeffries Wyman, who had kindly agreed to perform this office for me. The second edition yielded twelve hundred dollars, and the last edition one thousand dollars . . . . There is one feature of this book which is worthy of special notice. I refer to the fact that the description of the morbid anatomy of every organ in the body was preceded by an account of its healthy color, weight, size, and consistence, founded upon original investigation, a plan until then unknown in such works. The labor bestowed upon these investigations involved much trouble and painstaking. It was an important advance in the study of pathological structure . . . .

Among Gross's other important books are those dealing with history, including *History of American medical literature from 1776 to the present time* (Philadelphia: Collins, 1876) [G-M 6761], *Lives of eminent American physicians and surgeons of the nineteenth century* (Philadelphia: Lindsay & Blakiston, 1861), *Memoir of Valentine Mott* (New York: D. Appleton, 1868), and *Memorial oration in honor of Ephraim McDowell, the father of ovariotomy* (Louisville: Kentucky State Medical Society, 1879). In addition, he contributed a chapter to Edward Hammond Clarke's (1820–77) *A century of American medicine* (Philadelphia: H. C. Lea, 1876) [G-M 6586]. Among his important contributions to the periodic literature is one of the earliest articles on medical jurisprudence regarding manual strangulation [G-M 1737] and a lengthy account of the history of American surgery to 1876 [G-M 5795]. (See also GS19, GS34, GS46, GS49, OR2, and GU5.)

GS17. **USHER PARSONS** (1788–1868). *Boylston prize dissertations on: (1) inflammation of the periosteum; (2) eneuresis irritata; (3) cutaneous diseases; (4) cancer of the breast; also remarks on malaria.* 248pp. Boston: Little & Brown, 1839.

Parsons was a surgical naval hero in the War of 1812, having served on the frigate *Lawrence* under Commodore Oliver Hazard Perry (1785–1819). In later life, Parsons practiced in Rhode Island and was a founder of the American Medical Association. The Boylston Prize was awarded by Harvard University for dissertations on subjects connected with the medical sciences. A committee would compose questions which the medical community would then have the opportunity to answer in the form of a treatise. Parsons wrote four Boylston Prize-winning treatises, three of which were on surgical topics. Parsons's other books were *Sailor's physician, exhibiting the symptoms, causes and treatment of diseases incident to seamen and passengers in merchant vessels* (Cambridge: Hilliard & Metcalf, 1820) and *Directions for making anatomical preparations formed on the basis of Pole, Marjolin and Breschet* (Philadelphia: Carey & Lea, 1831).

GS18. **NATHANIEL CHAPMAN** (1780–1853). *Essays on practical medicine and surgery.* 2 vols. Philadelphia: Lea & Blanchard, 1841.

Chapman was on the faculty of the University of Pennsylvania, holding at various times the chairs of midwifery, materia medica, and the theory and practice of medicine. He was the first president of the American Medical Association and wrote the earliest book on therapeutics and materia medica in America, *Discourses on the elements of therapeutics and materia medica* (Philadelphia: James Webster, 1817). Although Chapman was not a surgeon, his writings frequently included surgical topics. These *Essays* are rather scarce and represent a compilation of many of his previously published articles. Among Chapman's other medical books are *Lectures on the more important eruptive fevers, hemorrhages and dropsies, and on gout and rheumatism* (Philadelphia: Lea & Blanchard, 1844), *Lectures on the more important diseases of the thoracic and abdominal viscera* (Philadelphia: Lea & Blanchard, 1844), and *A compendium of lectures on the theory and practice of medicine* (Philadelphia: Lea & Blanchard, 1846).

GS19. **SAMUEL DAVID GROSS** (1805–84). *Experimental and critical inquiry into the nature and treatment of wounds of the intestines.* 219pp. Louisville: Prentice & Weissinger, 1843. [G-M 3446]

Gross writes in his *Autobiography* (volume 1, pages 96–97) that after he assumed the chair of surgery in Louisville he began a series of experiments upon dogs:

> . . . with a view of determining more accurately than had hitherto been done the nature and treatment of wounds of the intestines. The investigations were commenced in the spring of 1841, and were continued, with various intermissions, for more than two years. The object was, in the first place, to inquire into the process employed in repairing such injuries; and secondly, and more particularly, to test the value of the more important methods of treatment recommended by surgeons from

the time of Ransdohr, a practitioner of the early part of the last century, down to our own. The experiments, upwards of seventy in number, were performed exclusively upon dogs, as the most eligible animals that could be procured for the purpose. The results, originally published in a series of papers in the *Western Journal of Medicine and Surgery*, were finally embodied in an octavo volume of two hundred and twenty pages, illustrated by wood-cuts and colored engravings. The work was exhaustive, and comprised an account of my own researches and a sketch of the literature of the subject. It was favorably noticed in a long review by the *British and Foreign Medico-Chirurgical Journal*, edited by Dr. Forbes, and was quoted approvingly by Mr. Guthrie in his work on Military Surgery. I have never seen any allusion to it in any of our own journals, or by any of our own writers. The labor spent upon these experiments was very great, and the expense itself was not inconsiderable, as I was obliged to pay for nearly all the dogs, and to hire a man to watch and feed them. My colleagues were kind enough to give me the basement rooms in the college for the accomodation of the poor creatures. The experiments besides, involved a great sacrifice of feeling on my part. I am naturally fond of dogs, and my sympathies were often wrought to the highest pitch, especially when I happened to get hold of an unusually clever specimen. Anesthetics had not yet been discovered, and I was therefore obliged to inflict severe pain . . . and if I were not thoroughly satisfied that the objects had been most laudable, I should consider myself a most cruel, heartless man, deserving of the severest condemnation . . . .

This volume, initially published in the January through March issues of the *Western journal of medicine and surgery* (1843), had only one edition and is the first textbook of experimental animal surgery to be published in America. (See also GS16, GS34, GS46, GS49, OR2, and GU5.)

GS20. **THOMAS DENT MÜTTER** (1811–59). *Syllabus of the course of lectures on the principles and practice of surgery.* 206pp. Philadelphia: Merrihew & Thompson, 1843.

These syllabi, of which several additional editions were printed in 1846, 1848, and 1855, were invaluable to the students at Jefferson Medical College. They provided an outline of the lectures which Mütter gave in his position as professor of surgery. Each syllabus was frequently interleaved with blank pages on which the student could take notes. The lectures were arranged under six headings: "Inflammation"; "Diseases of different tissues and organs"; "Various affections of regions"; "Tumours"; "Diseases peculiar to females"; and "Amputations." Mütter is remembered for having established the Mütter Pathological Museum at the College of Physicians of Philadelphia. (See also OR3.)

GS21. **HENRY HOLLINGSWORTH SMITH** (1815–90). *Minor surgery; or, hints on the every-day duties of the surgeon.* 303pp. Philadelphia: Ed. Barrington & Geo. Haswell, 1843.

Smith was lecturer on minor surgery at Philadelphia Hospital. He was later appointed to succeed William Gibson (1788–1868) as professor of surgery at the University of Pennsylvania. The first 275 pages of this volume present detailed instructions in the use of dressings and bandages and applications of apparatus for fractures and dislocations. The fourth part deals with minor surgical operations, including phlebotomy, blistering, and scarification. There are 189 figures but no plates. Smith writes in the preface:

> The shortness of the period usually allotted to a course of lectures on surgery, and the rapidity with which the lecturer is obliged to pass over the methods of dressing and the minor surgical operations, has left a deficit in the amount of knowledge required for daily practice, which every one commencing has more or less severely felt. With a view of filling up this, as well as in compliance with the repeated requests of several members of his class, the author has been induced to undertake the present work, not in the expectation of being able to offer any thing new or original on a subject which has so long engaged more or less of the attention of every one, but with the hope that he might afford a concise and methodical system of minor surgery, adapted to the wants of the student and young practitioner in the United States . . . .

Further editions were published in 1846, 1850, and 1859. (See also GS22.1, GS31, GS38, GS39, and GS55.)

GS22. **JOSEPH PANCOAST** (1805–82). *A treatise on operative surgery; comprising a description of the various processes of the art, including all the new operations;* exhibiting the state of surgical science in its present advanced condition. 380pp. Philadelphia: Carey & Hart, 1844. [G-M 5598]

Pancoast's *Treatise* is one of the most remarkable nineteenth-century American surgical textbooks. It went through two more editions in 1846 and 1852, and sold a total of 4,000 copies within nine years. With eighty quarto plates comprising 486 separate illustrations, the book's most distinguishing characteristics are the wonderfully executed lithographs, including some after Nicolas Jacob (1782–1871). The plates are exceedingly graphic, so much so that numbers 69 and 70 were often removed by religious purists because of their depiction of the female genitalia. A few copies of all three editions were issued with hand-colored plates. The colored plates were printed on thicker and finer paper and do not usually exhibit the foxing so often present on the plates of the regular edition. Copies with hand-colored plates are among the most magnificent of all American surgical books issued in the nineteenth century and are exceptionally rare. The original subscription price for regular copies was $10.00. In 1838, Pancoast was elected professor of surgery at Jefferson Medical College. However, in 1841 he was reassigned to the chair of general, descriptive and surgical anatomy. He remained in this position until his retirement from active teaching in 1874. The work contains four parts: "Elementary and minor operations"; "General operations"; "Special operations"; and "Plastic and subcutaneous operations." The latter section is among the earliest and most extensive published on plastic surgery in America. Pancoast's explanation for writing the *Treatise* appears in the preface:

> The necessity of thoroughly illustrating the operations of surgery, has been felt from the earliest periods of the art, as a means of rendering

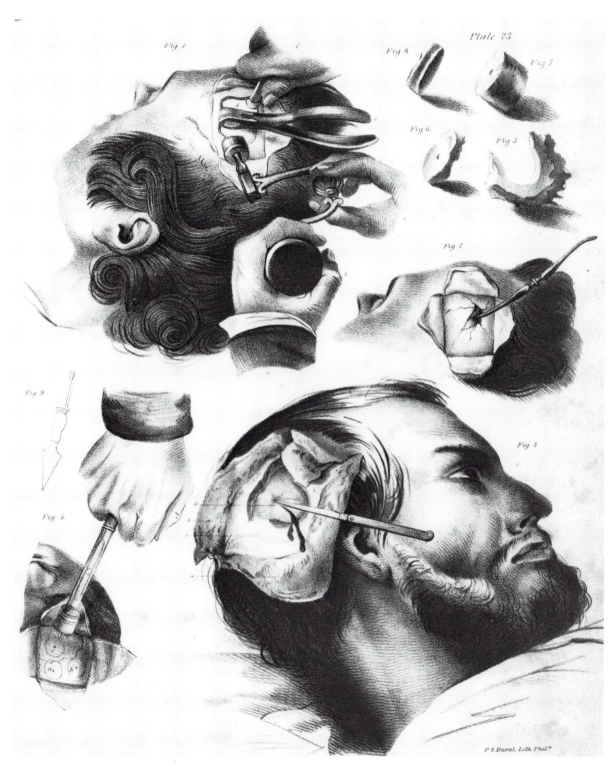

Fig. 8. (GS22) Pancoast's volume contained some of the most outstanding mid nineteenth-century American medical illustrations. This plate, figure 23 on page 102, shows trepanning, or trephining, of the cranium for a comatose patient. It was drawn on stone by S. Cichowski and P. S. Duval was the lithographer.

the processes for their performance, intelligible to the student . . . . having at hand the greater portion of the surgical works, which have recently appeared in various languages, and with the advantage which nine years continuous service in one of the largest hospitals of North America has given me, not only in comparing to a certain extent the value of the different methods, but in enabling me to obtain a large number of accurate drawings of operations which have been done by my own hand, I have endeavoured to furnish a work that shall represent, so far as its limits will allow, the operative surgery of the day . . . .

Pancoast was quite innovative, having devised operations for exstrophy of the bladder [G-M 4170] and tic douloureaux [G-M 4855].

GS22.1. **HENRY HOLLINGSWORTH SMITH** (1815–90). *Anatomical atlas, illustrative of the structure of the human body.* 200pp. Philadelphia: Lea & Blanchard, 1844.

Smith completed this book under the supervision of William E. Horner (1793–1853), professor of anatomy at the University of Pennsylvania. Smith and Horner enjoyed a lengthy relationship; while attending medical school in the late 1830s, Smith was Horner's private office student, and later married Horner's eldest daughter. On the title page Smith lists himself simply as a fellow of the College of Physicians and member of the Philadelphia Medical Society. This atlas was intended to accompany Horner's two-volume *Special anatomy and histology* (Philadelphia: Lea & Blanchard, 1843). Horner's book was first published in 1826 under the title of *A treatise on special and general anatomy*. It went through five editions, and the new two-volume set plus Smith's *Atlas* actually forms the sixth edition of Horner's original work. Smith notes in the preface that

the utility of drawings in illustration of a purely demonstrative branch, is now too well established to require any argument in its favour. Separated from the centre of instruction, and deprived of the advantages of the dissecting room, the ideas once so distinct, become confused and mixed. A recourse to plates, in the absence of dead bodies, is then the only means of refreshing our knowledge . . . .

There are 684 illustrations on 183 leaves. They are divided into five parts: "Bones and ligaments"; "Dermoid and muscular systems"; "Organs of digestion and generation"; "Organs of respiration and circulation"; and "The nervous system and senses." Most of the original drawings were completed by Pinkerton, and all the wood engravings were done by Gilbert. This work is especially notable for the early use of "microscopical observations on the anatomy of the tissues." (See also GS21, GS31, GS38, GS39, and GS55.)

GS23. **GEORGE McCLELLAN** (1796–1847). *Principles and practice of surgery.* 432pp. Philadelphia: Grigg & Elliot, 1848.

A founder of Jefferson Medical College, McClellan served as professor of surgery from 1826 to 1838 and was highly regarded as a promoter of medical education. He received his M.D. from the University of Pennsylvania in 1819 and was also a private student of John Syng Dorsey (1783–1818). Following McClellan's premature death, a son,

John H. B. McClellan (1823–74), posthumously published McClellan's lecture notes and other material as the *Principles*. McClellan's son writes in the preface: "Many of the accompanying pages were penned whilst suffering acutely from disease, and relief from pain was often sought by occupying his mind in recording the views contained in the present volume . . . . The work, therefore, necessarily bears the marks of haste and deficiency of arrangement . . . . " McClellan wrote a short author's preface just prior to his death:

> . . . I have now arrived at that period of life which I always thought entitled an educated and observing man to be heard; and my old friends and former pupils will give me no further indulgence in the way of resisting these demands . . . . When I first promised to undertake this publication, I must confess I thought it would be far easier to complete than it has since proved to be. In looking over the manuscript volumes of my best pupils I find they all mistook many important points and connections of ideas, and left too many gaps and interspaces among the different subjects to enable me to use them with any advantage. I have been obliged, therefore, to shut myself up occasionally from the world, at least for an hour or two at a time, and reproduce my former train of ideas and facts, as I was in the habit of giving them extemporaneously in the lecture room . . . .

The book proved to be an utter failure, both financially and professionally, although the description of shock (pages 13–20) remains a classic. The contents include: "Constitutional irritation"; "Effects of injuries upon the blood-vessels"; "Erysipelas"; "Furunculus"; "Anthrax"; "Absces-

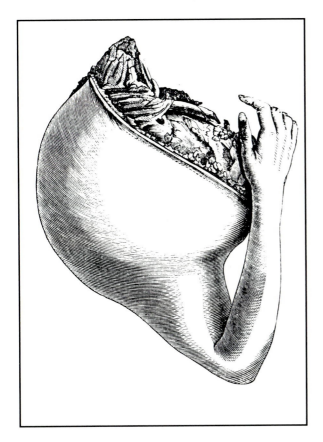

Fig. 9. (GS23) This engraving (number 15, page 412) was drawn from a preparation in which McClellan had removed the entire scapula and clavicle for a tumor. The procedure was performed in 1838 on a seventeen-year-old male, and according to the author's account was the "first if not the only case" to have ever been completed.

ses"; "Ulcers"; "Burns and scalds"; "Effects of cold"; "Wounds"; "Tetanus"; "Hydrophobia"; "Poisoned wounds"; "Syphilis"; "Morbid growths"; "Non-malignant tumors"; and "Malignant growths in general." This was the only edition. There are no plates and only fifteen rudimentary wood engravings. Another son was the famous Civil War general George B. McClellan (1826–85).

GS24. **JOHN NEILL** (1819–80) and **FRANCIS GURNEY SMITH** (1818–78). *A handbook of surgery, being a portion of an analytical compend of the various branches of medicine.* 122pp. Philadelphia: Lea & Blanchard, 1848.

Neill graduated in 1840 from the University of Pennsylvania. He served as a demonstrator in anatomy from 1845 to 1849 at his alma mater and later became the first professor of clinical surgery at the university. Smith was an obstetrician and physiologist who was professor of the institutes of medicine at the University of Pennsylvania. The authors published a series of handbooks on subjects such as anatomy, physiology, obstetrics, materia medica and therapeutics, chemistry, and the practice of medicine. It is said that Neill later regretted his connection with the project. Although the handbooks were a financial success, they attracted much criticism of their superficial treatment of medicine. The surgical manual discusses over seventy topics, devoting only one or two pages to each. There are fifty-one wood engravings. All seven manuals were published bound together under the title *An analytical compendium of the various branches of medical science.* This volume, in royal duodecimo, of over 900 pages and 350 illustrations sold for $4.00 in cloth and $4.75 in leather. The individual manuals were separately published concurrently using stout paper covers and sold for fifty cents each.

GS25. **FITZWILLIAM SARGENT** (1820–89). *On bandaging and other operations of minor surgery.* 379pp. Philadelphia: Lea & Blanchard, 1848.

This volume is divided into five parts: "On surgical dressing"; "On bandages and their application"; "Bandages and apparatus employed in the treatment of fractures"; "On the mechanical means employed in the treatment of dislocations"; and "On some of the minor surgical operations". *On bandaging* is significant because of its section (pages 359–64) on "Diminishing pain during operations." This is one of the earliest descriptions of the use of sulfuric ether and chloroform found in an American surgical textbook, coming less than twenty months after William T. Morton's (1819–68) startling demonstration. There is also an extensive appendix of medicinal formulae on pages 365–70. A total of 128 simple engravings are scattered throughout the text. Sargent writes in the preface:

> The object which the author has had in view in the preparation of the following pages, has been, to present to the younger surgeon and to the student, information relative to the art of bandaging, and to some other points of importance in the practice of surgery. These are subjects which are but slightly alluded to in systematic courses of lectures, or in most

of the published treatises on the science; yet the necessity of a familiar acquaintance with them will be readily acknowledged by every surgeon of experience . . . .

A revised edition was published in 1856, and in 1862 a third edition was printed with an additional chapter on military surgery. Sargent was an 1843 graduate of the University of Pennsylvania Medical School. He resided mainly in Philadelphia, where he was surgeon at Wills Eye Hospital from 1852 to 1858. He gave up his medical practice during the Civil War and lived in Europe for the remainder of his life. He is the father of John Singer Sargent (1856–1925).

GS26. JOHN COLLINS WARREN (1778–1856). *Etherization with surgical remarks.* 100pp. Boston: William D. Ticknor, 1848.

Warren's *Etherization* provides a fascinating account of the early use of sulphuric ether in surgery, including a detailed description of the epochal first operation using anesthesia, which he performed on October 16, 1846. *The life of John Collins Warren* describes this work (volume 1, page 387):

> *Etherization* was published in the latter part of 1847; giving the results derived from a year's experience of this agent, and from over two hundred cases in which it was used, or its employment witnessed, by Warren. It forms a neat little volume of one hundred pages, and gives an account of the operations of importance in which it had been used. At the hospital and in private practice, it had continued to be used with uniform success.

On pages 72–73 Warren proposes for the first time the use of ether "in regard to animal vivisection." Warren's other book-length works include *Cases of organic diseases of the heart* (Boston: Thomas W. Wait, 1809), *A comparative view of the sensorial and nervous systems in men and animals* (Boston: J. W. Ingraham, 1822), *The conchologist* (Boston: Odiorne & Metcalf, 1834), *Physical education and the preservation of health* (Boston: W. D. Ticknor, 1846), *The mastodon giganteus of North America* (Boston: William D. Ticknor, 1852), *The preservation of health, with remarks on constipation, old age, use of alcohol in the preparation of medicines* (Boston: Ticknor, Reed & Fields, 1854), and *Remarks on some fossil impressions in the sandstone rocks of Connecticut River* (Boston: Ticknor & Fields, 1854). (See also GS15, GS27.1, and OR1.)

GS27. DAVID L. ROGERS (1799–1877). *Surgical essays and cases in surgery.* 151pp. Newark: Daily Advertiser Office, 1849.

A pupil of William Andersen, Rogers graduated from the College of Physicians and Surgeons of New York in 1822. This volume contains sixteen essays dealing with such varied topics as "Aneurysm"; "Fractured spine"; "Osteosarcoma"; "Ovarian tumor"; "Urethral surgery"; "Pathological anatomy"; and "Surgical instruments." A slightly expanded second edition was published in 1850.

GS27.1. JOHN COLLINS WARREN (1778–1856). *Effects of chloroform and of strong chloric ether, as narcotic agents.* 66pp. Boston: William D. Ticknor, 1849.

Published as a small octavo volume, this brief work was an effort on Warren's part to make the public and the surgical community better aware of the dire consequences of using chloroform. According to *The life of John Collins Warren* (volume 1, pages 387–89):

> The introduction of chloroform produced an excitement scarcely less than that of the discovery of the narcotic effect of ether . . . . We were soon awakened from our dreams of the delightful influence of the new agent by the occurrence of unfortunate and painful consequences . . . . On hearing of the fatal cases under the use of chloroform, Dr. Warren was led to resume his experiments with chloric ether, prepared, by his order, in a highly concentrated state. The result of these experiments was favorable . . . . He always retained his preference for chloric ether. It does not seem, however, to have ever become a general favorite . . . . At this time, also, he published the *Effects of Chloroform and of Strong Chloric Ether as Narcotic Agents* . . . .

Because of Warren's great prestige, this work had considerable influence when it was published. Much of the text discusses ten deaths that had occurred due to the use of chloroform as an anesthetic. Warren recapitulates these cases in a fold-out chart opposite page 23. The second half of the text concerns other foreign and domestic reports regarding the dangers of chloroform anesthesia. One edition was printed, and the work is relatively scarce. (See also GS15, GS26, and OR1.)

GS28. **BENJAMIN LORD HILL** (1813–71). *Lectures on the American eclectic system of surgery.* 671pp. Cincinnati: W. Phillips, 1850.

Hill was professor of surgery and later professor of anatomy at the Eclectic Medical Institute of Cincinnati. This book is important because it was the first textbook of surgery to come out of the eclectic movement and the first nonallopathic surgical work to be published in America. Eclecticism was a botanical movement which flourished beginning in the 1840s; the last medical school to advocate eclecticism closed in 1939. The preface provides a rudimentary introduction to eclectic thought:

> Whatever fault may be found with this book, it cannot be said that it was not called for; or that it contains nothing but what may be found in other works on the same subject. Without the risk of presumption, as it regards himself, the author may safely claim that it presents the medical reader with more new and peculiar matter than any other surgical work, now in the hands of the profession. Mere novelty, however, on such a subject, would be a very questionable claim. The peculiarities of practice here recorded and recommended come with the sanction of experience. It may be necessary to apprise some of our readers that there are throughout this country, thousands of successful American practitioners . . . who do little but follow the guidance of their trans-atlantic authorities. The superior success of the Reformed or American Practice, is in no department more manifest than in that of surgery. This is acknowledged in every part of the country where a well informed Eclectic has established himself. Those who do not call him in for all cases of sickness, are apt to consult him in difficult surgical diseases, that have baffled the skill of others. Though he may not have had many opportunities to display mechanical dexterity in great operations, he is known as exercising the truly "healing art," which often renders operations

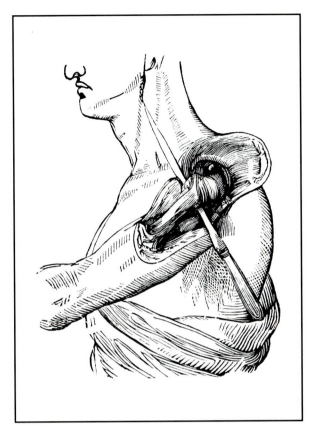

Fig. 10. (GS28) Most of the illustrations in Hill's work are rudimentary wood engravings. This engraving, figure 98 on page 581, demonstrates an amputation of the left arm at the shoulder joint.

unnecessary. This is the distinctive merit of our practice. So far as regards operative surgery, that is, the merely mechanical and destructive part of the practice, we cannot pretend to any very considerable improvement, except that of showing how, in a great many cases, we can dispense with operations altogether, even where they are usually looked upon as indispensable . . . . We cannot but condemn the ambitious eagerness of some old, as well as young surgeons, to cut, in preference of resorting to more rational as well as humane measures; and we desire to correct that wondering ignorance of society, which perpetuates the evil, by withholding the great need of approbation, which is due to the conservative surgeon, and often bestowing patronage and applause upon skillful but reckless operators, who really deserve the severest censure.

Unfortunately, this rare work has no table of contents, and the index is minimal at best. It contains sixty lectures covering a wide range of topics in addition to over a hundred illustrations. Among the more interesting subjects are anesthesia (pages 20–21) and an extensive appendix (pages 646–54) detailing numerous botanical formulae for medicines and external application. The last page has an interesting announcement concerning courses offered at the Eclectic Institute in addition to degree requirements and expenses.

In 1870, John Milton Scudder (1829–94) edited a revised version of the *Lectures* (Cincinnati: Medical Publishing), including a treatise on venereal disease. Hill's other medical books include *An epitome of the homoeopathic healing art, containing the new discoveries and improvements to the present time; designed for the use of families, for travelers on their journey, and as a pocket companion for the physician* (Cleveland: J. Hall, 1859) and *Illustrated midwifery; or lectures on obstetrics and the diseases of women and children* (Cincinnati: J. W. Sewell, 1860). (See also GS37.)

GS29. **HENRY BRYANT** (1820–67). *The radical cure of inguinal hernia; being a dissertation which obtained the Boylston prize for 1847, on the following question: "Is there any certain and safe manner of accomplishing the cure of common inguinal hernia?"* 70pp. Boston: W. Chadwick, 1851.

An 1843 graduate of Harvard Medical School, Bryant was an associate of Henry J. Bigelow (1818–90) and helped organize the Charitable Surgical Institute for Outdoor Patients in Boston. They encountered much professional jealousy, mostly because the institute offered free surgery and used billboard advertising. Bryant's surgical career was relatively brief because of his chronic poor health. The later part of his life was devoted to the study of ornithology. According to the biography of Bryant prepared by his son William Sohier Bryant (1861–1955) (New York: Craftsman Press, 1952), this short monograph was written after Bryant had returned to the United States from studying in Europe and reflects many of the principles he learned there.

GS29.1. **JOSEPH FOSTER FLAGG** (1789–1853). *Ether and chloroform; their employment in surgery, dentistry, midwifery, therapeutics, etc.* 189pp. Philadelphia: Lindsay & Blakiston, 1851.

Flagg was a graduate of Harvard Medical School (1815), but he considered himself primarily a dental surgeon and anatomical artist. In 1811, he became a private pupil of John Collins Warren (1778–1856) and later completed most of the drawings for the plates in Warren's *A comparative view of the sensorial and nervous systems in men and animals* (Boston: J. W. Ingraham, 1822). From 1833 on he was involved in treating dental problems and in the manufacture of mineral teeth. He also became interested in homeopathy and served as a major proponent of its teaching in the Boston area. In 1846, Flagg was entangled in the well-known ether controversy in which he opposed the patenting of ether, or "letheon" as it was then called. This brought him into bitter opposition to William Thomas G. Morton (1819–68), another dentist, who is generally credited with the discovery of ether anesthesia. Flagg writes in the introduction:

> In treating upon the discovery of the application of sulphuric ether in painful surgical operations as a discovery, I would observe, that I have no other interest or feeling in the matter, than what I believe to be a desire to elicit truth; making statements, or repeating such as may have reached me, with no further comment than the case seems absolutely to require; preferring that my readers should draw their deductions, and from conclusions from simple relation, rather than from party prejudice. It is much to be regretted, that several candidates should have appeared simultaneously for the exclusive honour of having first induced anaesthesia by inhalation; when the part allotted to each in its promulgation, would have been sufficiently meritorious to rank him

among the philanthropic of the age . . . . Having, from time to time, furnished various articles upon the subject of ether, for the purpose of giving information relative to many of its peculiarities, as well as to remove deep-rooted prejudice, it has been my object to collect and embody in this work, most of those writings, and to arrange them, with cases cited, as may serve to illustrate its usefulness in general; and if possible, to gain for it that attention which the subject demands at the hands of the medical world . . . .

Among the seventeen chapters are ones on "Sulphuric ether in surgery" (page 51ff.) and "Chloroform as a local anaesthesia" (page 119ff.); there were no illustrations. This was the only edition. Flagg's other booklength work is *The family dentist; containing a brief description of the structure, formation, diseases, and treatment of the human teeth* (Boston: J. W. Ingraham, 1822).

GS30. **RICHARD UPTON PIPER** (1816–97). *Operative surgery.* 384pp. Boston: Ticknor, Reed & Fields, 1852.

Piper, a graduate of Dartmouth Medical School, practiced medicine in Boston and Chicago. His textbook is one of the most comprehensively illustrated nineteenth-century American surgical works. It contains more than 1,900 engravings on 186 plates, most of which were completed by Piper himself. Fifty of the engravings are hand-colored (plates 10–16, 19, and 20). In the preface, Piper writes:

. . . almost every subject connected with practical surgery is covered . . . although it really contains ample illustrations of all the regular operations . . . the surgeon will also find here a large amount of useful and practical information, upon a wide range of collateral subjects connected with surgical manipulations . . . illustrations of a great number of irregular and special operations, are here for the first time brought together . . . .

In addition, Henry J. Bigelow's (1818–90) 1848 paper on anesthetic agents [G-M 5730] is included as an appendix. There is no table of contents, but the book does contain a detailed and lengthy index. This was the only edition and is the only book-length work on medicine that Piper wrote.

GS31. **HENRY HOLLINGSWORTH SMITH** (1815–90). *A system of operative surgery: based upon the practice of surgeons in the United States: and comprising a bibliographical index and historical record of many of their operations, during a period of two hundred years.* 698pp. Philadelphia: Lippincott & Grambo, 1852.

Smith wrote his first systematic textbook of surgery three years prior to his appointment as professor of surgery at the University of Pennsylvania. Comprehensive in scope, it was published in a second edition in 1856. Dedicated to Charles A. Pope (1818–70), professor of surgery at St. Louis University, the volume is particularly important to the photographic history of American medicine because it was the first American surgical textbook to have illustrations based on daguerreotypes. Smith wrote in the preface:

Having, from long intercourse with medical classes . . . learned that seeing an operation and performing it are very different acts, the author has wished to lead the reader to a more correct estimate of the means by which operative skill is to be acquired, and sought, in the following pages, to furnish him a guide which might also serve as an instructor, whilst performing for himself the operations which he desires to study

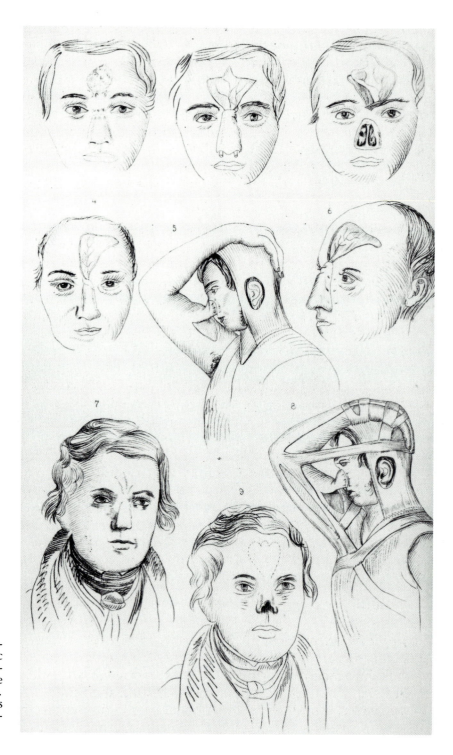

Fig. 11. (GS30) Some of the earliest examples of rhinoplastic operations in America are depicted in this black-and-white wood-engraved plate (No. LXXXV; page 144), from Piper's very extensively illustrated surgical text.

.... In selecting the illustrations, various sources have been resorted to, but upon none has the author relied more than on the beautifully finished plates of Messrs. Bernard & Huette. Wherever, in any instance, previous figures did not present such views as were desired, the aid of the Daguerreotype has been invoked, and original drawings made with all the accuracy of the scene at the moment ....

This is a massive work consisting of five major parts: "General duties and elementary operations"; "Operations on the head and face"; "Operations practiced on the neck and trunk"; "Operations on the genitourinary organs and rectum" and, "Operations on the extremities." There is an extremely important introductory section detailing the progress of American surgical history, a bibliographical index of American surgical writers and a list of their works by subject, and an extensive alphabetical list of American surgeons with the titles of their most important papers. The eighty steel-engraved plates were available either printed in sanguine or in the extremely rare form of "colored to life." The book sold for $7.50 or $15.00, respectively. (See also GS21, GS22.1, GS38, GS39, and GS55.)

GS32. **HENRY INGERSOLL BOWDITCH** (1808–92). *A treatise on diaphragmatic hernia.* 77pp. Buffalo: Jewett & Thomas, 1853.

Bowditch was a graduate of Harvard Medical School and professor of medicine at Harvard. He is recognized as one of the earliest physicians to specialize in diseases of the chest, having pioneered the operation for removal of pleural effusions with trocar and suction pump. He was a founder of the American Public Health Association and served as president of the American Medical Association in 1877. The occasion for writing his *Treatise* was the autopsy of a patient, which demonstrated a congenital diaphragmatic hernia. Bowditch was intrigued by this finding and determined to review all the medical literature on the subject. The result was a collection of eighty-eight cases published between 1610 and 1846. There are ten sections with several pages devoted to treatment. Under the heading "Operation" he states: "Finally, as a last resource, might not an operation for cutting the strangulated ring be attempted? It has never been done . . . having tried other means of relief without success, ought we not to undertake the more serious operation of the scalpel?" Bowditch's other medical books are *The young stethoscopist; or, the student's aid to auscultation* (New York: S. S. & W. Wood, 1846) and *Public hygiene in America* (Boston: Little & Brown, 1877).

GS33. **RALPH GLOVER** (1798–69). *A treatise on orthopedic surgery and hernia; containing directions for adjusting and applying trusses to every species of rupture, for the purpose of effecting radical cures by the use of an improved instrument.* 175pp. New York: A. Baptist, 1853.

Glover was an 1826 graduate of Jefferson Medical College, but he never held an academic position. On the title page of his *Treatise* he lists his credentials: "manufacturer of ladies' belts and abdominal supporters, shoulder braces, instruments for club-feet, spinal distortions, bow-legs, knock-knees, weak ankle joints, and every deformity of the human body." He founded the New York Truss and Bandage Institute, which adjoined the renowned American Museum of Phineas Taylor Barnum (1810–91). Only one edition was published, and copies are exceedingly scarce. There are numerous illustrations and plates depicting various trusses and orthopedic instruments. The first ninety-six pages are devoted to orthopedic surgery. The second portion contains chapters on "Hernia"; "Various body braces"; and "Deformities and distortions of the human body." Section 7 of chapter 3 (page 136ff.) contains an important observation on the use of chloroform as a new medical agent to enable the surgeon to "effect a reduction of strangulated hernia."

GS34. **SAMUEL DAVID GROSS** (1805–84). *A practical treatise on foreign bodies in the air-passages.* 468pp. Philadelphia: Blanchard & Lea, 1854. [G-M 3264]

Gross's *Treatise* was written when he was professor of surgery at the University of Louisville. He writes in his *Autobiography* (volume 1, page 95):

> My work was issued from the press of Blanchard & Lea in 1854, in an octavo volume of four hundred and sixty-eight pages, illustrated by fifty-nine engravings on wood. Its composition occupied me upwards of two years. It was the first attempt to systematize our knowledge upon the subject, and the work is therefore, strictly speaking, a pioneer work. My original intention was not to write a book, but to compose a short monograph for some medical journal. I had not, however, proceeded far before I discovered that I had formed a very imperfect idea of the enterprise, and that, in order to do it justice, much time and study would be required. If in the providence of God, the work shall be instrumental in saving the life of one human being, or even in ameliorating the sufferings of a single individual, I shall feel myself amply remunerated for the time I have bestowed upon its composition. If there be any situation better calculated than another to awaken our sympathy, it is when we see before us a fellow-creature who is threatened every instant with destruction, in consequence of the lodgment of a foreign body in the air-passages, without the ability to expel it or the power to inflate the lungs. It was this reflection which first induced me, many years ago, to turn my attention to the subject, and which has finally impelled me to write this treatise. This work has now been long out of print. A new edition, much abridged, might be made the basis of a complete treatise on the surgical affections of the air-passages.

The book is dedicated to George W. Norris (1808–75) and is " . . . designed as a contribution to statistical surgery, a subject which no one understands better than himself, because no one has studied it better."

There are seventeen chapters, including "General considerations"; "Immediate effects produced by the entrance of foreign bodies into the air-passages"; "Pathological effects"; "Symptoms"; "Diagnosis"; "Spontaneous expulsion"; "Medical treatment"; "Inversion of patient's body to promote expulsion"; "Surgical treatment"; "Laryngotomy"; "Tracheotomy"; "Laryngo-tracheotomy"; "Repetition of bronchotomy"; "Cases of bronchotomy in which no foreign body was found, although the symptoms were strongly denotive of its presence"; "Causes of death

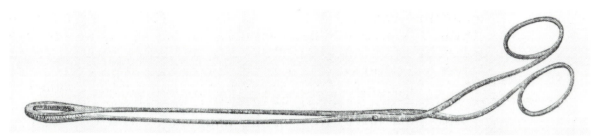

Fig. 12. (GS34) In this simple wood engraving (figure 20, page 252) Gross depicts his forceps used to extract foreign bodies from air-passages.

without operation"; and "Bronchotomy in the inferior animals." Using over 100 case reports, Gross presented principles concerning symptoms which remain fundamental to the care of pulmonary patients. (See also GS16, GS19, GS46, GS49, OR2, and GU5.)

GS35. **GEORGE HAYWARD** (1791–1863). *Surgical reports and miscellaneous papers on medical subjects.* 452pp. Boston: Phillips & Sampson, 1855.

Hayward is best known as the first American surgeon to perform a major surgical operation with ether anesthesia. As a member of the surgical staff at Massachusetts General Hospital, he completed an amputation of the thigh on November 7, 1846, (discussed on pages 230–31) less than a month after John Collins Warren's (1778–1856) epochal operation. The *Reports* is replete with important surgical topics, including ligature of the carotid artery, vesico-vaginal fistula [G-M 6030], hydrophobia, statistics on amputations, and the general use of anesthetic agents. In chapter 12, Hayward provides one of the earliest descriptions of pulmonary complications suffered in burn injury. His other book is *Outlines of human physiology; designed for the use of higher classes in common schools* (Boston: Marsh, Capen & Lyon, 1834).

GS36. **WILLIAM TOD HELMUTH** (1833–1902). *Surgery and its adaptation to homoeopathic practice.* 651pp. Philadelphia: Moss & Brother, 1855.

This work and Hill and Hunt's effort (GS37) were the first two American homeopathic surgical textbooks. They were both published in 1855 and reflect different schools within the homeopathic movement. Helmuth's volume is quite comprehensive. Its thirty-nine chapters cover a wide variety of topics and include 103 wood engravings. Many of the chapters contain a treatment section that outlines numerous homeopathic cures. Helmuth states in the preface:

> The author of this volume has a satisfactory reason for its publication at the present time, in the desire so urgently and generally expressed for a surgical work in connection with homeopathy. A perusal of its contents will satisfy the reader that the materials have been collected from a tolerably wide field of research. That much important matter has been overlooked is unhesitatingly admitted . . . . From the volume there is purposely excluded many surgical details, together with a large amount of material connected with surgery, but not with its practice;

the chief object of the publication having been the collection and arrangement of those materials which are considered as constituting the medical treatment of surgical diseases . . . . It would be foreign to the occasion as well as derogatory, to notice in a work devoted to a branch of medicine so essentially exalted in its nature as surgery, the very illogical objections so often repeated against everything connected with homeopathy. Its absurdity and impotency in the estimation of some are proven even in the fact, that homeopathic practictioners have recourse to mechanical means for the treatment of accidents, or the removal of mutilated or diseased parts; in other words, because medicines have not physical power to supply the place of cutting instruments, bandages, fracture boxes and pulleys, it is unworthy the attention of an intelligent mind. As this objection, however, applies equally to alleopathy, the two conflicting doctrines are thereby placed in the same position, and there the homeopathic physician may be quite satisfied in allowing them to remain . . . . "

Later editions of the book came out in 1873, 1878, 1879, and 1887 under the title *A system of surgery*. The most prominent homeopathic surgeon of his day, Helmuth was dean of New York Homoeopathic College and Flower Hospital. The present volume was written when he was just twenty-two years old. Helmuth was also a founder of and professor of surgery at the St. Louis College of Homoeopathic Physicians and Surgeons. Another of Helmuth's books is *Scratches of a surgeon* (Chicago: W. A. Chatterton, 1879). (See also GS53.1 and GU15.)

GS37. **BENJAMIN LORD HILL** (1813–71) and **JAMES GEORGE HUNT** (1822–?). *The homoeopathic practice of surgery, together with operative surgery.* Two volumes in one, 431pp. and 223pp. Cleveland: J. B. Cobb, 1855.

Hill had originally been professor of surgery at the Eclectic Medical Institute in Cincinnati. In the early 1850s, like many other physicians, he turned his attention to homeopathy and became professor of

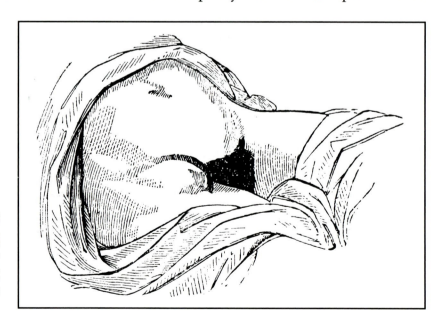

Fig. 13. (GS36) As with most of the early homeopathic texts, the figures in Helmuth's work were elementary wood engravings. In this drawing (figure 92, page 572) the artist has crudely attempted to depict a crural or femoral hernia.

obstetrics and diseases of females and later professor of surgery at Western Homeopathic College in Cleveland. Hunt, who was Hill's partner in practice, served as professor of surgery at the same college. This book is actually two volumes in one. The first has thirty-seven chapters, and the second has nineteen. There are 240 engravings. Along with William Helmuth's (1833–1902) work (GS36), this volume is the first of various homeopathic American surgical texts. However, in deference to Helmuth, whose textbook was written entirely within the field of homeopathy, Hill and Hunt's effort is actually a partial reprint (the major portion of volume 2 and a considerable portion of the description proper of diseases in volume 1) of Hill's earlier work on eclectic surgery (GS28). The present treatise has an interesting origin: it was written after a letter was distributed in January 1852 soliciting requests from numerous homeopathic physicians in America and Europe to provide information from their clinical experience. Portions of this letter read:

> Inasmuch as practical experience in our Science dates back but a short time in this country, it can not be supposed that any one man would have sufficient experience in surgical diseases (a considerable portion of which are of rare occurrence), to enable him alone to furnish the proper material for such a work . . . . For the accomplishment of this purpose, we have determined to ask some favors of our most learned and experienced practitioners, which, we hope, for the sake of the cause,

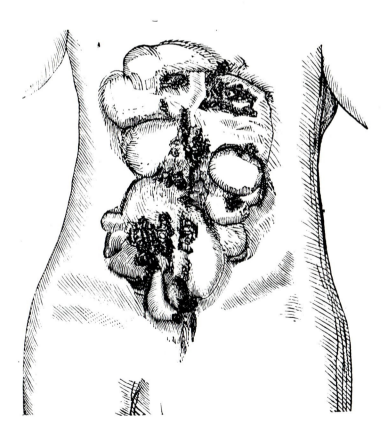

Fig. 14. (GS37) Hill and Hunt use this engraving (page 211) to demonstrate a forty-year-old female who had undergone surgical removal of a tumor of the abdominal wall. Shortly thereafter the tumor began to regrow and reached the size shown here. They applied a homeopathic preparation of arsenicum both internally and externally to the mass; the "cancer" eventually sloughed off in large pieces, and the wound healed by granulation.

will be granted. We are aware that it is asking much, but we hope, some time, to be able to render a suitable regard for the favor. We wish you to give us, in as full details as practicable, any very successful treatment you may have employed for the following affections: traumatic erysipelas, burns and scalds, frost-bites, irritable, indolent and varicose ulcers, necroses, scrofulous swellings and ulcers, chronic rheumatism, hip disease, lumbar abscess, white swelling, hydrops articuli, polypus of the nose and uterus, cancer of the womb, cancer in general, osteosarcoma, fungus haematodes, scald-head of children, fistula lachrymalis, fistula in ano, maxillary abscess, ophthalmis (purulent, scrofulous and gonorrheal in particular), amaurosis, nebula and leucoma, ulcers of the cornea and lids, cataract, dropsy of the eye, enlarged tonsils, goitre, mammary abscess, hernia, hydrocele, haematocele, orchitis, hemorrhoids, prolapsus ani, stricture of the rectum and urethra, spermatorrhea, gonorrhea, primary, secondary and tertiary syphillis . . . . We further ask that you will allow us the privilege of giving you credit in the book for what you contribute.

Volume 1 (pages 129–39) has an interesting and detailed list of numerous homeopathic treatments for ulcers. At the end of the volume there is an advertisement for the Western Homeopathic College and the Institution for the Treatment of Surgical Diseases in Berlin Heights, Erie County, Ohio. (See also GS28.)

GS38. **HENRY HOLLINGSWORTH SMITH** (1815–90). *Syllabus of the lectures on the principles and practice of surgery.* 115pp. Philadelphia: T. K. & P. G. Collins, 1855.

With his appointment as professor of surgery at the University of Pennsylvania in 1855, Smith had a syllabus of his surgical lectures printed for the use of the class. This was the only year in which it was done. The book was interleaved with blank pages to allow students to take notes. (See also GS21, GS22.1, GS31, GS39, and GS55.)

GS39. **HENRY HOLLINGSWORTH SMITH** (1815–90). *A treatise on the practice of surgery.* 828pp. Philadelphia: J. B. Lippincott, 1856.

This textbook was prepared as an adjunct to Smith's lectures on the principles and practice of surgery. He intended this volume to form a series with his *System of operative surgery* (GS31). It is illustrated by 274 engravings, many of which represent microscopic appearances of structure, marking one of the earliest uses of the microscope in an American textbook on surgery. The *Treatise* is dedicated to James Lawrence Cabell (1813–89), and Smith notes in the preface that this work, in conjunction with William Edmonds Horner's (1793–1853) *The United States dissector: or, lessons in practical anatomy* (Philadelphia: Lippincott & Grambo, 1854), which Smith had edited and completely revised, were intended to form one series on the science and art of surgery. The preface notes this intention:

> In the composition of the present Treatise, it has been the author's wish to present each subject as fully as was essential to its comprehension by the youngest of his pupils without entering into such details of the history, pathology, etc., of each as properly belongs to monographs. Such an extended treatise on each of the various affections that are daily

presented to the attention of the surgeon, would have enlarged this work beyond reasonable limits and destroyed the object of its formation . . . . As the present volume is intended to aid the inexperienced surgeon, the author has added, in various places throughout it, a few formulae of such combinations of medicinal articles as have proved useful; but he desires to express the wish that the reader will regard them only as applicable to certain conditions of diseased action, or to certain stages of the affections under which they are without a careful analysis of their adaptation to special cases, their use becomes empirical, and such as no intelligent surgeon would be willing to sanction.

The volume is divided into seventeen parts, including "Surgical pathology and therapeutics"; "Surgical pathology of the soft tissues"; "Pathology of the abnormal growths in the soft tissues"; "Of injuries of the soft tissues"; "Injuries and diseases of the bones"; "Injuries and diseases of the joints"; "Affections of the eyeball and its appendages"; "Diseases of the ear"; "Affections of the nose and its cavities"; "Affections of the throat and neck"; "Affections of the abdomen"; "Diseases of the genital organs"; "Affections of the kidneys and bladder"; "Affections of the testicle and cord"; "Diseases of the rectum"; "Affections of the blood vessels"; and "Affections of the extremities." (See also GS21, GS22.1, GS38, and GS55.)

GS40. **JOHN MURRAY CARNOCHAN** (1817–87). *Contributions to operative surgery, and surgical pathology.* 77pp. Philadelphia: Lindsay & Blakiston, 1857.

Carnochan was born in Savannah, Georgia, and received his M.D. from the College of Physicians and Surgeons in New York in 1836. Most of his professional career was spent in New York, where he was surgeon-in-chief to the State Emigrant Hospital on Ward's Island, then the largest hospital in the country. He is remembered for performing the first excision of the superior maxillary nerve for the treatment of facial neuralgia [G-M 4854], which he describes on pages 62–77. The initial *Contributions* consists of three parts, including "Descriptions of amputation of the entire jaw"; "Exsection of an ulna"; and "Restoration of the upper lip." The volume has eight magnificent chromolithographs and an intriguing introductory epistle to Valentine Mott (1785–1865). The preface states:

> While respect for life will dictate to the surgeon the greatest prudence— will counsel him to attempt no operation which he would not be willing to perform on his own child, it will also teach him, that if the extremes of boldness are to be shunned, pusillanimity is not the necessary alternative. The surgeon who has not sufficient courage to propose a useful operation and sufficient skill to perform it, is as open to censure as the reckless practitioner who is swayed by the unworthy lure of notoriety.

The exact publishing history of this work is difficult to establish. Additional parts totalling 127 pages were printed from 1858 through 1860. For unknown reasons no further parts were issued again until 1877. The 1877 edition is dedicated to Samuel David Gross (1805–84) and contains interesting sections on "Shock and collapse"; and "On the primary treatment of injuries" (pages 87–308). Eight parts were published through 1883, totalling almost 400 pages with sixteen colored plates. (See also OR6.)

GS41. **PAUL FITZSIMMONS EVE** (1806–77). *A collection of remarkable cases in surgery.* 858pp. Philadelphia: J. B. Lippincott, 1857.

Eve was internationally recognized as a lithotomist and eventually served as the eleventh president of the American Medical Association from 1857 to 1858. During the Civil War, he was chief surgeon to the Confederate Army. He was professor of surgery at the Medical College of Georgia, University of Louisville, and the University of Nashville. This volume, written when he lived in Nashville, presents unusual surgical problems grouped according to various divisions of the human body: "Head"; "Spinal column"; "Face"; "Neck"; "Chest"; "Abdomen"; "Pelvis"; "Genito-urinary organs"; and "Extremities." Among the "remarkable" cases are blindness from worms in the eye (pages 121–22) and an amputation of the head with the patient surviving thirty-six hours (pages 758–59). There is an extensive index of cases at the conclusion of the volume. This book provides some of the most enjoyable and entertaining reading to be found in any nineteenth-century American surgical text.

GS42. **WILLIAM HENRY COOK** (1832–99). *A treatise on the principles and practice of physio-medical surgery.* 714pp. Cincinnati: Moore, Wilstach & Keys, 1858.

Cook was professor of therapeutics and materia medica at the Physio-Medical College of Ohio at the time this work was published. He had previously served as professor of surgery in the same institution. Little else is known about him, but the preface does provide an explanation of physio-medical surgery:

> The distinguishing features of physio-medical surgery may be said to lie in these three points: 1st. That irritation, inflammation and fever, are purely vital demonstrations, opposing the encroachments of disease and never directly favoring the advance of death. 2d. That congestion, suppuration, ulceration and gangrene are processes of destruction, existing only when the life principle has lost its control over the tissues and the resolving power of chemical laws has usurped its place. 3rd. That no agent can be directly serviceable in the treatment of disease, unless it is essentially innocent in its qualities. These propositions lie at the very foundation of all surgical practice. It does not answer the purposes of truth to sneer at them as novelties, jilt them as speculations nor thrust them aside as verbal exactions. They are either wholly correct or totally false; and he who would pass them by without either establishing or refuting them, is rashly anxious to rush upon unknown ground. The physio-medicalist has the enviable satisfaction of knowing that his distinctive principles are in harmony with every fact in nature, that they are applicable to the minutest requirements of a bed-side practice, that they have stood the closest scrutiny for a period of seventy years and that they have saved thousands of limbs and thousands of lives that had otherwise been beyond the reach of human art . . . . As no book can supply a surgeon with mechanical skill, the description of

the several operations have been intentionally limited; and as unsettled questions are never helped to a solution by dogmatic pedantry, it has been deemed better and more just to confess a want of light where it was felt, than to attempt to establish a theory that had only plausibility to recommend it . . . .

The volume contains five sections: "Vital manifestations of disease"; "Processes of destruction"; "Accidents and injuries"; "Special affections of tissues and regions"; and "The operations of surgery." With forty-eight chapters and numerous engravings, the work is massive in scope. This was the only edition. Cook's other books are *Physiomedical dispensatory* (Cincinnati: private printing, 1869), *Man: his generative system and his marital relations* (Cincinnati: W. H. Cook, 1890), *A handbook of family medicine and hygiene* (Cincinnati: G. P. Houston, 1890), and *A compend of the new materia medica together with additional description of some old remedies* (Chicago: W. H. Cook, 1896).

GS43. **RICHARD MANNING HODGES** (1827–96). *Practical dissections.* 254pp. Cambridge: J. Bartlett, 1858.

A graduate of Harvard College and Medical School, Hodges was on the surgical staff of Massachusetts General Hospital. He was also a demonstrator in anatomy at Harvard under Oliver Wendell Holmes (1809–94), serving in that position for eight years. His dissecting ability was reputed to be second to none, and he is known for coining the term *pilonidal sinus.* This volume was a practical manual for both student and beginning surgeon. A second edition was published by Henry C. Lea in 1867. Among his other books is *A narrative of events connected with the introduction of sulphuric ether into surgical use* (Boston: Little & Brown, 1891). (See also OR8.)

GS44. **JAMES MARION SIMS** (1813–83). *Silver sutures in surgery.* 79pp. New York: S. S. & W. Wood, 1858. [G-M 5605]

Sims was one of the most prominent nineteenth-century American surgeons and was internationally renowned for his development of an operation for vesico-vaginal fistula [G-M 6037]. An 1835 graduate of Jefferson Medical College, he established the Women's Hospital in New York. Sims served as president of the American Medical Association in 1876. Introduction of silver sutures decreased wound sepsis and allowed Sims to develop numerous operative techniques [G-M 3625, 6049, 6050, and 6057]. The text for this volume is actually an anniversary address given on November 18, 1857, before the New York Academy of Medicine. Sims felt this would be a propitious occasion to advocate his technique for closing wounds that would prevent inflammation and save lives. He described a number of uses of silver sutures, including those for plastic surgery and gynecology. James Pratt Marr in his book *Pioneer surgeons of the Woman's Hospital* (Philadelphia: F. A. Davis, 1957) describes the lecture (pages 25–26):

> In February, 1854 Sims published a booklet on vesico-vaginal fistula cured by his silver-wire technique. Three years later, in delivering the Anniversary Oration at the New York Academy of Medicine, he made a plea for the use of silver wire as a suture material instead of silk or cot-

ton thread. He described his successes with silver wire in vesico-vaginal fistula; in old third-degree lacerations of the pelvic floor; in plastic surgery of the face, harelip and scalp wounds; in amputations of the breast or leg. He told of the number of cases thus treated wherein healing by primary union had taken place. He advocated tying the pedicle

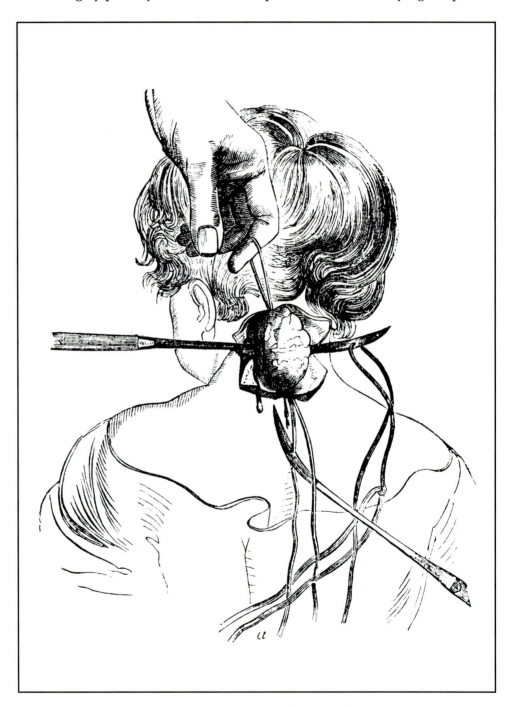

Fig. 15. (GS46) Although Gross's two-volume textbook has been called the most important surgical treatise of his time, there are no plates and all the illustrations consist of simple wood engravings. This particular engraving, figure 221 on page 973 in volume 1, depicts an "erectile" or benign vascular tumor of the posterior neck and demonstrates how to excise it by simple transfixation of its base.

of an ovarian cyst with silver wire rather than leaving a silk cord protruding from the wound to act as an avenue to intraperitoneal infection. He also spoke of suturing gunshot wounds of the large bowel with fine silver wire.

Sims closed his oration with a glowing picture of the Woman's Hospital-to-be with its new permanent building and its large and well-appointed staff. The new hospital had been unanimously endorsed by New York City's medical societies and university professors. Though Sims did not say so, his own efforts and zeal were in large part responsible for the enlarged institution becoming a reality . . . .

Among his other books is an autobiography, *The story of my life* (New York: D. Appleton, 1884). (See also GY12.)

GS45. **ELI GEDDINGS** (1799–1878). *Outlines of a course of lectures on the principles and practice of surgery delivered by E. Geddings, prepared by Thos. S. Waring and Samuel Logan.* 560pp. Charleston: S. G. Courtenay, 1858.

Geddings was professor of surgery at the Medical College of South Carolina. He was a well-known bibliophile, but events during the Civil War led to the destruction of his entire collection. Waring and Logan were students of Geddings who gained permission to publish his lectures. Since his talks were entirely extemporaneous, this volume was a monumental effort on their part. It consists of three sections ("General surgical diseases," "Structural affections," and "Regional or topographical surgery") divided into sixty-eight lectures and ten essays. There are no illustrations, and this was the only edition.

GS46. **SAMUEL DAVID GROSS** (1805–84). *A system of surgery; pathological, diagnostic, therapeutic, and operative.* 2 vols., 1162pp. and 1198pp. Philadelphia: Blanchard & Lea, 1859. [G-M 5607]

Gross's *Surgery* is considered one of the most important surgical treatises of its time and was a truly herculean effort. It went through five more editions, in 1862, 1864, 1866, 1872, and 1882. Bound only in leather, the set sold initially for $12.00. The first edition comprised two thousand copies. Gross describes his aims in the preface:

> The object of this work is to furnish a systematic and comprehensive treatise on the science and practice of surgery . . . . My aim has been to embrace the whole domain of surgery, and to allot to every subject its legitimate claim to notice in the great family of external diseases and accidents.

Its forty-seven chapters, 936 illustrations, and 2,360 pages attest to its encyclopedic scope. Referring to this work, Gross writes in his *Autobiography* (volume 1, pages 137–42):

> One of the chief motives which induced me to remove to Philadelphia was to get rid of a large and annoying family practice at Louisville and to write an elaborate System of Surgery, for the production of which my leisure in Kentucky was not sufficient . . . . I had determined to do my best to make it, if possible, the most elaborate, if not the most complete, treatise in the English language . . . . The heads of my lectures served me as a valuable guide, and I generally wrote with facility, as my knowledge

of the subject, from long study, practice, and contemplation, was extensive, and, in the main, accurate. I generally spent from five to eight
hours a day upon my manuscript, subject of course to frequent and
sometimes annoying interruptions by patients. In the winter I commonly sat up till eleven and half past eleven o'clock at night . . . . Unless I was greatly interrupted, I seldom wrote less than from ten to fifteen
pages of foolscap in the twenty-four hours, and I rarely retired until they
were carefully corrected. It was not often I rewrote anything . . . . The
edition cost a large sum of money, enough, as Blanchard & Lea assured
me, to have enabled them to open a respectable mercantile house on
Market Street . . . . What compensation does the reader think I obtained
for this hard work, this excessive toil of my brain, including original
composition, the correction and improvement of new editions, and the
proof-reading, in itself a horrible task, death to brain and eyes . . . .
Eighty-five cents a copy, all told, and no extra dividends! Two dollars
and a half ought to have been the price, or, what would have been more
equitable, an equal distribution of the profits from the sale of the work.
No wonder authors are poor and publishers are rich!

(See also GS16, GS19, GS34, GS49, OR2, and GU5.)

GS47. **SAMUEL WARD FRANCIS** (1835–86). *Report of Professor Valentine Mott's surgical cliniques in the University of New York, session
1859–60.* 209pp. New York: S. S. & W. Wood, 1860.

Francis was a member of Valentine Mott's (1785–1865) surgical staff
for two years. He then moved to Newport, Rhode Island, where he continued his practice of medicine. Francis is best remembered for the two
biographical works he wrote concerning American physicians: *Biographical sketches of distinguished living New York surgeons* (New York: J. Bradburn, 1866) and *Biographical sketches of distinguished living New York
physicians* (New York: G. P. Putnam & Son, 1867). Mott was one of the
premier surgeons of nineteenth-century America. His contributions
were numerous and included innovative vascular operations [G-M 2942,
2950–2953, and 2958] and oncologic procedures [G-M 3259, 4447, and
4452]. Unfortunately, Mott disliked writing and as a consequence never
wrote any surgical textbooks. His only book-length work is *Travels in
Europe and the East* (New York: Harper Brothers, 1842). Francis's work
comes closest to preserving, as he put it, " . . . some of the aphorisms of
one whose experience is as vast in the practice of surgery, as his reputation is great in the eyes of his countrymen." Although not organized
in a systematic fashion, the ninety-one cases provide a fabulous wealth
of information.

GS48. **JULIAN JOHN CHISOLM** (1830–1903). *A manual of military surgery,
for the use of surgeons in the Confederate States army; with an appendix of the rules and regulations of the medical department of the Confederate army.* 447pp. Richmond: West & Johnston, 1861.

A key figure in the medical hierarchy of the Confederate Army,
Chisolm was professor of surgery at the Medical College of South
Carolina. After the war he was appointed professor of operative surgery
and diseases of eye and ear at the University of Maryland. Chisolm's

Manual became the textbook of the Confederate surgeons. It was largely based on the experience he gained while observing the medical and surgical treatment of wounded soldiers in Italy in 1859. The initial printing of the *Manual* was published at varying locations, since Evans & Cogswell of Charleston, South Carolina, also published a first edition, as did West & Johnston. The *Manual* went through further editions in 1862 and 1864. The preface provides an explanation for Chisolm's writing of the work:

> In putting forth this *Manual of Military Surgery* for the use of surgeons in the Confederate service, I have been led by the desire to mitigate, if possible, the horrors of war as seen in its most frightful phase in military hospitals. As our entire army is made up of volunteers from every walk of life, so we find the surgical staff of the army composed of physicians without surgical experience. Most of those who now compose the surgical staff were general practitioners whose country circuit gave them but little surgery, and very seldom presented a gunshot wound. Moreover, as our country had been enjoying an uninterrupted state of peace, the collecting of large bodies of men, and retaining them in health, or the hygiene of armies had been a study without an object, and therefore without interest. Then the war suddenly broke upon us, followed immediately by the blockading of our ports, all communication was cut off with Europe, which was the expected source of our surgical information. As there had been no previous demand for works on military surgery, there were none to be had in the stores, and our physicians were compelled to follow the army to battle without instruction. No work on military surgery could be purchased in the Confederate States. As military surgery, which is one of expediency, differs so much from civil practice, the want of proper information has already made itself seriously felt. In times of war, where invasion threatens, every citizen is expected to do his duty to his state. I saw no better means of showing my willingness to enlist in the cause than by preparing a manual of instruction for the use of the army, which might be the means of saving the lives and preventing the mutilation of many friends and countrymen. The present volume contains the fruit of European experience, as dearly purchased in recent campaigning . . . .

The book is extremely scarce due to the poor quality of the paper it was printed on and the fact that it was so widely used by Confederate surgeons on the battlefield.

GS49. **SAMUEL DAVID GROSS** (1805–84). *A manual of military surgery; or hints on the emergencies of field, camp and hospital practice.* 186pp. Philadelphia: J. B. Lippincott, 1861.

Gross describes the occasion of this work in his *Autobiography* (volume 1, pages 142–43):

> At the outbreak of the war I wrote a little *Manual of Military Surgery*, a kind of pocket companion for the young surgeons who were flocking into the army, and who for the most part were ill prepared for the prompt and efficient discharge of their duties. It was composed in nine days, and published in a fortnight from the time of its inception . . . it passed through two editions of two thousand copies each. It was republished at Richmond, and was extensively cited by the Confederate

surgeons during the war. This little book was far more profitable to me, in a commercial point of view, considering the time and labor bestowed upon it, than any other of my productions. A translation of it in Japanese appeared at Tokio in 1874.

The book was available in cloth only for fifty cents. Gross writes in the preface:

> The sole object which prompts me to publish this little book is an ardent desire to be useful to the young physicians who have so hurriedly entered the volunteer service, perhaps not always with a full knowledge of the weighty responsibilities of their position . . . . It is essentially a book for emergencies . . . . The substance of it was originally intended as an article for the July number of the *North American Medico-Chirurgical Review*, and it was not until I had made considerable progress in its composition that the idea suggested itself to my mind that it might, if published separately, be of service to a part of my profession at this particular juncture in our public affairs . . . .

Gross goes on to provide an interesting exhortation regarding mutilating surgery:

> . . . take good care, not only of the lives of their countrymen, but also of their limbs, mutilated in battle. Conservative surgery has, at the present day, claims of paramount importance upon the attention of every military practitioner; for, in the language of good old George Herbert, Man is all symmetric, Full of proportion, one limbe to another,

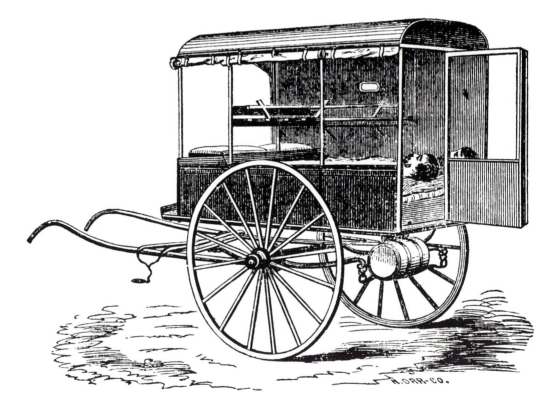

Fig. 16. (GS50) During the Civil War much progress was made in methods of conveying sick and wounded soldiers. Among the principal kinds of transportation were hand-litters, panniers, horse-litters, and wheeled ambulances. The two-wheeled ambulance shown in this engraving (page 133) was designed by R. H. Coolidge, a surgeon in the United States Army.

And all to all the world besides; Each part calls the furthest brother; For head with foot hath private amities; And both with moons and tides.

There are thirteen chapters, including "Importance of military surgery"; "Wounds and other injuries"; "Ill consequences of wounds and operations"; "Diseases incident to troops"; and "Feigned diseases." (See also GS16, GS19, GS34, GS46, OR2, and GU5.)

GS50. **FRANK HASTINGS HAMILTON** (1813–86). *A practical treatise on military surgery.* 234pp. New York: Bailliere Brothers, 1861.

Hamilton was a graduate of Union College in New York and received his M.D. in 1835 from the University of Pennsylvania. One of the most versatile of nineteenth-century American surgeons, he was professor of military surgery and of diseases and accidents incident to bones at Bellevue Medical College. Following the retirement of James R. Wood (1813–82), Hamilton was appointed professor of the principles and practice of surgery at Bellevue. His report on anaplasty was among the first to suggest treatment of leg ulcers by skin grafting [G-M 5747]. The purpose of his *Practical treatise* was to supply information on those areas in surgery, medicine, and hygiene that, although related to military and naval practice, were usually not considered in general surgical works. Within the fourteen chapters are discussions on "Bivouac"; "Accommodation of troops in tents"; "Conveyance of the sick and wounded"; "Amputations"; and "Hospital gangrene." The appendix on pages 215–19 contains information on camp and hospital cooking for large numbers of soldiers. In addition, pages 220–24 record the salary levels for physicians entering the military. There are approximately thirty illustrations scattered throughout the text. A second and much enlarged edition was published in 1865. Its new title was *A treatise on military surgery and hygiene,* and it contained 127 engravings. Among Hamilton's other medically related books are *Health aphorisms, and an essay on the struggle for life against civilization, luxury, and aestheticism* (New York: Bermingham, 1882) and *Conversations between Drs. Warren and Putnam on the subject of medical ethics, with an account of the medical empiricisms of Europe and America* (New York: Bermingham, 1884). (See also GS70, GS75, OP8, OR7, and OR37.)

GS50.1. **CHARLES THOMAS JACKSON** (1805–80). *A manual of etherization: containing directions for the employment of ether, chloroform, and other anaesthetic agents, by inhalation, in surgical operations, intended for military and naval surgeons, and all who may be exposed to surgical operations.* 134pp. Boston: J. B. Mansfield, 1861.

One of the most colorful and controversial figures in American medicine, Jackson received his M.D. from Harvard Medical School in 1829. During his professional life he is known to have suggested to William Thomas G. Morton (1819–68) that ether would render nerves insensible to pain. Later Jackson asserted his right to be considered the true discoverer of surgical anesthesia. In addition, Jackson claimed to have invented guncotton, and to have described to Samuel F. B. Morse (1791–1872) the essential features of the electric telegraph. During the

1830s and 1840s Jackson worked as a state and federal geologist, but frequently found himself in so much conflict with other geologists that he resigned from numerous positions. Jackson was frequently involved in bitter personal disputes and spent most of the last decade of his life in the McLean Asylum for the insane in Massachusetts. His *Manual* was written

> . . . with a view to interest both the surgeon and the soldier . . . as to the nature, effects, and management of anaesthetic agents . . . . It is not intended to place a small work, like this, in competition with more extended and elaborate treatises by others, but rather to fill up a space which no one has thus far occupied . . . . I would state that every allegation in this book is sustained by ample published evidence that has never been impeached in any quarter.

There are seven chapters, which are well summarized in an extensive table of contents on pages 128–34. Chapter 5 is almost entirely devoted to Jackson's attempts to have himself declared the discoverer of surgical anesthesia. Chapter 6 contains a lengthy discussion of etherization and its application to surgery. In it, Jackson makes the categorical statement that one should "never etherize a woman unless another of her sex is present." There are five rudimentary woodcut illustrations. There was only one edition.

GS51. **CHARLES STUART TRIPLER** (1806–66) and **GEORGE CURTIS BLACKMAN** (1819–71). *Handbook for the military surgeon: being a compendium of the duties of the medical officer in the field, the sanitary management of the camp, the preparation of food, etc.; with forms for the requisitions for supplies, returns, etc.; the diagnosis and treatment of camp dysentery; and all the important points in war surgery, including gun-shot wounds, amputations, wounds of the chest, abdomen, arteries and head, and the use of chloroform.* 121,xliipp. Cincinnati: R. Clarke, 1861.

An 1827 graduate of the College of Physicians and Surgeons in New York, Tripler was general director of the Army of the Potomac and organized all its medical services. Blackman was professor of surgery at the Medical College of Ohio. A second edition of the *Handbook* was published, also in 1861. The book was available in cloth covers for $1.00. It consists of ten chapters, which discuss such subjects as "Camp dysentery"; "Amputations"; "Use of chloroform"; and wounds of the chest, abdomen, head, and arteries. The publisher provides an explanation of the book's purpose in the preface:

> . . . the publishers requested Dr. Chas. S. Tripler, U.S.A., to consent to the issue of the lectures which for the last three years he has delivered in the Medical College of Ohio, by invitation of the professor of surgery in that institution. To this the doctor kindly consented. The publishers likewise requested Professor Blackman to supply the material for the chapters on wounds of the abdomen, head, and arteries . . . . A chapter on the use of chloroform has been added, taken from the valuable work of Mr. Macleod on the Crimean War.

Tripler's other book is *A manual of the medical officer of the army of the United States. Part 1. recruiting and the inspection of recruits.* (Cincinnati: Wrightson, 1858).

GS52. JOHN BUCHANAN (1852–1924). *The eclectic practice of medicine and surgery.* 860pp. 3rd edition. Philadelphia: J. Buchanan, 1867.

Buchanan was an eclectic and self-promoter who bordered on quackery. This volume has no table of contents, no index, and is particularly difficult to read. Most of the text extolls the virtues of Buchanan's numerous botanic remedies. He was later involved in granting bogus medical degrees.

GS53. STEPHEN SMITH (1823–1922). *Hand-book of surgical operations.* 279pp. New York: Bailliere Brothers, 1862.

Smith's *Handbook* was the most widely used surgical manual among the Union forces. It went through five editions within two years and proved a most valuable vade mecum for the field surgeon. Consisting of only six chapters, it discusses "Minor surgery"; "Arteries"; "Veins"; "Amputations"; "Resections"; and "Gunshot wounds." The first edition is exceptionally scarce due to its extensive wartime use. Smith was one of the most enterprising American surgeons of the nineteenth century. During the Civil War he was professor of principles of surgery at Bellevue Hospital Medical College. Interestingly, he did not gain his place in American medical history because of his career as a surgeon. Instead, Smith is remembered as a pioneer public health officer and sanitary reformer. He was New York City's commissioner of health from 1868 to 1875 and through this position helped found the American Public Health Association. He is also noted for his history of American surgery [G-M 5805]. Smith's other books related to medicine include *Principles of hospital construction* (New York: Holman, 1866), *Doctor in medicine, and other papers on professional subjects* (New York: William Wood, 1872), *The city that was* (New York: F. Allaben, 1911), and *Who is insane?* (New York: Macmillan, 1916). (See also GS95.)

GS53.1. WILLIAM TOD HELMUTH (1833–1902). *A treatise on diphtheria; its nature, pathology and homeopathic treatment.* 125pp. St. Louis: H. C. G. Luyties, 1862.

This little-known work was dedicated to William S. Helmuth (1801–80), the author's paternal uncle. The volume is intended to

> ... incorporate the observation of others with a somewhat extended experience of the author, and thus to produce a readable work upon a disease to which the attention of the whole medical profession has been directed, and which will ever occupy a conspicuous position in the medical history of the nineteenth century.

There are five chapters covering "Diphtheria"; "Description of the disease"; "Pathology"; "Treatment"; and "Surgical operations." Chapter 5 on operations (pages 97–123) is divided into three sections: "Ablation of the tonsils"; "Tracheotomy"; and "Tubage of the glottis." Helmuth is honest in stating, however, that (page 97):

in the treatment of diphtheria, surgical interference is, in the majority of instances, of doubtful utility; the use of instruments causes additional pain, and, in many cases, is absolutely uncalled for, and, in other instances, death is hastened by the blundering surgeon, who, disregarding the true nature of the disorder, seeks by mechanical means to arrest a local disease, while the patient is succumbing to constitutional poison . . . .

A second edition was printed in 1864. There are no illustrations. Interestingly, on the title page the Roman numeral for the year of publication is mistakenly printed MDCCCXLII (1842). (See also GS36 and GU15.)

GS54. **JOHN HOOKER PACKARD** (1832–1907). *A manual of minor surgery.* 288pp. Philadelphia: J. B. Lippincott, 1863.

One of the original members of the American Surgical Association, Packard was an 1853 graduate of the University of Pennsylvania Medical School. He never held a true academic position, but was on the surgical staff of the Episcopal Hospital and other Philadelphia institutions. He was the father of the well-known medical historian Francis Randolph Packard (1870–1950). The *Manual* has an interesting publisher's notice:

> The board appointed [by the surgeon-general of the United States] to examine and report upon the merits of a work on Minor Surgery, respectfully report that they have carefully examined this work . . . and are satisfied that it is a better text-book upon the subject than any of the treatises with which the American market has hitherto been supplied.

There are thirteen chapters dealing with a wide variety of surgical problems, including "Dressings"; "Fractures"; "Foreign bodies"; and "Disinfectants." Among Packard's other books related to medicine is *Sea-air and sea-bathing* (Philadelphia: P. Blakiston, 1880). (See also GS59 and GS71.)

GS55. **HENRY HOLLINGSWORTH SMITH** (1815–90). *The principles and practice of surgery, embracing minor and operative surgery; with a bibliographical index of American surgical writers from the year 1783 to 1860.* 2 vols., 826pp. and 769pp. Philadelphia: J. B. Lippincott, 1863.

This work represents a combining of new editions of Smith's *Minor surgery* (GS21), *Operative surgery* (GS31), and *Practice of surgery* (GS39) into an exhaustive textbook of surgery. Over five hundred pages of additional material were added. It is especially valuable since it contains a detailed history of surgery in the United States and a bibliography of American works on surgery from 1783 to 1860. It is illustrated with 400 woodcuts, 80 plates, and nearly 1,000 steel engravings. The text is divided into sixteen parts and over 100 chapters. At the conclusion of each chapter is an exhaustive list of important related papers by American physicians. (See also GS22.1 and GS38.)

GS56. **EDWARD WARREN** (1828–93). *An epitome of practical surgery for field and hospital.* 401pp. Richmond: West & Johnston, 1863.

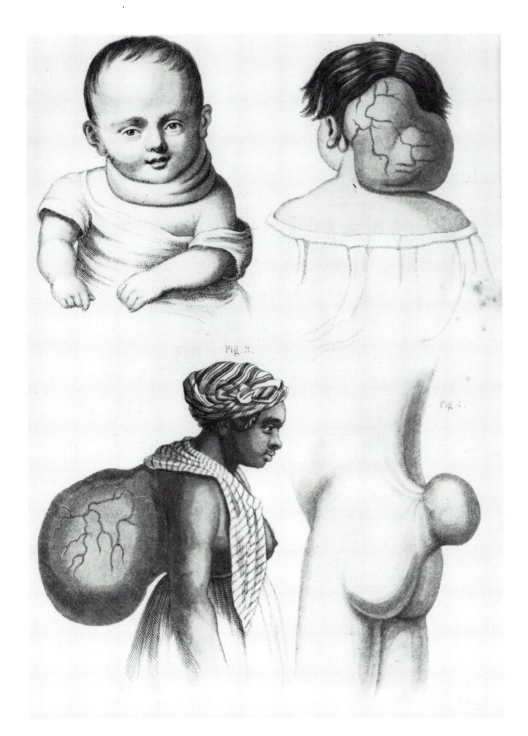

Fig. 17. (GS55) Smith uses this plate (number 48, page 45, volume 2) to show external characteristics of tumors of the back. Among those shown are a congenital tumor of the veins about the neck, a large hygroma of the back of the neck, sarcomatous tumor on the back, and spina bifida. A few copies of Smith's work have hand-colored versions of these steel engravings.

Warren was one of the most flamboyant of nineteenth-century American surgeons. An 1851 graduate of Jefferson Medical College, he served as professor of surgery at two small proprietary medical schools in Baltimore. In 1873 he left the United States for the Middle East, where he became chief surgeon of the general staff of the Khedive of Egypt.

Figs. 18–19. (GS56.1) These lithographed plates are signed by the publishers Ayres & Wade of Richmond, who operated the Illustrated News Steam Presses, and therefore had the technical capability to produce illustrations. Plates 4 and 5 graphically instructed the Confederate field surgeon on how to perform both resection and ablation of the radius and ulna as well as carpal and metacarpal resections.

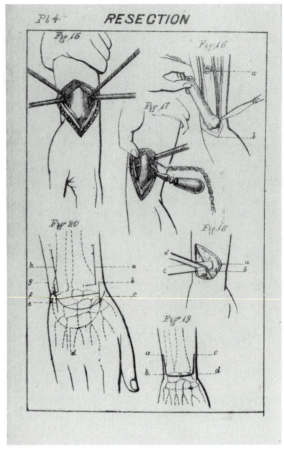

From 1875 to 1893 he practiced medicine in Paris. A rare and important work, Warren's *Epitome* was used by every Confederate medical officer. In writing it, Warren consulted a number of leading texts and made no claim to originality. In his autobiography, *A doctor's experiences in three continents* (Baltimore: Cushings & Bailey, 1885), Warren writes (pages 306–307):

> I devoted myself to the preparation of a manual of military surgery, such as my own experience with the medical officers of the Confederacy convinced me to be a desideratum. Pretending to no originality, I simply sought to describe the various operations in surgery according to the data furnished by the best authorities, and to show the appreciation to which they were entitled. The typographical execution of the book was very imperfect, as nearly all of the practical printers were in the army and the work had to be done by the merest tyros in the art, and yet it met with so cordial a reception as to necessitate immediate preparation for the issue of a second edition. It was entitled "Surgery for Field and Hospital," and though bearing the imprint of West & Johnston, of Richmond, it was really printed by some boys at Raleigh.

Despite the preparations for a second edition, the first edition was the only one that appeared.

Fig. 19.

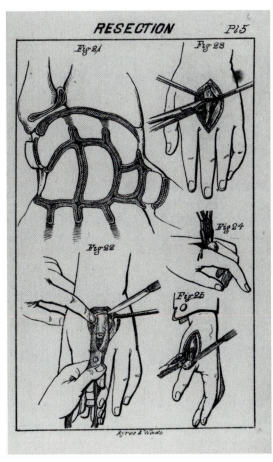

GS56.1. **SURGEON-GENERAL OF THE CONFEDERATE STATES.** *A manual of military surgery, prepared for the use of the Confederate States Army.* 297pp. Richmond: Ayres & Wade, 1863.

A scarce Civil War military manual, this volume was prepared by order of the Confederacy's surgeon-general. Written anonymously, the preface states:

> A convenient Manual has been much needed in the army of the Confederate States. To supply this deficiency, the Surgeon-General has directed the preparation of the present brief collection of papers. Unambitous of authorship, the officers to whom this duty was confided have sought only to supply, in the briefest possible period, the most comprehensive and, as near as they could, the most convenient handbook for the use . . . of medical officers in the field . . . . Throughout the work such opinions . . . have been derived from their personal experience . . . .

The book has neither a table of contents nor an index. The five chapters consist of "Surgical diseases"; "Gun-shot wounds"; "On the arteries"; "Amputations in general"; and, "On resections." Chapter II, which discusses gunshot wounds, is a condensation of Thomas Longmore's (1816–1895) contribution on the same subject to Timothy Holmes's (1825–1907) multivolume *System of surgery*. It is interesting that the surgeon-general of the United States Army also authorized the publication of Longmore's *A treatise on gunshot wounds* (Philadelphia: J. B. Lippincott, 1863) for the use of surgeons in field and general hospitals. Unlike its Southern counterpart, this Northern manual was taken essentially verbatim from Longmore's article and had no other authors. The southern *Manual* was well illustrated with thirty lithographed plates incorporating 174 figures. There was only one edition.

GS57. **WILLIAM ALEXANDER HAMMOND** (1828–1900). *Military medical and surgical essays, prepared for the United States Sanitary Commission.* 552pp. Philadelphia: J. B. Lippincott, 1864.

The Sanitary Commission was an organization that came into being through voluntary efforts to supplement the inept and inadequate services of the army medical corps during the Civil War. Hammond was surgeon-general of the United States during the war and is known for providing the first description of athetosis [G-M 4542]. These essays were completed between 1862 and 1864, and, as Hammond writes in the preface:

> The essays were prepared by gentlemen selected for their presumed acquaintance with the subjects upon which they were desired to write, and were originally published as separate monographs for gratuitous distribution to the medical officers of the army. The favor with which they have been received both at home and abroad, and the wish expressed in many quarters that they might be arranged in a more permanent form, have led to their collection and republication in one volume . . . .

Included in this relatively scarce work are papers by Valentine Mott (1785–1865) ("Pain and anesthestics"; "Hemorrhage from wounds, and the best means of arresting it"), Alfred Charles Post (1806–66) and William Holme Van Buren (1819–83) ("Military hygiene and therapeutics"), Stephen Smith (1823–1922) ("Amputations, foot and ankle joint"), Richard M. Hodges (1827–96) ("Excision of joints for traumatic cause"), Freeman J. Bumstead (1826–79) ("Venereal diseases"), and John Hooker Packard (1832–1907) ("Fractures in military surgery"). There are four full-page engravings in Mott's article on hemorrhage; the remaining illustrations are relatively crude and scattered throughout the text.

GS58. **SILAS WEIR MITCHELL** (1829–1914), **GEORGE READ MOREHOUSE** (1829–1905), and **WILLIAM WILLIAMS KEEN** (1837–1932). *Gunshot wounds and other injuries of nerves.* 164pp. Philadelphia: J. B. Lippincott, 1864. [G-M 2167]

This monograph is one of the acknowledged classics of nineteenth-century American medicine. It provided the first detailed study of traumatic neuroses and introduced the concept of causalgia. Extremely scarce, it was the forerunner to Mitchell's other classic work, *Injuries to nerves and their consequences* (Philadelphia: J. B. Lippincott, 1872) [G-M 4544]. Mitchell's son John Kearsley Mitchell (1859–1917) followed up his father's book by writing *Remote consequences of injuries of nerves, and their treatment; an examination of the present condition of wounds received 1863–1865* (Philadelphia: Lea Brothers, 1895). *Gunshot wounds* was based on the wartime research of the three authors, especially at the Battle of Gettysburg. Neither Mitchell nor Morehouse were surgeons. Keen had entered the army as a contract surgeon and eventually joined his coauthors on staff at the U.S. Army Hospital for Injuries and Diseases of the Nervous System in Philadelphia. He later held the chair of surgery at Jefferson Medical College. (See also GS154 and GS178.)

GS59. **JOHN HOOKER PACKARD** (1832–1907). *Lectures on inflammation.* 276pp. Philadelphia: J. B. Lippincott, 1865.

As a member of the College of Physicians of Philadelphia and its vice-president from 1885 to 1888, Packard gave the first Mütter lectures at that institution on the subject of inflammation. The series was completed over the course of a few months and later compiled in book form. It was dedicated to Samuel David Gross (1805–84). The book contains ten lectures discussing topics such as the "Causes of inflammation"; "Terminations of inflammation"; "The origin of lymph"; "Mode of development of new vessels in inflammatory lymph"; "The study of pus"; "Granulations"; and "The therapeutics of inflammation". (See also GS54 and GS71.)

GS60. **WILLIAM HOLME VAN BUREN** (1819–83). *Contributions to practical surgery.* 208pp. Philadelphia: J. B. Lippincott, 1865.

The son-in-law of Valentine Mott (1785–1865), Van Buren graduated from the University of Pennsylvania Medical School in 1840. For sixteen years he was professor of the principles of surgery at Bellevue Hospital Medical College. Van Buren's Contributions is a little-known work but was his first surgical text. At the time of its publication, he was professor of anatomy at the University of New York. The volume is a selection of his papers that had previously been published in medical journals. Most of the content is drawn from Van Buren's extensive clinical experience. Topics include "Amputation at the hip-joint"; "Tracheotomy"; "Inguinal aneurism"; "Malignant polypus of the nose"; "Rectal diseases"; "Urinary calculus"; "Popliteal aneurism"; "Dislocation of the femur"; "Strangulated hernia"; and "Salivary fistula." There was only one edition. (See also GS119, GU9, and CR6.)

GS61. **WILLIAM CANNIFF** (1830–1910). A manual of the principles of surgery, based on pathology. 402pp. Philadelphia: Lindsay & Blakiston, 1866.

Born in Ontario, Canniff received his M.D. from the University of the City of New York in 1854. He was acting assistant surgeon with the Army of the Potomac in 1865. The following year he became dean of the medical faculty of Victoria University in Toronto. In 1867, Canniff was instrumental in founding the Canadian Medical Association. During the early part of his career he was a lecturer on general pathology. This training, combined with his wartime experience, provided the basis for this volume. He states in the preface:

> This volume was commenced while the author was engaged in lecturing upon the Principles and Practice of Surgery. Finding that a single

Figs. 20–21. (GS63) These four albumen prints (Figs. 20–23) from the Surgeon General's Office and the Army Medical Museum (No. 167, 168, 169, 170) are a sample of the earliest published collection of clinical reference photographs. Depicted is an example of cheiloplasty, which was used to repair injuries suffered when a shell injury completely carried away the inferior maxillary bone and soft tissues.

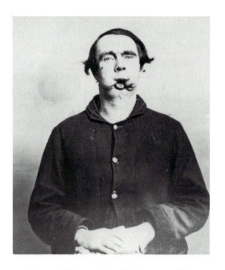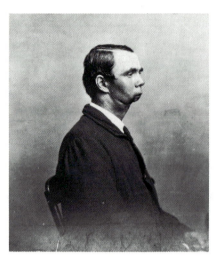

session, although of six months, was not sufficiently long to permit him to embrace in his course both the principles and the practice of the science, he proposed to himself to prepare a handbook of the principles for his class, that he might thereby be enabled to devote more time to the practical part of the subject. Circumstances having led to his withdrawal from the college, he has been induced to extend the limits of the work to the present size, in the hope that it may be found more useful. In doing so great attention has been devoted to surgical pathology, believing that it is most essential to a knowledge of all rational treatment.

The work consists of five divisions: "Inflammation, and diseases arising out of inflammation"; "The healing process, and diseases of the healing process"; "External injuries—contusions and wounds"; "Diseases of certain tissues, bones, joints (including fractures and dislocations), arteries, and veins"; and "Morbid growths." This was the only edition. Canniff also wrote *The medical profession in upper Canada, 1783–1850; an historical narrative including some brief biographies* (Toronto: William Briggs, 1894).

GS62. **GEORGE ALEXANDER OTIS** (1830–1881). *Histories of two hundred and ninety-six surgical photographs, prepared at the Army Medical Museum.* 296pp. Washington: Surgeon-General's Office, 1865–72?

Otis received an M.D. from the Universisty of Pennsylvania in 1851 and maintained a general medical and surgical practice in Richmond. The Civil War changed his life when in 1864 he was assigned as successor to John H. Brinton (1832–1907), then curator of the Army Medical Museum. Otis, who was also head of the surgical and photographic sections, spent the remainder of his life expanding the collection. The *Histories* provide a detailed description of the mutilating injuries which were suffered during the hostilities as they relate to photographs found in the surgical section of the Army Medical Museum. This volume was probably intended as a companion piece to GS63. Its actual publication date remains uncertain, and whether it was an integral part of the entire GS63 series or just an afterthought is unknown. (See also GS74, OR18, and OR23.)

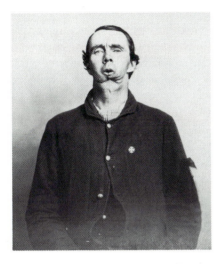 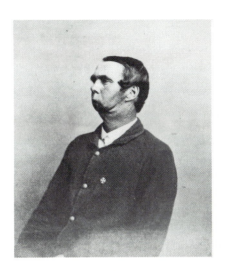

Figs. 22–23. (GS63) 46-year-old private Roland Ward received the wound at Ream's Station, Virginia, in August 1864. Two operations were eventually performed, both in the first half of 1865. He was discharged from Lincoln Hospital in June of that year having an oral-cutaneous fistula. The secretion of saliva was controlled by the use of a rubber button, which was adjusted to the fistulous orifice.

GS63. GEORGE ALEXANDER OTIS (1830–81). *Photographs of surgical cases and specimens: taken at the Army Medical Museum.* 7 vols. Washington: Surgeon-General's Office, 1865–72?

This is the major published photographic legacy of the Civil War and is among the rarest of American surgical texts. It is a huge and remarkable collection of early photographs depicting wounded Civil War soldiers and pathologic specimens. Each volume consists of approximately fifty tipped-in albumen photographs 4 inches by 6 inches or larger, with the history of each photograph on a printed slip mounted on the verso. All of the pictures were made from large glass plate negatives, mainly 10 inches by 12 inches, and most were taken by Army photographer, William Bell.

The most interesting question about this series concerns its publishing history. The volumes have no publication date on their title pages. However, an accompanying introductory letter, frequently found with the set, is dated June 1865. The letter states that the volumes were sent gratis from the Surgeon General's Office to various medical libraries and hospitals throughout the country. The initial set consisted of only four volumes. This is known because pages 573–76 of the *Catalogue of the Surgical Section of the United States Army Museum* (GS64) list all 181 photographs in the preliminary set. Therefore, the first four volumes were contemporaneous with the Civil War.

How many of these magnificent photographic albums were produced is a mystery. Because they were assembled by hand the number could not have been very large. Three more volumes were published after the war. Many more photographs must have been taken after hostilities had ceased (through 1872). However, these later volumes also contain some photographs similar to those found in the initial four. Unfortunately, unlike the first four albums, there are no published lists of the photographs in the final three. Therefore, it is possible that the order of photographs in these three albums varies from set to set. The seventh volume deals almost entirely with interesting civilian cases. All of these clinical photographs were distributed to medical officers and libraries throughout the United States as a form of educational instruction

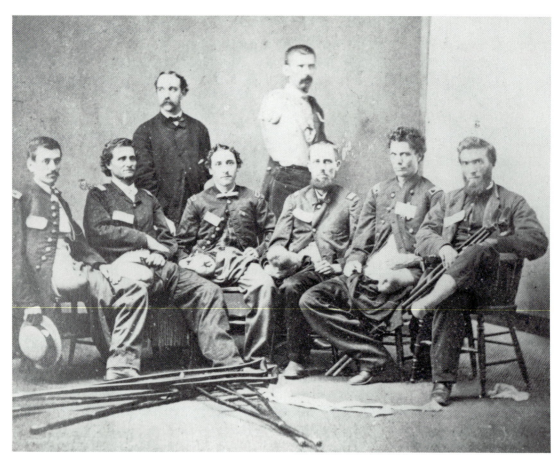

Fig. 24. (GS63) This remarkable photograph (number 101) shows a group of Northern officers who underwent various amputations for gunshot injuries. All of the wounds occurred in the spring or summer of 1865, and the men received treatment at Armory Square Hospital in Washington.

regarding various types of surgical trauma. Clearly, the initial four albums are the earliest examples of actual tipped-in silver-print photographs to be found in any American surgical work. It should be noted that over the years numerous copies have been made of these photographs, some as late as the early twentieth century, although they are usually so identified by markings on them. (See also GS62, GS74, OR18, and OR23.)

GS64. **ALFRED ALEXANDER WOODHULL** (1837–1921). *Catalogue of the Surgical Section of the United States Army Museum.* 664pp. Washington: Government Printing Office, 1866.

Thirty chapters of descriptions of 4,719 surgical specimens varying from cranium to tumors graphically detail the wounds suffered by thousands of soldiers during the Civil War. The attending physician's name is listed with each case. Many of these descriptions are specifically related to injuries which are further enumerated in the *Medical and surgical history of the War of the Rebellion* (GS68). This scarce volume is of major historical importance because it is the first American publication that actually gives an idea of the number and type of photographs taken by or for Army physicians during the Civil War. The book

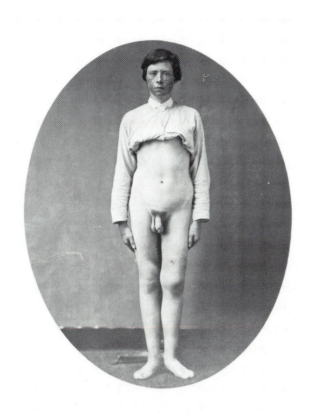

Fig. 25. (GS63) Private James O'Connor (photograph number 49; specimen number 4,982) was wounded at the Battle of Cold Harbor in June 1864 by a conoidal musket ball, which passed through his thigh three inches above the patella, fracturing his femur. No surgery was performed, although eight small fragments of bone were eventually removed though the exit site. His final physical impairment included an inch and a quarter shortening of that leg, but no angular deformity.

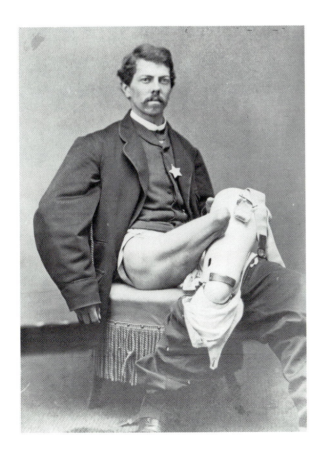

Fig. 26. (GS63) A cannon ball carried away the right leg of Captain Charles T. Greene (photograph number 134) in November 1863. An amputation of the lower third of the thigh was carried out on the battlefield under chloroform anesthesia. In May 1864, an artificial limb was applied and the patient resumed his duties as a staff officer.

lists (pages 577–79) 372 6 by 6 inch or larger format photographs of surgical cases and 49 surgical (pathologic) specimens as well as 1,064 cartes de visite photographs of surgical cases and 100 of surgical specimens. Woodhull was assistant surgeon and brevet major at the time of the Catalogue's completion. He was an 1859 graduate of the University of Pennsylvania Medical School. Following the war he continued in the military, specializing in hygiene.

GS65. EDWARD CARROLL FRANKLIN (1822–85). *The science and art of surgery, embracing minor and operative surgery; compiled from standard allopathic authorities, and adapted to homoeopathic therapeutics, with a general history of surgery from the earliest periods to the present*

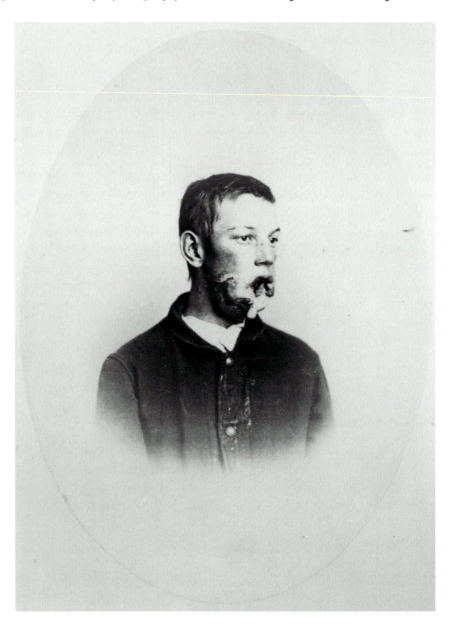

Fig. 27. (GS63) At the Battle of Weldon Railroad, Private William Coder was struck by a shell fragment which removed the anterior portion of his inferior maxillary bone (Ward 15, Bed 52). By October the wound was granulating well, although his voice was somewhat impaired. A plastic operation was advised but never performed.

time. 2 vols., 844pp. and 865pp. St. Louis: Missouri Democrat Book and Job Print, 1867–73.

Trained by Valentine Mott (1785–1865), Franklin became an adherent of homeopathic medicine after undergoing homeopathic treatment for a persistent fever that he contracted in Panama. A surgeon on the Union side during the Civil War, in 1862 he was appointed professor of surgery at Hahnemann Medical College of Chicago. Following the war he was nominated as professor of surgery at Homeopathic Medical College of Missouri and president of the Western Institute of Homeopathy. His textbook was the standard text in all the homeopathic colleges in the United States. The volumes are massive in scope and contain 448 figures. Pages 25–41 contain a general descriptive history of surgery with a specific section on surgery in the United States. The book includes a record of the most important surgical processes in America, arranged chronologically. Franklin had a certain disdain for the allopathic practitioner, and this prejudice is evident in the preface:

> The rapid increase of homeopathy, the constant demand made upon the science for additional laborers in this field of practice, the multiplication of medical colleges, and the continually-augmenting classes of students that throng these halls of learning, are sufficient evidences of the exalted position and standing of homeopathy in the social scale. Within the past few years, the adaptation of the law "similar" to the cure of surgical diseases has received a powerful and irresistible impulse by the labors of those who justly occupy a proud position in its ranks as accomplished and successful surgeons. The jeers and hackneyed jokes of allopathic practitioners, and their coarse denunciations of this system, have, like chickens in the proverb "come home to roost;" and homeopathic surgeons crowned with brilliant and successive triumphs, move onward, still onward, a giant now-"Excelsior" forever "graven" on its brow. The records of the late rebellion, the statistics of thousands of cases both in civil and military service, the published transactions of its literature, potently attest that homeopathic surgeons can not only perform surgical operations skillfully, but results prove that the success attending operative interference is largely in favor of the system of practice. Besides this, a number of diseases that under allopathic remedies are pronounced incurable, are readily and permanently cured by the principle of similars. The unbeliever, if he will, can find in the literature of the homeopathic school, abundant and well-attested evidences of the truth of this statement . . . .

An abridged one-volume version of this work was published in 1882. (See also GS107, GS108, OR35, and GU16.)

GS66. **ALBERT G. WALTER** (1811–76). *Conservative surgery in its general and successful adaptation in cases of severe traumatic injuries of the limbs; with a report of cases.* 213pp. Pittsburgh: W. G. Johnston, 1867.

Born in Germany, Walter emigrated to America in the late 1830s. Most of his professional life was spent in Pittsburgh, where he practiced until his death. He is best remembered for having been one of the first to perform exploratory laparotomy for traumatic injuries. His book is

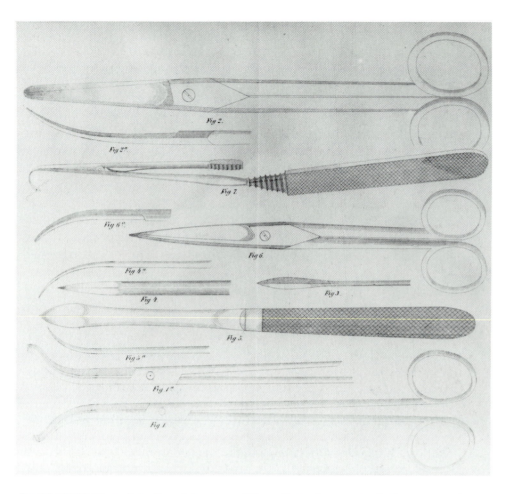

Fig. 28. (GS67) Warren's work contains some of the earliest references to plastic surgery in America. The instruments which he used to repair fissures of the hard and soft palates are shown in this fold-out plate, figure 1 on page 142, for which J. H. Bufford was lithographer.

significant in that he advocated the drainage of crushed limbs by long and deep incisions to release the "imprisoned" products. This early description of compartmental syndrome was quite accurate, and his method of treatment unique for the time. There was only one edition.

GS67. **JONATHAN MASON WARREN** (1811–67). *Surgical observations, with cases and operations.* 630pp. Boston: Ticknor & Fields, 1867.

The second son of John Collins Warren (1778–1856), Warren was a surgeon at Massachusetts General Hospital. He assisted his father in the operation for the first public demonstration of the use of ether for surgical anesthesia. Warren is particularly known for his procedure for fissure of the hard and soft palates [G-M 5745]. Warren's biography, *Memoir of Jonathan Mason Warren, M.D.* (Boston: private printing, 1886), describes his composition of this work (pages 255–56):

> . . . that Warren might develop and illustrate views and facts he published a work . . . to this he had given much time and thought during the final years of his life; and the book was in reality an epitome of his whole career, embodying, as it did, the more important results both of a large private practice and of his twenty years' experience . . . . In the

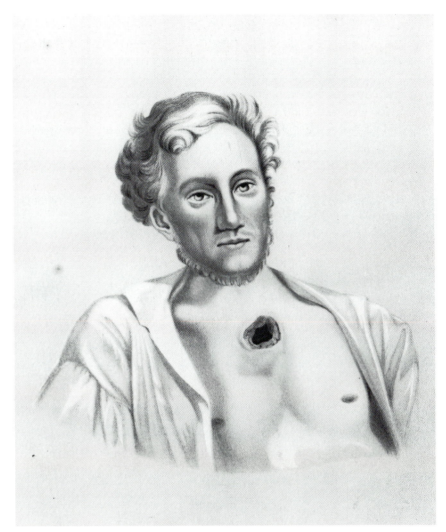

Fig. 29. (GS68) The surgical literature of the Civil War produced some of the most graphic of medical illustrations. This plate, figure 10 on page 486 in part 1 of volume 2, shows private Charles P. Betts of New Jersey, who sustained a penetrating gunshot wound of the anterior mediastinum. Unbelievably, the wound was not fatal and Betts recovered with minimal disability. This hand-colored plate was executed by Ed Stauch; T. Sinclair & Son was the lithographer.

preparation of this volume, which did not appear till nearly three months before his death, Warren found a certain indemnity for the pains he suffered while engaged upon it; . . . the criticisms that reached him caused him much satisfaction, and sufficed to show that his labor had not been in vain.

The book has fourteen chapters ("Head"; "Face"; "Neck"; "Chest"; "Abdomen"; "Anus"; "Genito-urinary organs"; "Extremities"; "Arteries and veins"; "Injuries and diseases of the nerves"; "Tumors"; "Gunshot wounds"; "Miscellaneous cases"; and "Anesthetics"), six plates, and thirteen woodcuts, but it is not meant to be a systematic treatise on surgery. The *Observations* contains some of the earliest American contributions to plastic surgery, including a section on rhinoplastic operations and restoration of the lower eyelid. Warren's work on palates is found on pages 126–42.

GS68. **JOSEPH K. BARNES** (1817–83). *The medical and surgical history of the war of the rebellion, 1861-1865.* 6 vols. Washington: Government Printing Office, 1870–88. [G-M 2171 and 5185]

This is one of the most remarkable works ever published on military medicine. It has been accurately called the "first comprehensive American medical book." These massive volumes containing thousands of pages of densely printed text present a detailed overview of medical and surgical conditions encountered by the Civil War surgeon and his patients. The introduction to the first surgical volume (pages xx-xxi) has an extensive list of American books and papers on military surgery. Surgical topics covered include every imaginable wartime injury with detailed summaries of each case. An index of operators and reporters appears at the end of the third surgical volume. This index makes it possible to look up any surgeon and find the patients he treated. The work was prepared under the direction of Barnes, who was surgeon-general of the Army, but it was actually written by Joseph J. Woodward (1833–84),

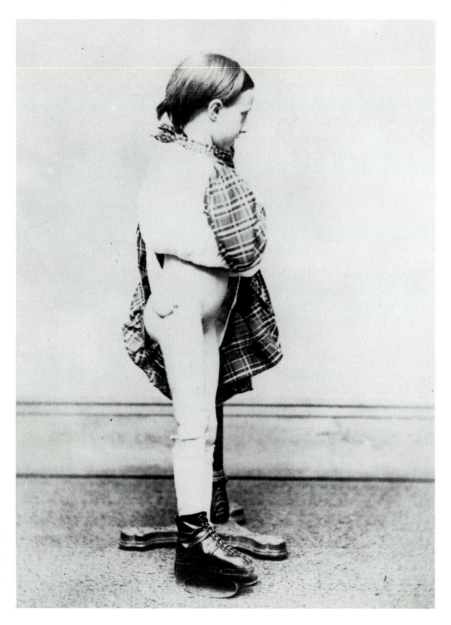

Fig. 30. (GS69) The wet-process of making albumen photographs was quite difficult. This early photograph on page 97 from Cheever's essay on excision of joints shows a side view of a hip excision.

Charles Smart (1841–1905), George A. Otis (1830–81), and David L. Huntington (1834–99). The initial press run was 5,000 copies, and a second printing was of a similar size.

The set is illustrated with hundreds of tinted lithographs primarily by Julius Bien after photographs by William Bell, E. J.Ward, and others. Also noteworthy are the numerous chromolithographs by Bien of histologic and pathologic studies by Edward Stauch, and other chromolithographs after paintings by Herman Faber. There are also more than 1000 engravings in the text.

The volumes are of historical importance because they are among the first American medical books to be illustrated with mechanical photographs. These Woodburytypes by the American Photo-Relief Printing Co. and heliotypes by Osgood & Co. were in some instances replaced by lithographs in the second printing.

GS69. **DAVID WILLIAMS CHEEVER** (1831-1915). *First medical and surgical report of the Boston City Hospital.* 688pp. Boston: Little & Brown, 1870.

Cheever's work is important because of its early use of photographs. The wet process of making albumen photographs was time-consuming and required mounting actual photographs by hand. Two such photographs are part of an article by Cheever on excision of joints (pages 71–107). Pages 665–88 contain extensive statistics related to the numbers of injuries treated and surgical procedures performed. In 1870, Cheever became staff surgeon at Boston City Hospital. He later succeeded Henry J. Bigelow (1818–90) as professor of surgery at Harvard Medical School. (See also GS158.)

GS70. **FRANK HASTINGS HAMILTON** (1813–86). *Surgical memoirs of the war of the rebellion; collected and published by the United States Sanitary Commission.* 2 vols. New York: U.S. Sanitary Commission, 1870–71.

This massive publication also concerns surgical problems during the Civil War. The first volume contains three lengthy articles by John Lidell (1823–83) on wounds of blood vessels, traumatic lesions of bone, and pyaemia. The second volume has an analysis of lower extremity amputations by Stephen Smith (1832-1922) and a treatise on hospital gangrene by Joseph Jones (1833–96). Hamilton was professor of the principles and practice of surgery and surgical pathology at Bellevue Hospital Medical College. (See also GS50, GS75, OP8, OR7, and OR37.)

GS71. **JOHN HOOKER PACKARD** (1832–1907). *A handbook of operative surgery.* 211pp. Philadelphia: J. B. Lippincott, 1870.

Conciseness was one of Packard's goals in preparing this volume. As a result, it has virtually no discussion of symptoms, diagnosis, or general treatment, except as they influenced the choice of a particular surgical operation. The fifty-four excellent plates depict a variety of surgical operations and pathologic conditions. The numerous text figures are primarily concerned with instruments. The twelve chapters include

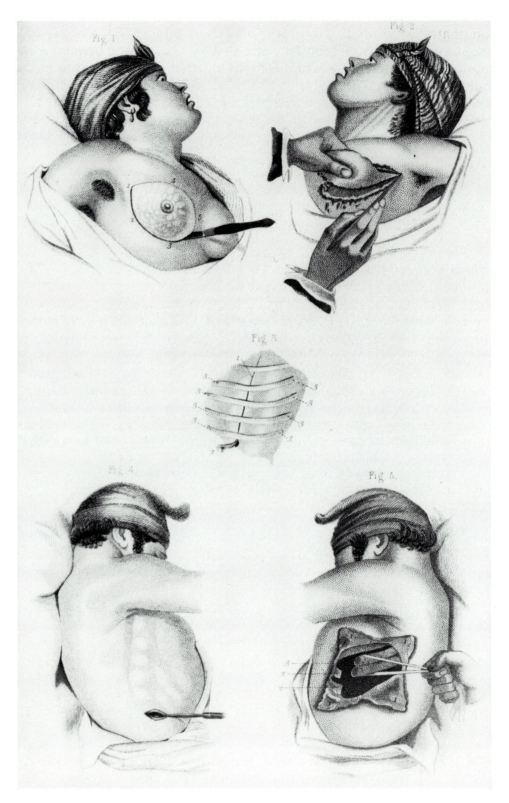

Fig. 31. (GS71) This steel-engraved plate, figure 25 on page 86 from Packard's best-known textbook, demonstrates an amputation of the breast and a paracentesis of the thoracic cavity.

operations on the eye (pages 29–48) and an extensive discourse on ligation of arteries in the limbs (pages 155–63). On pages 205–06, Packard
discusses transfusion of blood, noting that " . . . the blood being drawn
from a healthy person, is whipped with a little bunch of twigs (a piece
of a whisk or broom answers very well) . . . . " This work is one of many
unaccountably elusive nineteenth-century American surgical texts. (See
also GS54 and GS59.)

GS72. **JOHN ASHURST** (1839–1900). *The principles and practice of surgery.*
1,011pp. Philadelphia: Henry C. Lea, 1871.

Ashhurst was an 1860 graduate of the University of Pennsylvania
Medical School. At the time this work was published, he was surgeon at
the Episcopal Hospital in Philadelphia. In 1888 he was named Barton
Professor of Surgery at his alma mater. This textbook went through five
more editions, in 1878, 1882, 1885, 1889, and 1893, and remained a
standard reference work for many years. It is a massive treatise, containing forty-seven chapters, and provides a comprehensive review of all
facets of surgery. It was not designed as a reference text for specialists,
but as a source of broad general surgical knowledge for general practitioners and as a textbook for students. It was available in either cloth
($5.00) or leather covers ($6.00), and includes 533 engravings on wood.
Ashhurst notes in the preface:

> The object of this work is to furnish as concise a manner as may be com-
> patible with clearness, a condensed but comprehensive description of
> the modes of practice now generally employed in the treatment of sur-
> gical affections, with a plain exposition of the principles upon which
> those modes of practice are based . . . the author would for his work the
> character of being something more than a mere compilation from the
> writings of others . . . .

(See also GS100 and OR15.)

GS73. **JOSEPH WILLIAM HOWE** (1843–90). *Emergencies and how to treat
them; the etiology, pathology, and treatment of the accidents, diseases,
and cases of poisoning, which demand prompt action.* 265pp. New
York: D. Appleton, 1871.

Howe graduated from New York University Medical School in 1866,
and became clinical professor of surgery at his alma mater. This work
was an offshoot of his clinical experience as an attending physician in
the Outdoor Department (outpatient clinic) of Bellevue Hospital. It was
one of the earliest American texts to deal specifically with emergencies
and was quite useful to rural general practitioners, who did not have
surgeons available for consultation. It was originally published in cloth
for $2.50; further editions were printed in 1875, 1881, and 1884. His
other medical books are *The breath, and the diseases which give it a fetid
odor* (New York: D. Appleton, 1874), *Winter homes for invalids, an account
of the various localities in Europe and America, suitable for consumptives and
other invalids during the winter months* (New York: G. P. Putnam's Sons,
1875), and *Excessive venery, masturbation and continence* (New York:
Bermingham, 1883).

Fig. 32. (GS76) Some of the earliest examples of the photo-
relief process are found in this
book. The photograph on page
164 was taken on the eighteenth day after a mastectomy.
Hewsen was particularly proud
of his printing efforts and
provides a lengthy discussion
of the photorelief process on
pages ix–x in the preface.

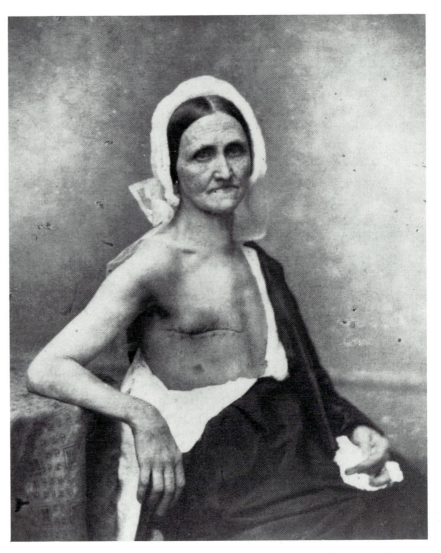

GS74. GEORGE ALEXANDER OTIS (1830–81). *A report of surgical cases treated in the army of the United States from 1865 to 1871.* 296pp. Washington: Government Printing Office, 1871.

This book is a scarce companion piece to the other volumes written by Otis about the surgical treatment of Civil War soldiers. The *Report* describes 1,037 cases in detail. Pages 287–89 contain a list of the surgeons whose cases were reported. There is also an alphabetical list of the patients treated (pages 290–94). A short table of contents appears at the conclusion of the monograph. The most interesting sections are those concerning arrow wounds of the head and neck, chest and abdomen (pages 144–63). They are described in graphic detail, almost all having been sustained in clashes with Indians on the Western frontier. There are three black-and-white engraved plates, which were taken from photographs by William Bell and Edward Ward. Otis prepared additional volumes, which dealt with the long-term follow-up of wounded Civil War veterans, but his premature death prevented any of them from being published. (See also GS62, GS63, OR18, and OR23.)

GS75. **FRANK HASTINGS HAMILTON** (1813–86). *The principles and practice of surgery.* 943pp. New York: William Wood, 1872.

Hamilton was professor of the practice of surgery with operations and of clinical surgery at Bellevue Hospital Medical College. Hamilton describes the purpose of the *Principles* as "to supply, within the compass of a single volume of moderate size, the instruction necessary to a full understanding of all the subjects belonging properly and exclusively to surgery . . . . " The *Principles* was a truly systematic textbook of surgery. The first part covers general surgery and the second part regional surgery. Although it contains 467 figures, few of them illustrate actual surgical operations. The book went through two further editions, the last in 1886. (See also GS50, GS70, OP8, OR7, and OR37.)

GS76. **ADDINELL HEWSEN** (1828–89). *Earth as a topical application in surgery, being a full exposition of its use in all the cases requiring topical applications admitted in the men's and women's surgical wards of the Pennsylvania Hospital during a period of six months in 1869.* 309pp. Philadelphia: Lindsay & Blakiston, 1872.

Hewsen graduated from Jefferson Medical College in 1850. After studying in Europe, he settled in Philadelphia, where he practiced general medicine and was surgeon at Pennsylvania Hospital from 1861 to 1867. His name has long been associated with "earth treatment" of wounds, contusions, inflammations, tumors and surgical dressings. Hewson wrote this book in an attempt to prove that spontaneously healing wounds could be cured by using external dressings. Hewson extols the use of earth applied as a treatment dressing preoperatively, intraoperatively and postoperatively. This volume is significant as one of the first American medical books to have photomechanical prints—in this case, Woodburytypes—and it was the first separate American surgical text to have mechanical photographs within the actual volume. The book is dedicated to Samuel D. Gross (1805–84). Hewsen writes in the preface:

> The following pages contain the results of clinical work done nearly three years ago, which have been delayed in their publication until now for the double purpose of weighing them by subsequent experience, and of interpreting their meaning by a careful study of the various subjects which they involve . . . . The illustrations, four in number, which I have introduced, for the purpose of giving a demonstration as strong as possible of my successes, have been made by the American Photo-Relief Printing Company, and are from photographs reproduced by a method that would seem to leave nothing to be desired as to permanency, as well as faithfulness and accuracy of representation.

The contents include ninety-three case histories and comments as to the importance of the contact of earth, including its effects on pain, its power as a deodorizer, its influence over inflammation and putrefaction, and its effect on the healing processes. The book is extremely scarce and provides unusual reading in light of today's terms *sepsis* and *antisepsis*. It must be assumed that the "earth" which Hewson utilized contained a type of mold which had an antibiotic effect. If more inquisitive and inventive minds had paid attention to Hewson's results, the development of antibiotics might have occurred earlier. A second edition was published in 1887. Hewsen's most lasting contribution to American surgury was his use of the ophthalmoscope to diagnose diseases of the eye.

GS77. **JOHN COLLINS WARREN** (1842–1927). *The anatomy and development of rodent ulcer; a Boylston Medical Prize essay for 1872.* 66pp. Boston: Little & Brown, 1872.

Son of Jonathan Mason Warren (1811–67), John Collins Warren was professor of surgery at Harvard from 1893 to 1907. He was president of the American Surgical Association in 1896. Early in his career he taught surgical pathology, and as he notes in his autobiography *To work in the vineyard of surgery* (Cambridge: Harvard University Press, 1958, page 176):

> As an illustration of the increased interest in scientific medicine, I may mention a private course of instruction which I gave in 1870 on the microscopical appearances and classification of tumors. This was offered in my improvised laboratory to members of the profession. The class was organized by no less a personage than Dr. David W. Cheever, who was then adjunct professor of anatomy. As a by-product of these activities I was able to produce a Boylston Prize Essay on the "Anatomy and Development of Rodent Ulcer," an ailment imperfectly understood at that time.

This disease process is actually a slowly enlarging ulcerated basal cell carcinoma, usually located on the face. Among Warren's other medical books is the two-volume *International textbook of surgery, by American and British authors* (Philadelphia: W. B. Saunders, 1900), written in collaboration with Alfred Pearce Gould (1852–1922). (See also GS127 and GS169.)

GS78. **JAMES GRANT GILCHRIST** (1842–1906). *The homoeopathic treatment of surgical diseases.* 421pp. Chicago: C. S. Halsey, 1873.

Gilchrist was an 1863 graduate of Hahnemann Medical College in Philadelphia. At the time this volume was written, he was editor of the surgical department of *The medical investigator.* This was his first textbook, and Gilchrist writes in the preface:

> At the time this little book was projected, so far as my knowledge extended, there was not one line, outside of our periodical literature, that taught the application of our therapeutic principles to the treatment of so-called "surgical diseases." A work on this subject has been sorely needed, and our accumulated experience demands a gathering together of this scattered material . . . . It may be objected (and I allow that the objection has weight) that works of this character are apt to encourage superficial study of the Materia Medica, and, perhaps, tend to perpetuate the absurd custom of treating diseases by name rather than symptoms. It has been the main object of this work to teach, unmistakably, that apart from mechanical injuries (and these are not diseases) there can be no such thing as a local disease. Tumors, ulcers, and all kinds of abnormal growths, are simply symptoms; peripheral symptoms of a generally diseased organism . . . . The student of homeopathy finds one difficulty in studying the Materia Medica in connection with surgical diseases. Surgical diseases may be called those which are chiefly

recognized through objective symptoms. A new form of tumor is found, i.e., new to the student, and where in our bulky Materia Medica will he find its simile? It is not there. A remedy has never developed a tumor during a proving. Applying remedies for symptoms apparently unconnected with this tumor, we have now and then succeeded in causing a disappearance of the growth, and in time the fact creeps into the symptomatology as a "clinical symptom." Many of these clinical symptoms are only to be found in our periodicals, and many more in private case books. It has been my task to gather as many of these as possible, and thus reduce the number of remedies to be consulted from four hundred in number to a very few. When the objective symptoms are found in the following pages, the Materia Medica must be consulted for those which are subjective, the union of the two making the true similar, which is the only agent that will cure . . . .

The table of contents lists twenty-seven chapters, each treating the diseases of specific organs. Included is an interesting chapter on diseases of the mind (pages 19–21) dealing with shock and traumatic delirium. Further editions were published in 1876 and 1880. (See also GS101, GS117, and GS166.)

GS79. **GEORGE WASHINGTON NORRIS** (1808–75). *Contributions to practical surgery.* 318pp. Philadelphia: Lindsay & Blakiston, 1873.

As John Rhea Barton's (1794–1871) successor at Pennsylvania Hospital, Norris later became professor of clinical surgery in the University of Pennsylvania (1848–57). The *Contributions* is actually a compilation of papers which had been previously published in medical periodicals. To this collection Barton "added a paper on compound fractures, a large amount of new material on the occurrence of false joints, and numerous clinical histories . . . . " Perhaps the most interesting section presents statistical tables of the mortality following arterial ligations (pages 220–313). Norris's only other book concerns medical history and is titled *The early history of medicine in Philadelphia* (Philadelphia: private printing, 1886).

GS80. **JOHN ALLAN WYETH** (1845–1922). *A handbook of medical and surgical reference.* 279pp. New York: William Wood, 1873.

An 1869 graduate of the University of Louisville School of Medicine, Wyeth practiced in New York and founded the Polyclinic Medical School and Hospital. This was the first postgraduate school of medical education in United States. Wyeth served as president of the American Medical Association in 1901. Written when Wyeth was just twenty-eight years old, the *Handbook* provides a cursory look at surgical diseases. Little information about actual operative surgery is included. Among Wyeth's other medical textbooks is *Surgery* (New York: M. S. Wyeth, 1908). (See also GS96 and GS132.)

GS81. **EUGENE PEUGNET** (1836–79). *The nature of gunshot wounds of the abdomen, and their treatment; based on a review of the case of the late James Fisk, Jr., in its medico-legal aspects.* New York: 96pp. William Wood, 1874.

Peugnet graduated from the College of Physicians and Surgeons in New York in 1858 and later became surgeon at North-Western Dispensary. Dedicated to Willard Parker (1800–84), this monograph was first read before the Medico-Legal Society of New York City to demonstrate the necessity of changing the manner of conducting criminal investigations and introducing expert testimony. There are five chapters, including "A detailed history of the case of James Fisk"; "Description of shock"; "Penetrating gunshot wounds of the abdomen"; "The physiological and toxical actions of morphine"; and "The medical jurisprudence of the Stokes case including accounts of three separate trials." An extensive bibliography of works dealing with gunshot injuries appears on page 93.

GS82. CHARLES BROOKS BRIGHAM (1845–1903). *Surgical cases*. 110pp. Cambridge: H. O. Houghton, 1876.

An 1870 graduate of Harvard Medical School, Brigham was one of the earliest practitioners of surgery in California. While still in medical school, he won the Boylston Prize in 1868 for work on diabetes mellitus. His *Surgical cases* reflects some of the time (1873–74) that he spent as professor of orthopedic and military surgery at the University of California. When Brigham wrote the *Surgical cases*, he was surgeon at the French Hospital in San Francisco. Among the twenty-six chapters are "Congenital naevus of the face"; "Removal of upper jaw"; "Gunshot wound of neck"; "Aneurism of wrist"; "Gangrene of foot"; and "Sponges in surgical dressings." Twelve photographic plates taken in San Francisco (1873–76) are included. They are some of the earliest examples of mechanical photographs included in an American surgical text.

GS83. GURDON BUCK (1807-77). *Contributions to reparative surgery; showing its application to the treatment of deformities produced by*

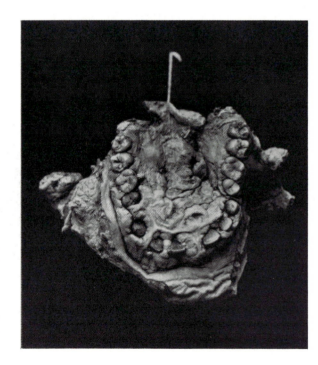

Figs. 33–34. (GS82) These two remarkable heliotypes (number 3, page 22, and number 11, page 78) are among the earliest examples of mechanical photographs used in a surgical textbook. Bingham's removal of an entire upper jaw for malignant disease in a 26-year-old man was a prodigious surgical feat. The injury of the perineum, scrotum, and penis of a seventeen-year-old boy by a threshing machine is unique in that extensive skin grafting led to a satisfactory recovery.

destructive disease or injury; congenital defects from arrest or excess of development; and cicatrical contractions from burns. 237pp. New York: D. Appleton, 1876.

Buck was surgeon at New York Hospital for almost forty years. He performed one of the earliest successful ligations of the femoral artery [G-M 2960], treated cancer of the larynx by a thyrotomy [G-M 3263], and was an active orthopedist [G-M 4324 and 4419]. His *Contributions* dealt with reconstructive surgery and was the first American text to do so. Twenty-nine operations are described in detail, illustrated with almost 100 engravings. The illustrations are among the earliest engravings in an American surgical text to be made from photographs. Buck photographed his plastic surgery cases both before and after surgery. In this way he was able to demonstrate his results to anyone wishing to consult them. This scarce volume was available only in cloth for $3.00. Among the most famous cases is that of Carleton Burgan, whose history was initially reported in the *Medical and surgical history of the War of the Rebellion* (see GS68) and is considered Buck's greatest reconstructive triumph.

GS84. **ANDREW JACKSON HOWE** (1825–92). *The art and science of surgery.* 886pp. Cincinnati: Wilstach & Baldwin, 1879.

Howe was considered the foremost surgeon of eclectic medicine in America. He received his M.D. from Worcester Medical Institute in 1855, and in 1861 he was named to the chair of surgery at the Eclectic Medical

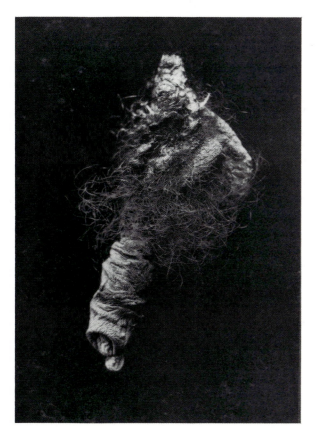

Fig. 34.

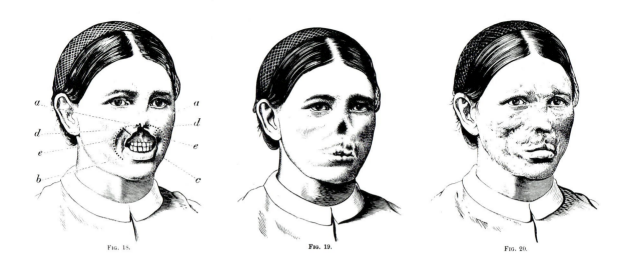

Figs. 35 – 37. (GS83) Buck wrote in the preface that his book used the "indispensable aid of pictorial illustration" and the "skill of Ferdinand Froning of Vienna who executed all the principal figures from photographs." Buck used photographs extensively to show operative results, and these three engravings from a photograph (numbers 18, 19, and 20 on pages 64, 69, and 74, respectively) were among the first such illustrations ever to appear in a surgical work. Jane Tucker was twenty-six years old when the first illustration was made. She had been "addicted to constantly picking her nose with her fingers" since the age of seven. As a consequence a "destructive ulceration eventually followed." In March 1866, Buck commenced a series of eight operations lasting through June 1870. The figures readily demonstrate his skills as a plastic surgeon. Buck made the actual albumen prints available to anyone wishing to consult them, and for that purpose had duplicate photographic albums deposited in the U.S. Army Medical Museum and the Pathological Museum of the New York Hospital (presently located as part of the Webster Collection at the Health Sciences Library of Columbia University).

Institute in Cincinnati. His textbook was the most widely accepted eclectic text and is quite comprehensive in scope. Howe operated mainly in the days prior to surgical asepsis, but was remarkably successful in his treatment of surgical diseases. Although he disagreed with many details of Joseph Lister's (1827–1912) method, Howe was a firm believer that infection was the most important problem facing the surgeon. Howe writes in the preface:

> The position I have held for the last twenty years as a teacher of anatomy and surgery has placed me under obligations to numerous friends who have frequently requested me to prepare a work on the principles and practice of surgery. When my manuscript and illustrations were nearly completed, a fire swept away the toil of years, but not discouraged by the seemingly untoward event, I undertook at once to reproduce what had been lost . . . . When my *Treatise on Fractures and Dislocations* was published, the design was that in time it should become part of a general work on surgery; and such continued to be the understanding when the *Manual of Eye Surgery* made its appearance; but the work as a whole embraces fifteen hundred pages, therefore the three parts would make a book inconveniently large. To carry out the original plan it has been my aim to bring this volume into as small a compass as the nature of the material would allow . . . . It has been my endeavor to make this work, a textbook for students, and a reliable reference for physicians engaged in the general practice of their profession, therefore I have dealt largely in essentials, and occupied little space with what might be regarded as theoretical or transcendental . . . . In the preparation of this

work I have avoided partisan views, and striven to be as positive in expressing myself as is becoming in a surgical author. The productions of the most reputable writers and teachers have been consulted, and occasionally drawn upon; but in the main I have given expression to ideas based upon knowledge gained by personal experience . . . . The illustrations are not especially numerous, nor are all of them executed in the highest style of art; yet as far as they go they serve the purpose for which they were designed; and in no instance is an old cut introduced to occupy space or to swell the number employed in the work. The pictures are mostly from my own sketches . . . .

There is a rather cursory table of contents which lists twenty chapters. Among these are "Tumors"; "Tuberculosis"; "Venereal diseases"; "Vascular lesions"; "Plastic surgery"; "Amputations"; "Diseases of the anus"; and "Deformities of the hands and feet." This was the only edition. Many of Howe's contributions to medical journals were collected by his wife in *Miscellaneous papers by Andrew Jackson Howe, M.D.* (Cincinnati: Robert Clarke, 1894), which also contains a short biography. (See also OP21, OR25 and GY37.)

GS85. **GREENSVILLE DOWELL** (1822–81). *A treatise on hernia: with a new process for its radical cure, and original contributions to operative surgery, and new surgical instruments.* 206pp. Philadelphia: D. G. Brinton, 1876.

Dowell was professor of surgery at Texas Medical College in Galveston, having graduated from Jefferson Medical College in 1846. Dowell wrote in the preface: "The number of sufferers from hernia is immensely large, and too often the inadequate knowledge of their attending physicians leads them to the nets of the charlatans who advertise trusses and bandages." This point was true in Dowell's time, and it is still true today. Unfortunately, Dowell's method of hernia operation (pages 48–71) leaves much to be desired. He nevertheless concludes this section by stating that " . . . giving about all that is known on the subject, . . . there will never be a better method invented than the author's . . . . " There were seventy-six illustrations and six full-page plates. It was initially available in cloth for $2.00. Dowell's other medical book is *Yellow fever and malarial diseases embracing a history of the epidemics of yellow fever in Texas: new views on its diagnosis, treatment, propagation and control* (Philadelphia: Medical Publication Office, 1876).

GS86. **HOMER IRWIN OSTROM** (1852-?). *A treatise on the breast and its surgical diseases.* 180pp. Philadelphia: J. M. Stoddart, 1877.

Ostrom was a homeopathic physician who practiced in New York City. The *Treatise* was originally written for the *American journal of homeopathic materia medica* and appeared in that periodical in May, June, July and August 1876. Because serial publication excluded much valuable material, it was decided to publish a definitive textbook. Accordingly, this is the first surgical work written in the United States dedicated solely to breast disease. There is an interesting homeopathic repertory on pages 332–47. Chapter 7 provides homeopathic therapeutics for

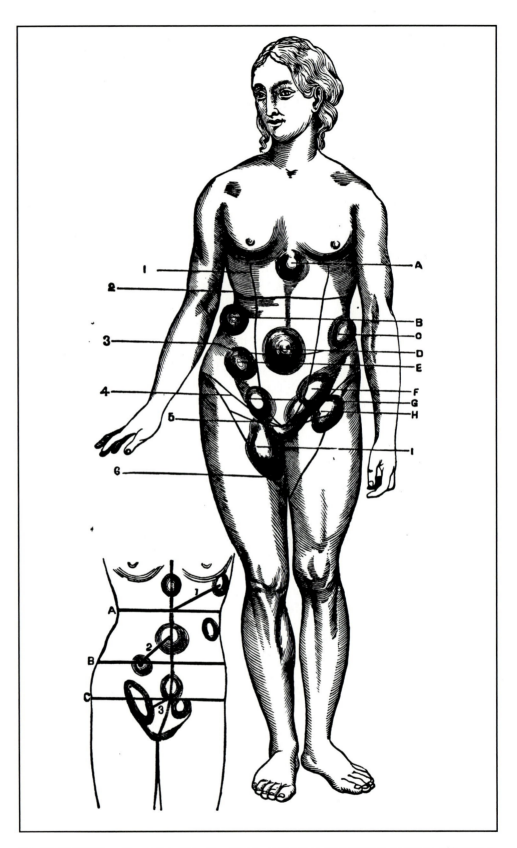

Fig. 38. (GS85) Dowell uses this plate (number 1, page 13) to demonstrate positions of hernia in the abdominal region.

treatment of the breast. A second edition was published in 1885. Among Ostrom's other medical books are *The diseases of the uterine cervix* (Philadelphia: Boericke & Tafel, 1904) and *Leucorrhoea and other varieties of gynaecological catarrh; a treatise on the catarrhal affections of the genital canal of women; their medical and surgical management* (Philadelphia: Boericke & Tafel, 1910). (See also OT41.)

GS87. HUGH HUGER TOLAND (1806–80). *Lectures on practical surgery.* 520pp. Philadelphia: Lindsay & Blakiston, 1877.

Toland received his M.D. from Transylvania University in Lexington and practiced surgery in California. He was surgeon at San Francisco City and County Hospital for many years. At the time this volume was published, he was professor of the principles and practice of surgery and clinical surgery in the medical department of the University of California. Toland organized his own medical school shortly after the Civil War, but it was relatively short-lived. Toland notes in the preface:

> Before the Toland College was transferred by the Trustees to the Regents of the University of California, and thereby became the medical department of that Institution, the students requested me to write a textbook; I told them that my engagements were so numerous that I could not find time to write a book with the scientific accuracy of some that had been published, but that if they were willing, I would talk a book that would contain the principles of surgery, with illustrations from my own experience . . . .

There are forty-nine chapters with numerous illustrations. A second edition was published in 1879.

GS88. DAVID HAYES AGNEW (1818–92). *Principles and practice of surgery, being a treatise on surgical diseases and injuries.* 3 vols., 1062pp., 1066pp, and 784pp. Philadelphia: J. B. Lippincott, 1878–83.

Agnew was professor of surgery at the University of Pennsylvania. He was attending surgeon to President James Garfield when Garfield was shot in 1881. J. Howe Adams writes in his *Life of D. Hayes Agnew, M.D., LL.D.* (Philadelphia: F. A. Davis, 1892, pages 160–64):

> Agnew wrote the entire book with his own pen . . . . He was engaged many years upon the work, doing it at odd times, such as working late into the night and getting up early in the morning, working before his early breakfast . . . it is a medical diary of his professional life for fifty-one years . . . . It is written in much the same manner as he lectured . . . in 1889 he revised his work . . . after his death the publishers of the work feeling that there was a necessity again for its revision, suggested that the work be done . . . but at the wishes of Mrs. Agnew, who felt that this monument to his life-work should stand as he had erected it, they decided, permanently, that it should go down to posterity as it had been written . . . being the most complete and exhaustive description of one man's surgical experiences in the history of the world.

Agnew notes in the preface:

> In the composition of its pages, while I have expressed my own views independently on all subjects, I have also endeavored, as far as was consistent with the scope and limits of the work, to record those of other

> writers, not only that the student and the practitioner may be made familiar with the literature of their profession, but also that they may be able in their observation and practice to contrast different plans of treatment, and in this way draw their own conclusions in regard to the relative merits of the various modes of managing surgical disease. Whatever may be the defects of the work,—and none can be more sensible of these than myself,—I have endeavored most conscientiously to furnish a safe and reliable guide for the surgical practitioner.

The work is massive: volume 1 has ten chapters and 897 illustrations, volume 2 has thirteen chapters and 790 illustrations, and volume 3 has thirteen chapters and 512 engravings. There is no index to the work as a whole, each volume having its own index. The treatise was translated into Japanese and published in Tokyo in 1888. Agnew was also a medical historian and wrote the *History and reminiscences of the Philadelphia Almshouse and Philadelphia Hospital* (Philadelphia: Deltre, 1890). (See also GY19.)

GS89. **JAMES EWING MEARS** (1838–1919). *Practical surgery: including surgical dressing, bandaging, ligations and amputations.* Philadelphia: 279pp. Lindsay & Blakiston, 1878.

A charter member of the American Surgical Association and its president in 1894, Mears was a graduate of Jefferson Medical College. He was among the first to suggest Gasserian ganglionectomy for trigeminal neuralgia [G-M 4857]. Mears's *Surgery* was dedicated to Samuel David Gross (1805–84), who was his mentor. Mears writes in the preface:

> This book has been written in response to the request of students who have been from time to time under the instruction of the author, and who have expressed a desire for a work which should embrace in a condensed form the subjects herein treated of. It has been the endeavor of the author to present these subjects in as concise a manner as possible, and at the same time to omit nothing which might be deemed necessary to render the instruction complete. While he has aimed to embody chiefly the results of his own experience as a teacher and as a practitioner, he has not hesitated to make use of the standard text-books on surgery, and of such works as are devoted to the consideration of the special topics presented in this.

There are four parts, as noted in the title, and 227 illustrations. Further editions were published in 1885 and 1889.

GS90. **GEORGE HENRY NAPHEYS** (1842-76). *Modern surgical therapeutics: a compendium of current formulae, approved dressings and specific methods for the treatment of surgical diseases and injuries.* 587pp. Philadelphia: D. G. Brinton, 1878.

Within four years of graduating from Jefferson Medical College in 1866, Napheys had authored one of the most popular medical books of the post-Civil War era. Napheys's *Therapeutics* eventually went through seven editions. The work consists of "favorite prescriptions" gathered from a number of authorities. An advertisement for the book states:

> The diseases are arranged alphabetically, under the proper nosological classes. Under each its treatment is given, first, by several leading

authorities of this country and Europe, and their differences carefully set forth; nexpert tereatment in several prominent hospitals is recorded, and any especial formulae claimed, on good authority, to be of peculiar efficacy; finally, an abstract or resume is added, setting forth, alphabetically, the more important drugs and remedial measures used in the disease, their doses, indications, and most successful combinations . . . . There is a complete Table of Contents, and three elaborate indices, one of authors, a second of remedies and remedial measures, and a third of diseases.

Napheys had previously written a volume dealing with medical therapeutics entitled *Modern therapeutics: a compendium of recent formulae and specific therapeutical directions* (Philadelphia: S. W. Butler, 1870). An editor notes in the preface to *Surgical therapeutics*:

> Its chief purpose is to set forth the medical aspects of surgery. While there are abundant treatises on operative, mechanical and minor surgery, there is none which aims to collect in one book the therapeutics of surgery in the stricter sense of the word . . . . This was the aim of the talented author of the present work, who, however, was called from his labors before he had completed them . . . . The work grew out of the author's "Modern Therapeutics," and is an amplification of the surgical portion of that work . . . .

The seventeen chapters include "Inflammation"; "Anesthetics"; "Wounds"; "Lesions from heat and cold"; "Connective and muscular tissue"; "Bones and joints"; "Circulation"; "Digestion"; "Urination"; "Reproduction"; "Special senses"; "New growths"; "Scrofula"; "Skin"; and "Venereal diseases." Napheys was among the most prolific nineteenth-century physicians, having also written *The transmission of life: counsels on the nature and hygiene of the masculine function* (Philadelphia: J. G. Fergus, 1871), *The prevention and cure of disease: a practical treatise on the nursing and home treatment of the sick* (Springfield: W. J. Holland, 1872), *The physical life of women: advice to the maiden, wife, and mother* (Philadelphia: J. F. Fergus, 1873), *The body and its ailments: a handbook of familiar directions for care and medical aid in the more usual complaints and injuries* (Philadelphia: H. C. Watts, 1876), and *Handbook of popular medicine, embracing the anatomy and physiology of the human body; with over 300 choice dietetic and remedial recipes* (Philadelphia: H. C. Watts, 1878). Unfortunately, Napheys died prematurely and so was unable to enjoy his success.

GS91. **LEWIS ATTERBURY STIMSON** (1844–1917). *A manual of operative surgery*. 477pp. Philadelphia: Henry C. Lea, 1878.

Stimson graduated from Bellevue Hospital Medical College in 1874. He occupied numerous academic positions in New York medical schools, but was most closely affiliated with New York Hospital. When Cornell University Medical College was organized in 1898, Stimson became its first professor of surgery. His intensive efforts assured the close association that Cornell's medical school shared with New York Hospital. The

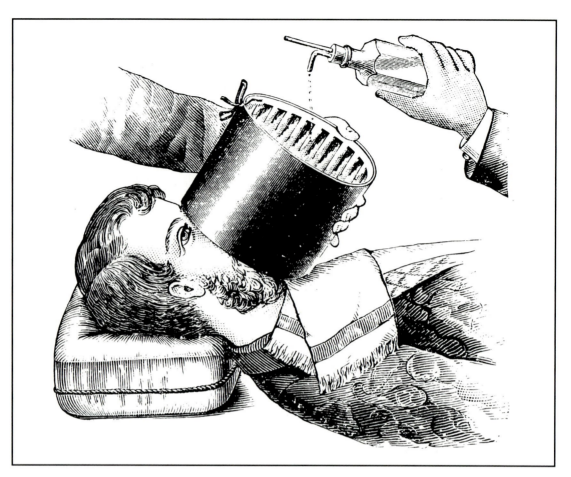

Fig. 39. (GS93) In this illustration (number 7, page 33) Turnbull shows the ether inhaler designed by Oscar H. Allis with modifications by Snowden. The figure demonstrates the mode of using the completed apparatus, its application to the patient's mouth, and a protective towel placed across the chest in case of nausea and vomiting.

Manual reflects Stimson's extensive clinical expertise and went through further editions in 1885, 1895, and 1900. It was meant to serve as both a work of reference and a handy guide to operative surgery. It therefore stressed the details of operations and the different ways of performing them. The work initially sold in cloth for $2.50. Stimson's son, Henry L. Stimson (1867–1950), was secretary of war under President Taft and secretary of state under President Hoover. (See also OR40, OR45, and OR61.)

GS92. **JOHN OSGOOD STONE** (1813–76). *Clinical cases, medical and surgical.* 230pp. New York: G. P. Putnam's Sons, 1878.

An 1836 graduate of Harvard Medical School, Stone never held an academic position. He practiced in New York City, where he was surgeon at Bellevue Hospital. Throughout his professional career, Stone kept a careful record of all cases in his practice. During the last year of his life he wrote out those cases which seemed of most interest to him. They had been intended for publication in *The New York Medical Journal*, but after his death the manuscript was found essentially ready for publication. It was at the request of many of his physician friends that this volume was issued. The work covers eighty-two cases, including such topics as "Croup treated by the probang and caustic"; "Amputation of both thighs"; "Hydrocele of the neck cured by seton"; and "Lithotomy."

GS93. **LAURENCE TURNBULL** (1821-1900). *The advantages and accidents of artificial anaesthesia. Being a manual of anaesthetic agents, and their modes of administration, considering their relative risk, test of purity, treatment of asphyxia, spasm of the glottis, syncope, etc.* 210pp. Philadelphia: Lindsay & Blakiston, 1878.

Turnbull was an aural surgeon at Jefferson College Hospital and was best known for his writings on hearing and the ear. This volume was the first work by an American surgeon to discuss anesthesia and its applications in depth. Turnbull writes in the preface:

> This little work was originally written by the author as a report for a medical society, and was subsequently extended to its present form to supply a want that evidently exists at the present day, for a convenient handbook, on the administration of the various anesthetics . . . . Many valuable books have, unquestionably, been written on the subject of anesthetics, but, as far as the writer's observation extends, none of a practical character have appeared within the last few years . . . .

The advantages contains eleven chapters of text and twenty-five illustrations. There is an interesting list of agents that "will produce anesthetic sleep" on page 16. A second edition was published in 1879 and a third in 1890. (See also GS124, OT12, and OT30.)

GS94. **AMBROSE LOOMIS RANNEY** (1848–1905). *A practical treatise on surgical diagnosis.* 386pp. New York: William Wood, 1879.

Ranney received his M.D. from the University of the City of New York in 1871. At the time this volume was written, he was adjunct professor of anatomy and lecturer on minor surgery at his alma mater. He omitted questions of etiology, pathology and treatment from this work. There are no illustrations, and its eight sections deal exclusively with physical diagnosis of surgical diseases: "Diseases of the blood-vessels"; "Joints"; "Bone"; "Dislocations"; "Fractures"; "Male genitals"; "Abdominal cavity"; and "Tissues." A second edition was published in 1881 and a third in 1884. Among Ranney's other medical texts are *The applied anatomy of the nervous system* (New York: D. Appleton, 1881), *The topographical relations of the female pelvic organs* (New York: William Wood, 1883), *Practical suggestions respecting the varieties of electric currents and the uses of electricity in medicine; with hints relating to the selection and care of electrical apparatus* (New York: D. Appleton, 1885), and *Lectures on nervous diseases from the standpoint of cerebral and spinal localization, and the latter methods employed in the diagnosis and treatment of these affections* (New York: F. A. Davis, 1888). (See also GS109 and OP76.)

GS95. **STEPHEN SMITH** (1823–1922). *Manual of the principles and practice of operative surgery.* 689pp. Boston: Houghton & Osgood, 1879.

The *Manual* contains sixty chapters and over 730 illustrations, providing an exhaustive review of all aspects of surgery. Smith wrote in the preface to the *Manual*:

> The Handbook . . . prepared by the writer in 1862, though specially designed for military practice, was received with much favor. The request has often been made, by both medical practitioners and students, that the plan of the work should be enlarged so as to include the general operations of surgery in civil practice. The present work is the result of an effort to realize that object within the limits assigned, namely, general operations in surgery, the organs of special sense being excluded.

On page 13, Smith provides an interesting rationale for choosing the proper month, day, and hour for an operation. Further editions were published through the 1880s. (See also GS53.)

GS96. **JOHN ALLAN WYETH** (1845–1922). *Essays in surgical anatomy and surgery.* 262pp. New York: William Wood, 1879.

In 1876, Wyeth won a $100 prize offered by the Bellevue Hospital Medical College Alumni Association for an essay on the surgical anatomy of the tibio-tarsal articulation. Two years later, he was awarded the first and second prizes of the American Medical Association for papers on the surgical anatomy and history of the carotid and innominate and subclavian arteries. These winning essays and another on the obturator artery form the contents of his *Essays.* (See also GS80 and GS132.)

GS97. **SAMUEL WEISSELL GROSS** (1837–89). *A practical treatise on tumors of the mammary glands, embracing their histology, pathology, diagnosis, and treatment.* 246pp. New York: D. Appleton, 1880.

Son of Samuel David Gross (1805–84), Samuel W. Gross was an 1857 graduate of Jefferson Medical College. He served on the surgical faculty at Jefferson, and is also well known for writing the first comprehensive work on bone sarcoma [G-M 4346]. Dedicated to his father, the *Treatise* argued that breast tumors could be operated on successfully if the disease had not metastasized. The twenty-eight figures provide extensive descriptions of microscopic appearances of breast tumors. Gross writes in the preface:

> . . . so far as I know, tumors of the mammary gland have not, up to the present time, constituted the subject of a systematic and strictly accurate treatise. To fill this void, I have studied their minute structure, investigated their general pathology, and applied the principles which are fairly deducible from their anatomy and their history to their differential diagnosis and to their rational treatment . . . . Not the least important part of the work is that in which the view is sought to be maintained by an abundant array of facts, that carcinoma may be permanently relieved by thorough operations practised in the early stages of its evolution. I am aware that this doctrine will not meet with general acceptance on the part of those purely mechanical surgeons who believe that freedom from recurrence denotes an innocent neoplasm . . . .

The thirteen chapters include "Classification and relative frequency of tumors of the mammary gland"; "Evolution and transformation of mammary neoplasm"; "Etiology of neoplasms of the mammary gland"; "The anatomy of the connective tissue neoplasms"; "Fibroma"; "Sarcoma"; "Myxoma"; "Carcinoma"; "Cysts"; "Diagnosis of tumors of the mammary gland"; "Treatment of tumors of the mammary gland"; and "Tumors of the male mammary gland." (See also GU13.)

GS98. **THOMAS GEORGE MORTON** (1835–1903) and **WILLIAM HUNT** (1825–96). *Surgery in the Pennsylvania Hospital, being an epitome of the practice of the hospital since 1756; including collations from the surgical notes, and an account of the more interesting cases from 1873 to 1878.* 348pp. Philadelphia: J. B. Lippincott, 1880.

Morton graduated from the University of Pennsylvania Medical School in 1856 and was professor of clinical and operative surgery at the Philadelphia Polyclinic for Graduates. Both he and Hunt, who graduated from the University of Pennsylvania in 1849, were attending surgeons at Pennsylvania Hospital. Morton is remembered for being among the first to deliberately operate on and remove an inflamed appendix after a correct diagnosis [G-M 3569] and for providing the first complete description of anterior metatarsalgia [G-M 4341]. Their *Surgery* is important because from the founding of the Pennsylvania Hospital in 1752, its physicians preserved notes of almost all the operations completed. This record is unique in American surgical history, and their text provides an in-depth look at colonial and early to mid nineteenth-century surgical practices. In addition, a table on page 349 lists all surgical cases

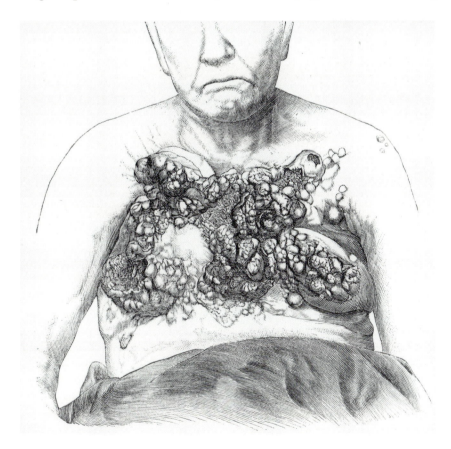

Fig. 40. (GS97) Gross's illustrations were elementary wood engravings. This engraving, figure 26 on page 149, demonstrates a disseminated simple carcinoma of the breast.

for the five-year period from May 1873 to May 1878. The table reveals that even by the 1870s there were few actual operations; most surgery was the treatment of fractures, strictures, and wounds. Morton also wrote *A history of the Pennsylvania Hospital, 1751–1895* (Philadelphia: Time Printing House, 1895).

GS99. **JOHN BINGHAM ROBERTS** (1852-1924). *Paracentesis of the pericardium, a consideration of the surgical treatment of pericardial effusions.* 100pp. Philadelphia: J. B. Lippincott, 1880.

Roberts was a house officer at Pennsylvania Hospital when he wrote his first paper on pericardial effusions. He updated this report by publishing his *Paracentesis*, which reviewed sixty cases. His major conclusion was that paracentesis of the pericardium is indicated in every case of pericardial effusion which does not respond readily to medical care. Roberts was an 1874 graduate of Jefferson Medical College. Active in numerous organizations, he was president of the American Surgical Association and the American College of Surgeons. Roberts also introduced the push-back procedure or backward displacement of the velum to ensure adequate speech [G-M 5757.3]. Among Roberts's other books are *The doctor's duty to the state; essays on the public relations of physicians* (Chicago: American Medical Association Press, 1908), *Surgery of deformities of the face including cleft palate* (New York: William Wood, 1912), and *Treatise on fractures* (Philadelphia: J. B. Lippincott, 1916). (See also GS102, GS143, OR53, OR60, and NS1.)

GS100. **JOHN ASHURST** (1839–1900). *The international encyclopedia of surgery; a systematic treatise on the theory and practice of surgery by authors of various nations.* 6 vols., 717pp., 754pp., 760pp., 987pp., 1207pp. and 1272pp. New York: William Wood, 1881–86.

These volumes played an important role in American surgery because they introduced the concept of a multiauthor surgical textbook. Previous surgical texts were based on the cumulative experience of one individual. However, Ashhurst's *Encyclopedia* showed that a textbook written by many surgeons could be a publishing success. The list of contributors was a who's who of world surgery. Among the prominent American names are David Hayes Agnew (1818–92), Jacob DaSilva Solis Cohen (1838–1927), John H. Packard (1832–1907), and John A. Wyeth (1845–1922). Foreign surgeons include William Allingham (1829–1908), Henry Trentham Butlin (1845–1912), William Watson Cheyne (1852–1932), Christopher Heath (1835–1905), Henry Morris (1844–1926), Louis Ollier (1825–1901), Antonin Poncet (1849–1913), and Frederick Treves (1853–1923).

Due to his efforts, Ashhurst became recognized as the greatest authority in the world on surgical bibliography. An 1860 graduate of the University of Pennsylvania Medical School, he was named John Rhea Barton Professor of Surgery at his alma mater in 1888. (See also GS72 and OR15.)

GS101. **JAMES GRANT GILCHRIST** (1842-1906). *Surgical principles and minor surgery.* 205pp. Chicago: Duncan Brothers, 1881.

At the time this volume was published, Gilchrist was in the middle of changing academic positions from lecturer on surgery at the Homeopathic Medical College of the University of Michigan to professor of surgical pathology and therapeutics at the State University of Iowa. He writes in the preface:

> When the last edition of an exceedingly defective book—*Surgical Diseases*—became exhausted, my publishers supposed that a new and improved one would be well received, and suggested the revision and re-writing of the work. The errors, inaccuracies, and crudities of the old edition, however, were soon found to be so numerous, that it was impossible to use to advantage any portion of the text, or even to follow the arrangement of the original work . . . . Considering the present volume, then, as the initial volume of a series on surgical topics, a scheme has been arranged with some reference to an ideal collegiate course of instruction, embracing four volumes, at least, if not five . . . . To supply a text-book for each of these college years, has been my desire; the present volume being intended for the first year; the volume on Therapeutics, already before the profession, answering for the second, until a thorough revision can be had; a volume on Surgical Emergencies, now in press, for the third; and a volume of Surgical Operations will be prepared as a text-book for the last or fourth year . . . . The reader will note the absence of all allusion to cauteries, as a therapeutic agent, hypodermic injections, blisters, and the like. They have no place in our armamentum chirurgie, and require no notice at our hands . . . .

There are nineteen chapters, with the majority concerning bandaging. Other topics include "Vaccination"; "Tongue-tie"; "Bleeding"; and "Catheterism." The work includes ninety illustrations; most demonstrate various bandages. There was only one edition. (See also GS78, GS117, and GS166.)

GS101.1 **HENRY MUNSON LYMAN** (1835–1904). *Artificial anaesthesia and anaesthetics.* 338pp. New York: William Wood, 1881.

Lyman was born in the then Kingdom of Hawaii. He graduated from Williams College in 1858 and received his M.D. from the College of Physicians and Surgeons in New York in 1861. Most of his professional life was spent in Chicago, where he was appointed to the chair of chemistry at Rush Medical College in 1871. From 1877 to 1890 he held the chair of physiology and diseases of the nervous system and from 1890 until 1900 was professor of medicine. In 1891 Lyman was president of the Association of American Physicians, and in 1892 he became president of the American Neurological Association. Although not a surgeon, Lyman was influential in the early clinical application of surgical anesthesia. This influence was not only due to *Artificial anaesthesia* but because he was a frequent contributor to surgical textbooks, primarily in the form of chapters on anesthesia. The most prominent of these contributions was in John Ashhurst's (1839–1900) six-volume *International encyclopedia of surgery* (GS100). *Artificial anaesthesia* was written with much assistance from Moses Gunn (1822–87), who was professor of surgery at Rush Medical College. It was the second comprehensive textbook on anesthesia to be written by an American. The most interesting section of the book (pages 98–329) provides in-depth discussions of forty-seven anesthetic agents. There is also a short chapter (page 330ff.) on anesthesia by electricity. A striking feature of this volume is the large number of kymographs utilized throughout the text. This instrument was first developed by Karl Ludwig (1816–95) in 1847, and Lyman's book was among the first American works to use it. This text is volume 17 in Wood's Library of Standard Medical Authors. It has no plates, and only one edition was published. Among Lyman's other books are *The practical home physician* (Chicago: Western Publishing House, 1884), *Insomnia and other disorders of sleep* (Chicago: W. T. Keener, 1885), *A textbook of the principles and practice of medicine* (Philadelphia: Lea Brothers & Co., 1892), and *The book of health* (Providence: W. P. Mason, 1898).

GS102. **JOHN BINGHAM ROBERTS** (1852-1924). *The compend of anatomy, for use in the dissecting room, and in preparing for examinations.* 191pp. Philadelphia: C. C. Roberts, 1881.

In 1882, Roberts proposed and assisted in the establishment of the Philadelphia Polyclinic and College for Graduates in Medicine, serving as secretary. Eight years later, he became president and opened the Polyclinic Hospital. He resigned in 1899 but continued as professor of anatomy and surgery at the college until its merger into the Medico-Chirurgical College Graduate School of Medicine, University of Pennsylvania, in 1918, when he became professor of surgery at the new school. Roberts's *Compend* grew out of lectures which he gave in his capacity as professor of surgery. They were intended solely for students and young surgeons. A second edition was printed in 1881 and a third in 1885. (See GS99, GS143, OR53, OR60, and NS1.)

GS103. **CHARLES H. VON TAGEN** (1835–?). *Biliary calculi; perineorrhaphy; hospital gangrene and its kindred diseases, with their respective treatments.* 154pp. New York: Boericke & Tafel, 1881.

Von Tagen was a homeopathic surgeon who graduated from Pennsylvania Homeopathic College in 1858. He later was appointed professor of operative surgery at the Homeopathic Hospital College, Cleveland. Most of his written contributions were in the form of articles in medical periodicals. This volume is his only textbook and consists of articles previously published in journals.

GS104. **JOSEPH HUCKINS WARREN** (1831–91). *Hernia, strangulated and reducible, with cure by subcutaneous injections, together with suggested and improved methods for kelotomy; also an appendix giving a short account of various new surgical instruments.* 280pp. Boston: C. N. Thomas, 1881.

Warren received his M.D. in 1853 from Bowdoin Medical College. He practiced surgery in Boston but never held an academic position. This scarce volume was initially published in London in 1880; the

American edition followed in 1881. The book was dedicated to Joseph Pancoast (1805–82), Henry Thompson (1820–1904), and John Collins Warren (1778–1856). Warren writes in the preface:

> There seemed to me a great need for a work like the one now issued, giving a short sketch of the various operations for the cure of hernia that are most worthy of mention, in order that the busy practitioner could refer to them without wading through whole volumes. Much labour has been bestowed upon the little monograph, and very many authors consulted. I have striven, with the time at my command, to make a trustworthy work of reference on Hernia, although it is far from being as perfect or as extended as I should like. It will be found to contain much that is original with the author (the result of the study of Hernia for many years), and never before given to the profession in a printed form. Besides this will be found a condensation of many operations from the French, German, and English. A short bibliography is given to indicate some of the work that has been devoted in previous years to the subject under consideration . . . .

There are nine chapters with much material on the subcutaneous injection method of curing hernia. Warren states in an appendix to the American edition that " . . . from information which I have obtained from records and documents, and other sources, I am convinced that the honor of the discovery of the subcutaneous operation and method of curing hernia, by injection, belongs rightly to my esteemed and distinguished fellow-countryman, Professor Joseph Pancoast . . . . " There are seventy-four wood engravings but no plates. A second, greatly enlarged edition was published in 1882 as *A practical treatise on hernia*; it contains three plates. (See also GS120.)

GS105. **EDWARD JOHN BERMINGHAM** (1853–?). *An encyclopaedic index of medicine and surgery.* 934pp. New York: Bermingham, 1882.

This extremely scarce volume was edited by Bermingham. He writes in the preface:

> This is an age of "Encylopaedias" and "Systems" in medical literature, but it seems to have been the aim of both the editors and publishers of those that have appeared to endeavor to make them as large as possible—to stretch them out volume after volume. Many of these are valuable reference books, but the price places them beyond the acquisition of the majority of practitioners, and even though they be in the library, they cannot be conveniently consulted on account of the bulk and the arrangement of the subjects. In the present volume an effort has been made to avoid these objectionable features. The arrangement of the subject is alphabetical, with cross references for all synonymous terms. Each article is a comprehensive account of the disease . . . . The entire field of the science and practice of both medicine and surgery is covered . . . the aim of the editor having been to produce a book which should be pre-eminently useful . . . The work, being in one volume, can lie on the desk, for constant use and ready reference.

The book sold for $6.00. The surgical contributors included Nathan Bozeman (1825–1905) [G-M 4221 and 6085], Frank H. Hamilton (1813–86), Willard Parker (1800–84), Oren D. Pomeroy (1834–1902), Henry B. Sands (1830–88) [G-M 3272 and 3565], and Theodore Gaillard Thomas (1832-1903). Among Bermingham's other books are *The disposal of the dead, a plea for cremation* (New York: Bermingham, 1881), *Practical therapeutics: a compendium of selected formulae and practical hints on treatment* (New York: J. R. Bermingham 1885), and the 45-page pamphlet *Chronic nasal catarrh, and what the general practitioner can do for it* (New York: Chambers Print, 1893).

GS106. **JOHN BUTLER** (1844–85). *Electricity in surgery.* 111pp. New York: Boericke & Tafel, 1882.

Born in Ireland, Butler was a homeopathic physician who practiced in New York. This volume was

> ... intended as a practical guide for the use of the specialist and general practitioner, and aimed at showing the necessity of attaining accuracy of detail in all electro-surgical operations. The scope of the work precludes the possibility of more than cursory allusion to clinical cases, but is based almost entirely upon the author's own personal experience, and is for the most part composed of articles written from time to time for different periodicals, revised and condensed ....

Among the contents are discussions of "Hydrocele"; "Aneurism"; "Permanent removal of superfluous hairs"; "Burns"; "Lateral spinal curvature"; "Amputation of the tongue"; "Prolapse of the rectum"; and "Cautery as a haemostatic." This last chapter (page 86ff.) is an interesting forerunner to Harvey Cushing (1869–1939) and W. T. Bovie's classic paper on electrocoagulation in neurosurgery [G-M 4897.1]. Butler's other medical book is *A text-book of electro-therapeutics and electro-surgery* (New York: Boericke & Tafel, 1878) .

GS107. **EDWARD CARROLL FRANKLIN** (1822–85). *A complete minor surgery.* 423pp. Chicago: Gross & Delbridge, 1882.

Franklin was a homeopathic surgeon who held the title of professor of surgery at the University of Michigan. This volume was dedicated to John Nickoleius Eckel (?-1901), a homeopathic physician from San Francisco. Franklin notes in the preface:

> As a teacher of surgery, and the various processes and methods of treatment connected with it, I have been repeatedly requested by students of Homeopathic colleges to prepare a treatise on minor surgery. An early effort in this direction was presented in my *Science and Art of Surgery*, which, though confessedly imperfect, may be justly claimed as the pioneer work in this department of our literature. Since then the range of minor surgery has been continually extending, including much that pertains to accessory treatment and the general management of the sick-room, till now it forms in itself a distinct and systematic branch of study. The authors of our large work on surgery have assumed much of this preliminary knowledge; and, as a consequence, many important and interesting details have been omitted, or else too briefly mentioned to satisfy the requirements of the profession. The present volume, therefore, is written with the intention of occupying this ground, and of furnishing the student and the busy practitioner with the teachings of Homeopathy upon the different subjects considered, in as complete and concise a form as possible.

There are almost 200 illustrations. The book is divided into four parts: "General surgical semeiology"; "Bandaging, and other points of minor surgery"; "Venereal and sexual diseases"; and "Dietary table for the sick." This was the only edition. (See also GS65, GS108, OR35, and GU16.)

GS108. **EDWARD CARROLL FRANKLIN** (1822–85). *The practitioner's and student's manual of the science of surgery.* 187pp. Ann Arbor: S. C. Andrews, 1882.

This volume is a compendium of the course of lectures which Franklin delivered before the junior classes of the Homeopathic College of the University of Michigan in his position as professor of surgery and clinical surgery. The preface states:

> . . . they are the notes or guides to the instruction I have given on the various subjects . . . . Being more comprehensive than a syllabus, and less prolix than the greater works on surgery, they possess that concise and sharp-cut distinctiveness that appeals directly to the understanding . . . . It is not to be expected that in a work like this, written for the purpose of condensing rather than augmenting the sphere of surgical science, that I should give to the student all that is valuable for a thorough understanding of this complex study . . . .

There are eleven chapters dealing with a wide range of subjects. The table of contents is labeled "Vol. I.," and Franklin had intended to complete a series of compendia related to his surgical lectures. However, he became ill and died within three years, never completing his project. (See also GS65, GS107, OR35, and GU16.)

GS109. **AMBROSE LOOMIS RANNEY** (1848–1905). *Practical medical anatomy; a guide to the physician in the study of the relations of the viscera to each other in health and disease, and in the diagnosis of the medical and surgical conditions of the anatomical structures of the head and neck.* 339pp. New York: William Wood, 1882.

Although Ranney was not known as a surgeon but as an anatomist and neurologist, his *Anatomy* was important because of its emphasis on the head and neck and on the surgical diseases related to this area. He early recognized the connection of eyestrain as a cause of functional nervous disorders, and many of his writings concern this relationship. At the time of this publication, he was adjunct professor of anatomy at the University of the City of New York, having previously served as lecturer on genitourinary and minor surgery at the same institution. This work was the seventh volume in Wood's Library of Standard Medical Authors. Ranney comments in the introduction:

> This volume is an indirect outgrowth of two courses of lectures delivered by me before students . . . during the winters of 1879 and 1880 . . . . The pages, such as they are, have cost me many hours of research to write . . . some hints that properly pertain to physiology and surgery cannot be omitted, if the aim of this work is to be fully attained, although the limited size of this volume will preclude the insertion of but scattered hints in this direction. It is not to be inferred, however, that this work pretends to cover the ground, either

of physiology or of operative surgery, since but a small portion of the former science treats of the vessels and nerves, while the latter department embraces remedial measures for every existing condition demanding surgical interference . . . .

The work contains four chapters in part 1 on the head and six chapters in part 2 on the trunk. No plates are included, but there are 156 wood engravings. A second edition appeared in 1888. (See also GS94 and OP76.)

GS110. **DAVID TOD GILLIAM** (1844–1923). *The essentials of pathology.* 296pp. Philadelphia: P. Blakiston & Son, 1883.

An 1871 graduate of the Medical College of Ohio, Gilliam was a gynecologist renowned for his treatment of uterine prolapse [G-M 6111]. In 1877 he settled in Columbus, Ohio, where he held the chair of pathology at Columbus Medical College. The *Pathology* was published after Gilliam had assumed the chair of physiology at Starling Medical College. He writes in the preface:

> The object of this little book is to unfold to the beginner the fundamentals of pathology in a plain, practical way, and by bringing them within easy comprehension to increase his interest in the study of the subject. It is not, therefore, intended to supplant more pretentious works by allaying, but rather to lead up to them by kindling, a thirst for pathological investigation . . . . I have, in great measure, purposely avoided the discussion of unsettled questions, and have occasionally stated dogmatically that which admits of question. This has been done with a view to prevent confusion in the mind of the student, and to impart clear-cut conceptions of the generally accepted doctrines of to-day.

The *Pathology* has thirty-three chapters, including discussions of "Histology"; "Death"; "Tumors"; and "Cysts"; the last fourteen focus on various organ systems. This book is significant because it was the first textbook devoted solely to pathology to be written by an American surgeon. In addition, the forty-seven wood engravings show the early use of a microscope to view histologic preparations. Among Gilliam's other medical works is *A text-book on practical gynecology for practitioners and students* (Philadelphia: F. A. Davis, 1903).

GS111. **CHARLES WINSLOW DULLES** (1850–1921). *What to do first in accidents and emergencies; a manual explaining the treatment of surgical and other injuries in the absence of the physician.* 2nd edition. 119pp. Philadelphia: P. Blakiston & Son, 1883.

Dulles practiced surgery in Philadelphia for over forty years. He never held an academic title, but was consulting surgeon at Rush Hospital and lecturer on the history of medicine at the University of Pennsylvania from 1893 to 1908. His *Manual* was initially published in 1880, but the first edition had less emphasis on surgical problems than did later editions. The second edition in 1883 and those that followed it in 1888, 1892, 1897, 1904, and 1909 contained in-depth discussions of surgical first aid.

GS112. **WILLIAM BARTON HOPKINS** (1853–1904). *The roller bandage.* 95pp. Philadelphia: J. B. Lippincott, 1883.

An 1874 graduate of the University of Pennsylvania Medical School, Hopkins was a surgeon in the outpatient departments of the Pennsylvania and Episcopal hospitals in Philadelphia. He also held the title of assistant demonstrator of surgery at his alma mater. The intent of the book is described in the preface:

> The plan which has been adopted in this book, . . . is to teach by numerous illustrations rather than by elaborate description the method of applying the roller bandage. In order that the student may most readily familiarize himself with this very important subject, a series of illustrations are presented which were made in the following manner: each bandage was applied to a living model, and whenever the roller pursued a course which the author has found in his association with students was the cause of any uncertainty, it was at once photographed. From these photographs accurate drawings were made . . . . In this way it is hoped that the intricate course traversed by the roller in the most complex dressing has been made sufficiently plain to enable the student to apply it for himself almost unaided by the text. The latter will be found very brief and devoid of everything but the rule for application and the use to which the dressing is commonly put.

There are seventy-three illustrations demonstrating how to bandage every conceivable area of the body. Further editions were published in 1886, 1891, 1897, and 1902.

GS113. **ORVILLE HORWITZ** (1859–1913). *A compend of surgery.* 133pp. Philadelphia: P. Blakiston & Son, 1883.

Horwitz was a surgeon who practiced in Philadelphia. He never held an academic position but often lectured on surgery at various institutions. The *Compend* discusses numerous topics, including "Hectic fever"; "Hospital gangrene"; "Erysipelas"; "Chancroid"; "Chancre"; "Bubo"; "Shock"; "Hernia"; "Dislocations"; "Fractures"; "Housemaid's knee"; "Whitlow"; and "Drowning". The text includes fifty-one illustrations. This volume was the ninth in Blakiston's Quiz-Compends Series, which were meant to be used in quiz-classes and examination rooms. The pocket-sized volumes were based on popular textbooks and lectures of prominent professors. The clothbound edition cost $1.00, and an interleaved edition for taking notes was available for $1.25. There were other editions in 1885, 1887, 1890, 1893, and 1907.

GS114. **LEWIS STEPHEN PILCHER** (1845–1934). *The treatment of wounds; its principles and practice, general and special.* 391pp. New York: William Wood, 1883.

The first editor of *The annals of surgery* (1885 to 1934), Pilcher was an 1866 graduate of the University of Michigan Medical School. He served as president of the American Surgical Association in 1919. In the preface to his *Treatment*, Pilcher writes:

> I have attempted to state, first, the principles upon which the treatment of wounds should be based; then, to describe the means which are available to the surgeon for satisfying the demands of these principles; and,

lastly, to point out the particular modifications which the peculiarities of special wounds may require . . . .

The *Treatment* consists of twenty-one chapters with 116 figures, and was the first American work to deal thoroughly with this topic. In his autobiography, *A surgical pilgrim's progress, 1845–1925; reminiscences of Lewis Stephen Pilcher* (Philadelphia: J. B. Lippincott, 1925, pages 217-18), Pilcher briefly mentions the genesis of this work: "Shortly after I was elected a member of the newly formed New York Surgical Society, the most prominent medical book publisher of New York solicited me to undertake the writing of a book on the subject then uppermost in the surgical world, viz: the treatment of wounds . . . . " There was only one edition of the *Treatment*; it formed volume 22 in Wood's Library of Standard Medical Authors. Among Pilcher's other medical books are *Odium medicum and other addresses and studies in medical life and affairs* (Philadelphia: J. B. Lippincott, 1910), *The commander's year* (Philadelphia: J. B. Lippincott, 1914), and *Fractures of the lower extremity or base of the radius* (Philadelphia: J. B. Lippincott, 1917). Pilcher was a well-known bibliophile, and in 1918 he published an annotated bibliography of his own

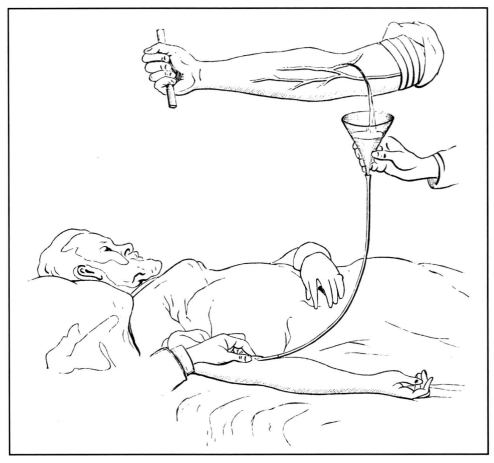

Fig. 41. (GS114) This figure (number 36, page 131) is one of the earliest depictions of direct blood transfusion by hydrostatic pressure in an American surgical textbook. Pilcher was a major proponent of this new procedure and was well aware of the accompanying problems with air and blood emboli.

collection, *A list of books by some of the old masters of medicine and surgery, together with books on the history of medicine and on medical biography* (Brooklyn: private printing). (See also GS190.)

GS115. **SEABORN FREEMAN SALTER** (?-?). *Principles and practice of American medicine and surgery.* 621pp. Atlanta: J. P. Harrison, 1883.

Salter was professor of principles and practice of medicine and clinical medicine at the College of American Medicine and Surgery in Atlanta. The preface of this extremely scarce volume states:

> In the absence of any standard textbook on practice, suited to the student and practitioner of American medicine, I have undertaken the preparation of this volume. Originality in the descriptive text is not claimed . . . . In treatment I claim originality, having given that which years of practical experience have proved worthy of confidence . . . .

In this work, Salter discusses numerous surgical problems but describes little in the way of operative surgery. The book is difficult to read, but there is an extensive index on pages 617-21.

GS116. **JOSEPH DECATUR BRYANT** (1845–1914). *Manual of operative surgery.* 2 vols., 307pp. and 285pp. New York: Bermingham, 1884.

Bryant graduated from Bellevue Hospital Medical College in 1868. He rose to prominence not only as a surgeon but also as sanitary inspector and health commissioner of New York City, and commissioner of the New York State Board of Health. In 1907 he was president of the American Medical Association. Bryant is perhaps best remembered for having performed a "secret" operation on President Grover Cleveland for sarcoma of the left upper jaw in 1893. Bryant's *Manual* was written when he was professor of anatomy and clinical surgery at Bellevue Hospital Medical College. It was intended

> . . . to aid the student in acquiring established facts, rather than to add to the art itself. The works of Ashhurst, Gross, Erichsen, Holmes, Packard, Smith, Esmarch, Stimson, and others, have been fully consulted, and in some instances their language has been employed or paraphrased . . . . The operations peculiar to the female, and the eye and ear, have not been considered, since they are, in the opinion of the author, entitled to a far more extended consideration than the intentional scope of this work will admit of.

There is no table of contents. With 705 figures and an abbreviated index, this work does provide a comprehensive look at surgical operations. Further editions were published in 1887, 1899, and 1905. All of these were issued by D. Appleton, with the two volumes being combined into one. The second edition was available in either cloth ($5.00) or sheepskin ($6.00). Bryant's other medical work is the eight-volume *American practice of surgery; a complete system of the science and art of surgery, by representative surgeons of the United States and Canada* (New York: William Wood, 1906–11). [G-M 5805]

GS117. **JAMES GRANT GILCHRIST** (1842-1906). *Surgical emergencies and accidents.* 599pp. Chicago: Duncan Brothers, 1884.

A homeopathic physician, Gilchrist was professor of surgical pathology and therapeutics at the State University of Iowa. He writes in the preface:

> The systematic study of accidents of all kinds, the indications for treatment, both instrumental and medicinal, with particular reference to prognosis as affected by Homeopathic therapeutics will form the subjects for our present enquiry. Some attempt has been made to treat the subjects presented in an exhaustive manner, in fact on a plan somewhat different from that of any work in our school at least, with which the writer is acquainted. In this the third volume in the series, the student is introduced to what should constitute the studies for the third year of his pupilage . . . . No extended instruction has been given on principles of dressing, or ordinary pathological processes, as the work is supplementary to its predecessors. Major operations, and the principles of operative surgery, have also been briefly alluded to, as a later volume is designed to cover this field as thoroughly as the author's ability will permit . . . .

There are twenty-eight chapters and almost seventy illustrations. This was the only edition. (See also GS78, GS101, and GS166.)

GS118. **CHARLES HUNTOON KNIGHT** (1849–1913). *A year-book of surgery for 1883.* 197pp. New York: G. P. Putnam's Sons, 1884.

A graduate of the College of Physicians and Surgeons in New York, Knight was among America's earliest laryngologists. He held the chair of professor of laryngology at the New York Post-Graduate Medical School from 1892 to 1898, when he was elected professor of diseases of the throat and nose at Cornell University Medical College. Knight's *Year-book* reflects his training as a general surgeon, although by 1884, his major professional interest was in diseases of the upper air passages. The last paragraph of the preface states: "From this brief review it would seem that the year has not been remarkably fruitful in important additions to surgical resources, yet it is hoped that enough material has been gathered to give interest to the present volume." The work consists of five parts: "General surgery and surgery of the extremities"; "Surgery of the head and neck"; "Surgery of the chest and abdomen"; "Surgery of the genito-urinary organs"; and "Venereal diseases." These sections consist of reviews of numerous journal articles which present current information on a particular topic. No illustrations are included. Knight's other important medical book is *Diseases of the nose and throat* (Philadelphia: P. Blakiston's Son, 1903).

GS119. **WILLIAM HOLME VAN BUREN** (1819–83). *Lectures on the principles of surgery.* 588pp. New York: D. Appleton, 1884.

As professor of the principles and practice of surgery at Bellevue Hospital Medical College, Van Buren was one of America's most respected surgeons. This volume presents lectures that he delivered at Bellevue. However, it was published after Van Buren's death and reflects the vigorous editing of Lewis Stimson (1844–1917), who gathered the lectures into book form. Stimson writes in the preface:

> During the last fifteen years of his life Dr. Van Buren was Professor of Surgery in the Bellevue Hospital Medical College, and for nearly twenty years previously he had been Professor of Anatomy and of Clinical Surgery in the University of the City of New York. His success was as great in this field as it was in others, and was earned by the most thorough and careful preparation for every course and every lecture. It was always his practice to prepare a syllabus, and often to write out a lecture in full before its delivery. During the last years of his life he wrote and rewrote many of these lectures, arranged them, and added to them in such a way as to make them a systematic exposition of the subject as he sought to present it to his classes. From these manuscripts this book has been printed, without other changes than a few verbal ones, and without addition. It is offered, not as a complete treatise on the principles of surgery, prepared with the thoroughness and attention to detail that all have recognized and learned to expect whatever Dr. Van Buren gave to the press, but simply as that presentation of them which he, in his large experience as a teacher, thought best fitted to be of service to the student and to the practitioner who returned to take his place upon the benches of the lecture-room. And, in thus giving to these notes a permanent form, Dr. Van Buren's friends feel that they not only pay a proper tribute to his memory, but also do a service to the profession, and especially to those who have received their surgical education from him.

There are twenty-six chapters ranging over a number of subjects, although the greatest concentration is on inflammation and infectious surgical diseases. There are only eighteen rudimentary illustrations and no plates. The volume is difficult to read because it lacks an index and has only a simplified table of contents. This work was available in either cloth ($4.00) or sheepskin ($5.00). (See also GS60, GU9, and CR6.)

GS120. **JOSEPH HUCKINS WARREN** (1831–91). *A plea for the cure of rupture; or, the pathology of the subcutaneous operation by injection for the cure of hernia.* 117pp. Boston: J. R. Osgood, 1884.

This scarce treatise contains six papers, some of which had been previously published in medical journals in England, Scotland, and the United States. Included are "Inflammation and its relation to tissue repair"; "Permanent cure of hernia by subcutaneous injections"; "History of my connection with the method of subcutaneous injections for hernia"; "A plea for operative measures for the relief and cure of hernia"; "The proper fitting and wearing of a truss"; and "Causation of hernia." The last chapter contains an interesting form (pages 113–17) used to obtain follow-up statistics on patients treated for hernias. (See also GS104.)

GS121. **JAMES LEONARD CORNING** (1853–1923). *Local anesthesia in general medicine and surgery, being the practical application of the author's recent discoveries.* 103pp. New York: D. Appleton, 1885.

Corning was a New York neurologist who performed some of the earliest experiments with local, regional, and spinal anesthesia. He completed a spinal block within a year following the demonstration of the anesthestic property of cocaine and only ten months after the invention of conduction anesthesia [G-M 5680]. In 1885, at the same time that William Halsted (1852–1922) was conducting his research on local infiltration anesthesia [G-M 5679], Corning showed experimentally that cocaine had a prolonged anesthetic effect when it was administered subcutaneously. This discovery led to Corning's use of it on patients. These initial research trials were published in this volume. In this book Corning reports that cocaine anesthesia could be indefinitely prolonged by decreasing the circulation in the part anesthesized by means of a tourniquet. Only one edition was printed; it sold in cloth for $1.25. Halsted, in a letter dated August 23, 1918, to William Osler (1849–1919), recalled: "Corning's book on cocaine anesthesia was based almost entirely on my work. He was a student of mine and followed my work with cocaine closely . . . . " Corning's other books consist of *Brain-rest* (New York: G. P. Putnam's Sons, 1883), *Brain exhaustion, with some preliminary considerations on cerebral dynamics* (New York: D. Appleton, 1884), *A treatise on headache and neuralgia, including spinal irritation and a disquisition on normal and morbid sleep* (New York: E. B. Treat, 1888), *A treatise on hysteria and epilepsy, with some concluding observations on epileptic insomnia* (Detroit: G. S. Davis, 1888), and *Pain in its neuro-pathological, diagnostic, medico-legal and neuro-therapeutic relations* (Philadephia: J. B. Lippincott, 1894).

GS122. **WILLARD PARKER** (1800–84). *Cancer: a study of three hundred and ninety-seven cases of cancer of the female breast, with clinical observations.* 61pp. New York: G. P. Putnam's Sons, 1885.

A graduate of Harvard Medical School in 1830, Parker served as professor of the principles and practice of surgery at the College of Physicians and Surgeons of Columbia University. An ingenious surgeon, he is remembered for innovations in vascular [G-M 2962 and G-M 4169] as well as urologic [G-M 4169] surgery. He was also the first American surgeon to operate for appendicitis [G-M 3564]. Although a voluminous contributor to the medical periodicals, and the collector of a vast and important medical library formerly at the Brooklyn Academy of Medicine but now widely dispersed, Parker never wrote a true textbook on surgery. Following his death, *Cancer* was compiled by his son using manuscript notes that had been in preparation. Parker's son notes in the preface to the work:

> During the few years preceding his death, my father, relieved in large part from the arduous labors of active professional life, occupied himself in gathering together and classifying the cases of mammary cancer that had come under his observation, amounting in all to nearly four hundred. Before the work, however, had been completed to his satisfaction, his health and strength broke down, and he was able to do but little in its revision. As it was his wish that the record should be published, I give it to the public nearly in the form in which he left it, and would ask that it be regarded, not as an elaborate work, but as embodying some of the observations made and conclusions reached during a long and busy professional life, by one who combined with an exceptionally large experience, strong, practical common-sense.

At the conclusion of the volume is a twenty-page table listing all 397 cases.

GS123. **GEORGE HERBERT TAYLOR** (1821–96). *Pelvic and hernial therapeutics. Principles and methods for remedying chronic affections of the lower part of the trunk, including processes for self-cure.* 282pp. New York: J. B. Alden, 1885.

Taylor was an 1852 graduate of the New York Medical College. Having studied for a year in Stockholm in 1858–59, he became an early vigorous advocate of mechano-therapy, which is now known as Swedish massage. The mechano-therapy movement had many advocates, including surgeons who were beginning to specialize in orthopedic surgery. The volume contains thirty-seven illustrations and is divided into three parts: "Principles"; "Processes"; and "Practice." The last section contains chapters 19 and 20, which deal with hernia. There was only one edition. Among Taylor's most important other medical books are *An exposition of the Swedish movement cure* (New York: Fowler & Wells, 1860), *The movement-cure in every chronic disease; a summary of its principles, processes, and results* (New York: R. Larter, 1861), *Paralysis and other affections of the nerves; their cure by vibratory and special movements* (New York: S. R. Wells, 1871), *Health by exercise. what exercises to take and how to take them, to remove special physical weakness; embracing an account of the Swedish methods, and a summary of the principles of hygiene* (New York: American Book Exchange, 1880), *Health for women, showing the causes of feebleness and the local diseases, resulting therefrom; with full directions for self-treatment* (New York: J. B. Alden, 1883), *Massage, principles and practice of remedial treatment by imparted motion; description of manual processes* (New York: Fowler & Wells, 1884), and *Mechanical aids in the treatment of chronic forms of disease* (New York: G. W. Rogers, 1893). (See also GY16.)

GS124. **LAURENCE TURNBULL** (1821-1900). *The new local anaesthetic; hydrochlorate of cocaine (muriate of cocaine), and etherization by the rectum.* 76pp. Philadelphia: P. Blakiston & Son, 1885.

Turnbull was an aural surgeon at Jefferson Medical College Hospital. This small volume represents a continuation of his research on anesthetic agents. He was one of the first American surgeons to write about and actively use many of the different anesthesia techniques then available. Among the contents of this book are several chapters dealing with cocaine and its use in rhinology, pharyngology, and laryngology. Other chapters include "Minor and general surgery"; "Dermatology"; "Gynecology"; "Genitourinary surgery"; "Dental surgery"; and "Otology." The second part contains detailed lists of cases where etherization via the rectum had been utilized. Turnbull also included six pages (pp. 67-72) of objections to this method. (See also GS93, OT12, and OT30.)

GS125. **ROBERT TUTTLE MORRIS** (1857-1945). *How we treat wounds today; a treatise on the subject of antiseptic surgery which can be understood by beginners.* 162pp. New York: G. P. Putnam's Sons, 1886.

Morris, the son of a governor of Connecticut, graduated from the College of Physicians and Surgeons in New York in 1882. He began a private surgery practice in New York City and made numerous contributions to surgical literature. The *Treatise* was based largely on his experience during his study in Europe in 1884–85. Morris was later house surgeon at Bellevue Hospital and consulting surgeon at the Woman's Hospital of Brooklyn when the book was published. The text reveals a supercilious attitude and is written in a sarcastic style. A review of it in the *Medical bulletin* (March 1886) stated:

> The author of this bombastic book is fully imbued with his own importance and the importance of dressing wounds according to his method or the method of his friends. He announces "that the time has come when it is best for the general practitioner to have as little as possible to do with surgery." In our opinion the time has come when the general practitioner should have as little as possible to do with all such egotistical specialists, or would-be specialists.

Morris recounts the writing of this work on pages 70–72 of his autobiography, *Fifty years a surgeon* (New York: E. P. Dutton, 1936):

> Upon my return to New York I found that bitter controversy was still raging in America over the subject of antiseptic surgery . . . . So, fresh from Europe, I sat right down to a duty task and in a week or less tossed off the material for a little brochure entitled *How We Treat Wounds To-day*. Before offering the manuscript for publication, I consulted Dr. Shrady, Editor of the *Medical Record*. He advised me in a fatherly way not to publish the book. He said that it would hurt me with the sort of men upon whom a younger man was to look for advancement and security in professional position. The manuscript was then taken to Dr. Weir, who said, "Publish the book but be prepared to take the consequences of your show of syllogistic fists." That sounded like good sport of the football kind. The book went rapidly through several editions and into French and Russian translations. It was adopted by our Surgeon General's office at Washington for use at army posts . . . . Dr. Shrady had been quite right in his prophecy. Two or three physicians of established position who had seemed to be on the point of asking me to share their offices hesitated about making a definite offer because of my display of radical attitude and because of its repercussions.

Regardless of the controversy, the book was well received and went through further editions in 1886, 1887, and 1890. It was initially available in cloth for $1.00. Morris also wrote two books of medical essays: *Dawn of the fourth era in surgery and other articles* (Philadelphia: W. B. Saunders, 1910) and *A surgeon's philosophy* (New York: Doubleday & Page, 1915). (See also GS167.)

GS126. **CHARLES BEYLARD GUERARD DE NANCREDE** (1847-1921). *Essentials of anatomy including the anatomy of the viscera.* 352pp. Philadelphia: W. B. Saunders, 1887.

An 1869 graduate of the University of Pennsylvania Medical School, Nancrede initially was in practice in Philadelphia, where he eventually served as professor of general and orthopedic surgery at the Philadelphia

Polyclinic. His *Anatomy*, based on Henry Gray's (1827–61), was intended for students and was arranged in the form of questions and answers. This volume, which contains over 100 illustrations, was the third in Saunders's Question Compends Series and was available for $1.00 in a cloth binding and $1.25 interleaved for notes. The textbook was updated in new editions in 1889, 1890, 1891, 1895, 1899, and 1904. (See also GS185.)

GS127. **JOHN COLLINS WARREN** (1842–1927). *The healing of arteries after ligature in man and animals.* 184pp. New York: William Wood, 1886.

Warren was assistant professor of surgery at Harvard Medical School when this monograph was written. The physiologic and pathologic response of ligated arteries was an extremely important subject to the nineteenth-century American surgeon. Warren notes in the preface:

> The attempt has been made here to study the question from a more comprehensive standpoint, to observe not only the behavior of the various tissues concerned in the process of repair, but also the different phases through which the vessel passes from the moment of ligature until the condition is reached after which no further change occurs.

A lengthy review of the history of the subject preceded a section reporting the results of experiments in animals. Warren studied in Europe in 1869, and during this time he met briefly with Joseph Lister (1827-1912). It is believed that this short meeting stimulated a lasting interest in the topic of arteries and led to Warren's thorough and detailed monograph. (See also GS77 and GS169.)

GS128. **GEORGE RYERSON FOWLER** (1848–1906). *Syllabus of a course of lectures on first aids to the injured, arranged for the medical officers of the second brigade, National Guard of the State of New York.* 57pp. New York: A. Coffin & Rogers, 1887.

Fowler was an 1871 graduate of Bellevue Hospital Medical College. He practiced in Brooklyn and New York City and is remembered for completing the first thoracoplasty [G-M 3179] and for describing Fowler's position for treatment of diffuse septic peritonitis [G-M 5623]. While in Europe in 1884, Fowler was introduced to the practice of stationing ambulances in various parts of England to aid the seriously injured. On his return he decided to establish classes for instruction in first aid to the injured in America. His prominent rank in the National Guard enabled him to present the matter to the military authorities, and his first classes were given in 1885. First aid instruction was afterward given at all armories and to all National Guard organizations, since knowledge of first aid was regarded as an essential part of a soldier's training. Fowler was also one of the organizers and first president of the Brooklyn Red Cross Society in 1890. Among Fowler's other medical books are the two-volume *A treatise on surgery* (Philadelphia: W. B. Saunders, 1906) and *The operating room and the patient* (Philadelphia: W. B. Saunders, 1906). (See also GS160.)

GS129. **JASPER JEWETT GARMANY** (1859–1947). *Operative surgery on the cadaver.* 150pp. New York: D. Appleton, 1887.

Garmany dedicated this volume to James R. Wood (1813–82) for " . . . acts of kindness during my three years' pupilage, and while interne of Bellevue Hospital . . . . " An attending surgeon to the Out-door Dispensary of Bellevue Hospital, Garmany was only twenty-eight years old when *Operative surgery* was published. He writes in the preface: "It is my endeavor to present a guide to the manipulative procedures of the ordinary surgical operations. Acknowledgment of indebtedness is chiefly due to Stephen Smith's Operative Surgery." Although the book has virtually no illustrations, its eleven chapters provide a thorough review of most major operations.

GS130. **JOHN HOMANS** (1836–1903). *Three hundred and eighty-four laparotomies for various diseases, with tables showing the results of the operations and the subsequent history of the patients. A resume of the writer's experience in abdominal surgery during the last fifteen years.* 56pp. Boston: N. Sawyer, 1887.

Homans was a pioneer ovariotomist who graduated from Harvard Medical School in 1862. After serving in the Civil War, he returned to Boston and began to practice at a number of hospitals. Homans's only academic appointment was as clinical instructor in the diagnosis and treatment of ovarian tumors at Harvard Medical School. He did little writing, this volume being his only major text. It details his experience in abdominal surgery over a fifteen-year period. He writes:

> Of my first five unantiseptic ovariotomies all died. Of my antiseptic ovariotomies 248 have recovered and 34 have died. About one quarter, probably, of all the fatal cases are to be attributed to some error or carelessness of mine, or perhaps to a slightly suppurating hang-nail or other sore on my hands, or to something that might have been avoided. Perhaps this comes from too much operating within a given time. Deaths for which I am inclined to think I am at fault, have occurred generally towards the end of many daily ovariotomies, when I may have been tired or possibly unclean.

An interesting aspect of this monograph is the twenty-six foldout tables which accompany the text. Homans was the father of John Homans (1877-1954) [G-M 1160, 2722, and 3894].

GS131. **EDWIN HARTLEY PRATT** (1849–1930). *Orificial surgery and its application to the treatment of chronic diseases.* 139pp. Chicago: W. T. Keener, 1887.

Pratt was professor of orificial surgery in the Chicago Homeopathic Medical College and surgeon at Cook County Hospital. A definition of orificial surgery appears in his introductory chapter:

> In all pathological conditions, surgical or medical, which linger persistently in spite of all efforts at removal, from the delicate derangements of brain-substance that induce insanity, and the various forms

of neurasthenia, to the great variety of morbid changes repeatedly found in the coarser structures of the body, there will invariably be found more or less irritation of the rectum, or the orifices of the sexual system, or of both.

The book contains nine chapters, but there is no table of contents and only an abbreviated index. The most interesting aspect of this work is the early use of forty-nine photographs of operations on the rectum and male and female sexual organs. An enlarged edition was published in 1890. Pratt's other medical book is *The composite man as comprehended in fourteen anatomical impersonations* (Chicago: New Age Publishing House, 1900).

GS132. **JOHN ALLAN WYETH** (1845–1922). *A text-book on surgery, general, operative, and mechanical.* 777pp. New York: D. Appleton, 1887.

Dedicated to J. Marion Sims (1813–83), whose youngest daughter was Wyeth's wife, this monumental work was Wyeth's major contribution to American surgical literature. He recalls in his autobiography, *With sabre and scalpel* (New York: Harper Brothers, 1914, page 377):

> In 1884 an agent of the publishing firm of D. Appleton & Co. called upon me with a proposition to write a text-book on surgery for that firm; but we failed to agree on terms. I was very desirous of writing such a book, for much of the work I had already done was directly in that line. I insisted on a new style of illustration in colors which was more than ordinarily expensive, and told the Appletons it was not worth while to bring out a new book unless it could be made more attractive than any other book on surgery. The cost was thought to be too great, and for the time being the matter rested there as far as they were concerned; but I went on with the surgery without saying a word to any one, for I felt that I would find a publisher. The next fall the Appleton agent came back and said, "Well, what about the surgery?" I replied, "Nothing, unless your firm will give me carte blanche on illustrations," and, to my delight, he said: "All right; I am authorized to close the contract now. Can you do it in a year?" I said, "In less time, if you are in a hurry." We signed the contract, and then I told him the book was written, and I could give him the manuscript as fast as he wanted it. As I had anticipated, the beautiful illustrations in three colors, which had never before been used in a text-book on this subject, proved very attractive. I was to be at no expense and to receive ten per cent of the gross sales, which for the various editions amounted to between two and three hundred thousand dollars.

The work is massive in scope and covers almost every conceivable surgical topic. Colored illustrations of particular operations with reference to the arteries were an important feature of the work. Updated editions were published in 1890, 1898, and 1908. The original purchase price was $7.00 for buckram with uncut edges, $8.00 for sheepskin, and $8.50 for half morocco. Wyeth also published two books related to military history, *Life of General Nathan Bedford Forrest* (New York: Harper Brothers, 1899) and *History of La Grange Military Academy and the cadet corps* (New York: Harper Brothers, 1914). (See also GS80 and GS96.)

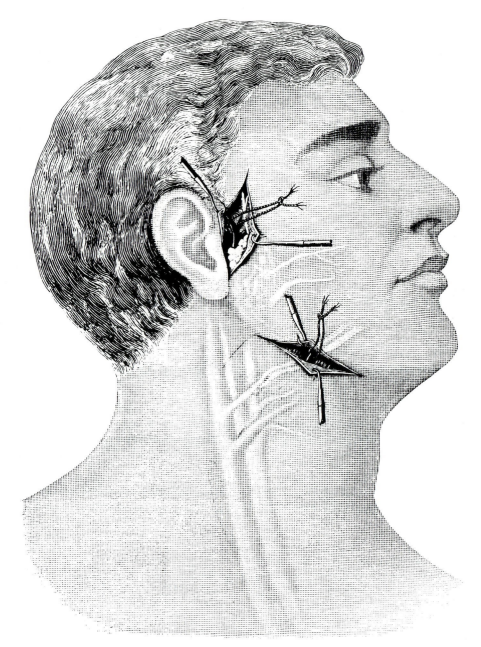

Fig. 42. (GS132) Wyeth was proud of his use of color illustrations. In this example, figure 290 on page 247, he depicts ligation of the posterior temporal vessels at the zygoma and of the facial vessels upon the inferior maxilla; the arteries are red and the veins blue.

GS133. **ARPAD GEYZA GERSTER** (1848–1923). *The rules of aseptic and antiseptic surgery.* 332pp. New York: D. Appleton, 1888.

Gerster, who was born in Hungary, arrived in America in 1873. He is credited with being the first physician in New York City to practice surgery exclusively. A fellow of the American Surgical Association, he was its president in 1911. He was also professor of surgery at New York

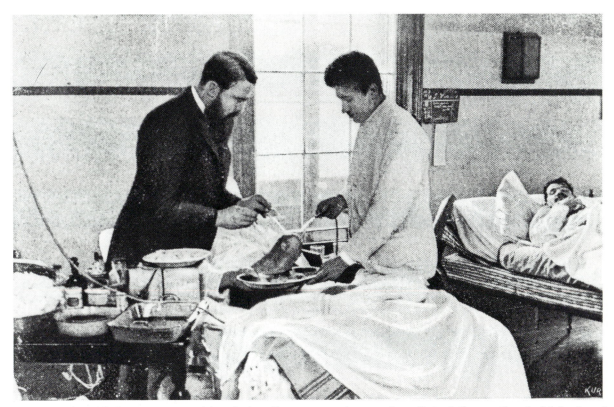

Fig. 43. (GS133) Gerster was one of America's earliest amateur photographers. He took the negatives for his book and had William Kurtz reproduce them using a halftone phototypographic process. This engraving, figure 4 on page 21, shows Gerster performing a change of dressing after amputation of the thigh.

Polyclinic Hospital and visiting surgeon at Mount Sinai Hospital. Gerster's *Rules* was the first American surgical text based on Listerian principles. The book caused a furor, for at that time suppuration was considered a natural sequence of every surgical procedure. The book was immensely popular and passed through further editions in 1888 and 1891. However, its importance was not only in its content but also the efforts that were expended in its production. It was printed on heavy calendered paper with many halftone illustrations, which were then rare in scientific books. Gerster had mastered the technique of photography and made his own plates at a time when photography by an amateur was unusual. The contents include five parts: "Asepsis"; "Antisepsis"; "Tuberculosis"; "Gonorrhoea"; and "Syphilis." Gerster comments in his autobiography, *Recollections of a New York surgeon* (New York: Paul B. Hoeber, 1917, pages 236–38):

> The work of writing was begun in October, 1885, and on December 17th the contract with Daniel Appleton & Company was signed. They were liberal and helpful publishers. For the illustrations the adoption of the new Meisenbach process, then an untried innovation, was proposed, to which the firm assented, on condition, that the cost must not exceed $2,500. The author was to furnish the photographs . . . . The actual writing of the first draft was done in about three months. This result was achieved only because everything had been properly assembled and classified beforehand, and because a carefully prepared skeleton plan

was strictly followed. The book appeared in October, 1887, but at the request of the firm was postdated to 1888 . . . the cost of illustrations was kept well below $2,000, a feat which raised the author in the publishers' estimation higher than either his literary or his surgical skill . . . . There were three editions, the second following the first within three months. Altogether, a few less than 11,900 copies were sold . . . .

GS134. **EDWARD MARTIN** (1859–1938). *Questions and answers of the essentials of surgery: together with a full description of the handerchief and roller bandages.* 314pp. Philadelphia: W. B. Saunders, 1888.

An 1883 graduate of the University of Pennsylvania Medical School, Martin was John Rhea Barton Professor at his alma mater from 1910 to 1918. A founding member of the American College of Surgeons, he is remembered for performing a cordotomy for the relief of intractable pain [G-M 4883]. When he wrote this text, he was an assistant to David Hayes Agnew (1818–92). Not meant as a definitive treatise on surgery, it was oriented more to the needs of the student or beginning surgeon and is listed as No. 2 in the Saunders series of Question Compends. The volume contained ninety illustrations. Each volume in the Saunders series was arranged in question-and-answer form and bound in a convenient size (5 x 7 inches) so it could be carried in a pocket. Most of the Saunders Question Compends were so popular that they went through six or seven editions. This text could be bought with interleaving for student's notes for $1.00. Among Martin's other books is *Surgical diagnosis* (Philadelphia: Lea & Febiger, 1909). (See also GS142, GS147, GU31, and GU38.)

GS135. **OTIS KIMBALL NEWELL** (?-?). *The best surgical dressing; how to prepare it and how to use it; with a consideration of Beach's principle of bullet-wound treatment.* 179pp. Boston: Cupples & Hurd, 1888.

Newell was assistant demonstrator of anatomy at Harvard Medical School and surgeon to the out patients at Massachusetts General Hospital. He writes in the preface:

> . . . few of us have found time to become familiar with the true chemistry, physiological action, and best surgical use of iodoform. Four years ago I had daily opportunities to see results of the clinical tests which its use as a surgical dressing furnished at the clinic of Professor Billroth . . . . I am happy to say that the great value of iodoform, when properly used, has been proved beyond a doubt . . . . It is well to remember that the practised surgeon of to-day seldom needs any dressing as far as the result in fresh wounds of operation is concerned, since there he almost invariably has a wound which goes on to complete union without any suppurative action. When, however, the wound comes to him in a septic condition, or through some unavoidable accident becomes in its later progress a septic one, then the great desideratum is that form of dressing which will, since its insoluble basis is not rapidly diluted and washed away by the discharge, remain as a permanent protection to the surface exposed. For this purpose nothing thus far discovered, can stand comparison with iodoform . . . .

In the text Newell recommends that surgeons "never disturb a bullet wound unless there are positive indications of the necessity of doing so." Pages 16–119 consist of a translation of the work of Johann von Mikulicz-Radecki (1850–1905), "The use of iodoform in surgery," *Wien klin. 1 heft*, January, 1882. Beach's method of bullet wound treatment, along with several case reports, appears on pages 123–79.

GS136. **HAL C. WYMAN** (1852-1908). *Abdominal surgery.* 87pp. Detroit: G. S. Davis, 1888.

Wyman was professor of surgery and operative surgery at the Michigan College of Medicine and Surgery. This volume is part of G. S. Davis's Physicians' Leisure Library. This series was produced each year beginning in 1886 and usually consisted of a dozen volumes on various medical and surgical topics. *Abdominal surgery* was part of the third library series and was priced at twenty-five cents in paper and fifty cents in cloth. The entire series cost $5.00. This particular volume deals mainly with experimental surgery. There is no table of contents and only a limited index, which makes reading it a difficult task. The preface is perhaps the most interesting portion of the book:

> The purpose of this work is to aid students and practitioners in the elementary study of abdominal surgery by a plain presentation of facts . . . . While literary excellence will be sought to the very best of my ability, I shall always have my doubts as to results in that direction . . . . The firm and unquestionable position attained by abdominal surgery within the past few years, renders this branch of surgical science of vital interest to every practitioner who is ambitious to keep abreast of the times. It has secured a footing which renders it imperative that all practitioners should familiarize themselves with the technical details of the work. Realizing this proposition to be a true one, my mind was attracted to a consideration of the facilities and opportunities for acquiring such knowledge. Where can the necessary material be obtained? For answer, I say, search the kennels and the hutches about you. Hunt up those oft tried, faithful and most efficient martyrs who give their lives to the cause of science— the dogs and rabbits . . . . Dogs have rendered inestimable aid in evolving the numerous great surgical discoveries which have added so much to the years and comfort of mankind. With the aid of dogs hundreds of ambitious, enthusiastic surgeons have been enabled to make successfully the studies necessary for an understanding of the means by which nature repairs damage. Parenthetically, I wish to state that I have great faith in the life-saving value of abdominal surgery, yet I do not believe I am a "crank" on the subject. No man is more firmly set than myself, against that blood-loving, chance-taking recklessness so sententiously if not elegantly expressed by the phrase; "belly rippers." Abdominal surgery, as I believe, should be practiced (in its present state of development at least) as a last resort, and so practiced the most successful operator, in my opinion, will be the one who is quickest to decide accurately when death is at hand, when the "last-resort-opportunity" is offered.

(See also GU23.)

Fig. 44. (GS138) This simple black-and-white illustration on page 471 demonstrates various methods of intestinal anastomosis and Senn's modification of Jobert's suture.

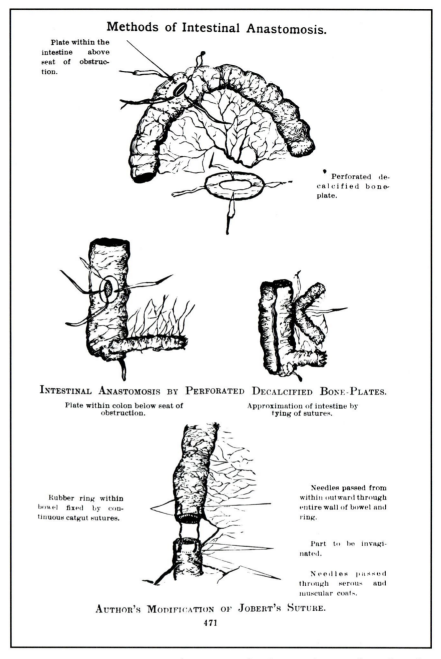

Methods of Intestinal Anastomosis.

Plate within the intestine above seat of obstruction.

* Perforated decalcified bone-plate.

INTESTINAL ANASTOMOSIS BY PERFORATED DECALCIFIED BONE-PLATES.

Plate within colon below seat of obstruction.

Approximation of intestine by tying of sutures.

Rubber ring within bowel fixed by continuous catgut sutures.

Needles passed from within outward through entire wall of bowel and ring.

Part to be invaginated.

Needles passed through serous and muscular coats.

AUTHOR'S MODIFICATION OF JOBERT'S SUTURE.

471

GS137. **HENRY ORLANDO MARCY** (1837-1924). *A treatise on hernia, the radical cure by the use of the buried antiseptic animal suture.* 251pp. Detroit: G. S. Davis, 1889.

Marcy graduated from Harvard Medical School in 1864, and was Lister's first American pupil. Upon his return to America, Marcy was the first to introduce antiseptic methods in surgery. He practiced in Massachusetts, where he established a private hospital in Cambridge for the treatment of surgical diseases of women. He was president of the American Medical Association in 1892. Marcy devoted many years to a continuous study of microorganisms in wounds, which culminated in his use of antiseptic ligatures in the radical cure of hernia [G-M 3594]. In the preface to the *Treatise* he comments:

> This little book is offered the profession, as the outgrowth of special studies upon the subject of hernia for the last eighteen years. In 1870 I first operated for the radical cure of hernia by the open wound method, and the closure of the parts by the use of the buried animal suture. Based upon a series of experimental studies upon animals, . . . it was believed to be demonstrated that aseptically applied animal sutures became so incorporated into the vital structures as to be, in large measure, replaced by connective tissue. The result of these investigations taught that the application of animal sutures, for the cure of hernia, is clearly of the first importance.

The twelve chapters cover a wide range of material, including various types of surgical operations and instrumentation. This monograph, part of Series III of Davis's Physicians' Leisure Library, was a forerunner to Marcy's classic textbook on hernia [G-M 3601]. (See also GS155.)

GS138. **NICHOLAS SENN** (1844–1908). *Experimental surgery.* 522pp. Chicago: W. T. Keener, 1889. [G-M 5620]

Senn's *Surgery* is an early attempt to establish the experimental foundation on which future American surgical successes would occur. This extremely scarce book is a collection of Senn's articles from various medical journals; only one edition appeared. Among the papers are ones dealing with rectal insufflation [G-M 3494] and pancreatic surgery [G-M 3629]. A chapter on intestinal surgery reports some of Senn's earliest research on gastrointestinal anastomosis [G-M 3511]. Senn was an 1868 graduate of Chicago Medical School. Unhappy with his medical training, he studied at the University of Munich and received a Ph.D. in 1878. He returned to Chicago and eventually became professor of the principles of surgery and surgical pathology at Rush Medical College. Senn's work has special significance to the bibliophile because he bequeathed his own valuable surgical library to the Newberry Library in Chicago. It was later transferred to the John Crerar Library, which merged with the University of Chicago. Senn had been a passionate collector of medical books and in 1886 purchased the rather large collection which Wilhelm Baum (1799–1883), professor of surgery at the University of Göttingen, had been assiduously gathering for over fifty years. Among Senn's other books are *Practical surgery for the general practitioner* (Philadelphia: W. B. Saunders, 1902), *A nurse's guide for the operating room* (Chicago: W. T. Keener, 1902), *War correspondence (Hispano-American War); letters from Dr. Nicholas Senn* (Chicago: American Medical Association Press, 1899), *Medico-surgical aspects of the Spanish American War* (Chicago: American Medical Association, 1900), *Around the world via Siberia* (Chicago: W. B. Conkey, 1902), *Surgical notes from four continents and the West Indies* (Chicago: private printing, 1903), *Around the world via India, a medical tour* (Chicago: American Medical Association Press, 1905), and *In the heart of the arctics* (Chicago: W. B. Conkey, 1907). (See also GS139, GS140, GS144, GS162, GS168, OR49, and GU36.)

GS139. **NICHOLAS SENN** (1844–1908). *Intestinal surgery.* 269pp. Chicago: W. T. Keener, 1889.

Included in this collection of papers are "The surgical treatment of intestinal obstruction"; "An experimental contribution to intestinal surgery, with special reference to the treatment of intestinal obstruction"; and "Rectal insufflation of hydrogen gas, an infallible test in the diagnosis of visceral injury of the gastro-intestinal canal in penetrating wounds of the abdomen." Senn writes in the preface:

> There are few subjects in practical surgery on which opinion is more unsettled than on the best method of treating intestinal obstruction and injuries of the gastro-intestinal canal . . . . The first part of the book contains a resume of the best literature on the surgical treatment of intestinal obstruction . . . . The second part represents the author's own original work . . . . One of the principal objects in publishing these papers in book form is a desire to stimulate the young men in our profession to enter the field of original investigation, as the author is firmly convinced that experimental research constitutes the shortest and safest route to the perfection of the principles and practice of intestinal surgery.

(See also GS138, GS140, GS144, GS162, GS168, OR49, and GU36.)

GS140. **NICHOLAS SENN** (1844–1908). *Surgical bacteriology.* 270pp. Philadelphia: Lea Brothers, 1889.

Senn published this volume after returning from a trip to Europe, where he had studied bacteriology in its relation to surgery. The book is worthy of mention for several reasons. It provides a very thorough and exhaustive review of current literature on that part of bacteriology relating to surgery. Unfortunately, even with excellent discussions of surgical and wound infections, Louis Pasteur (1822–95) is mentioned but once and Joseph Lister (1827–1912) not at all. The volume was indispensible to the student, but its chief value was its compilation, which made it possible for the busy practitioner to become conversant with the most advanced ideas of surgical pathology and bacteriology. A second edition was published in 1891. (See also GS138, GS139, GS144, GS162, GS168, OR49, and GU36.)

GS141. **JAMES KELLY YOUNG** (1862-1923). *Synopsis of human anatomy; being a compend of anatomy, including the anatomy of the viscera and numerous tables.* 393pp. Philadelphia: F. A. Davis, 1889.

Young was an instructor in orthopedic surgery and assistant demonstrator in surgery at the University of Pennsylvania. He also served as an attending orthopedic surgeon to the outpatient department of University Hospital. This work was prepared especially for students, although sufficient descriptive portions were added to make it valuable to the practitioner, particularly sections on the viscera, special senses, and surgical anatomy. It included a complete account of osteology, articulations and ligaments, muscles, fascias, and the vascular, nervous, alimentary, vocal and respiratory, and genitourinary systems. In addition, tables were included to facilitate the reader's understanding of anatomy. There were seventy-six wood engravings. The book was bound in blue cloth and cost $1.40. It was No. 3 in Davis's Physicians' and Students' Ready-Reference Series. (See also OR51.)

GS142. **EDWARD MARTIN** (1859–1938). *Essentials of minor surgery and bandaging, with an appendix on venereal diseases. Arranged in the form of questions and answers.* 166pp. Philadelphia: W. B. Saunders, 1890.

This volume is No. 12 of Saunders's Question Compends Series. In some respects, it is a partial condensation of Martin's previous book in this series (GS134). The most important addition is the presentation of an entire section on venereal diseases. Several editions of this work were published in the 1890s and after the turn of the century. (See also GS134, GS147, GU31, and GU38.)

GS143. **JOHN BINGHAM ROBERTS** (1852-1924). *A manual of modern surgery; an exposition of the accepted doctrines and approved operative procedures of the present time.* 800pp. Philadelphia: Lea Brothers, 1890.

Roberts was professor of surgery at the Woman's Medical College of Pennsylvania. In his words:

> This treatise is the result of an effort to give the profession, in a condensed form, the accepted doctrines and approved procedures of modern surgery. I have endeavored to write a practical work, giving the surgical principles and operative methods generally accepted and practiced by the leading surgeons of the world at the present time. The opinions of the best authorities, the methods of the most practical surgeons, and the well-established facts of surgical science are discussed; but the consideration of theories, historical questions, traditional views and operations, and innovations of undecided value has been rigidly avoided.

With 501 illustrations and twenty-seven chapters, the *Manual* includes a wide range of information. However, it is disappointing in that neither Pasteur nor Lister is mentioned. A second edition was published in 1899. (See also GS99, GS102, OR53, OR60, and NS1.)

GS144. **NICHOLAS SENN** (1844–1908). *Principles of surgery.* 611pp. Philadelphia: F. A. Davis, 1890.

Senn writes in the preface:

> The many treatises on surgery, by American and English authors, which have made their appearance in rapid succession during the last ten years or more, are replete with valuable practical information, but most of them are defective in those parts relating to the matter treating of the fundamentals of the art and science of surgery. It has been my aim to write a book for the student and general practitioner which should, at least in part, fill this gap in surgical literature, and which should serve the purpose of a systematic treatise on the causation, pathology, diagnosis, prognoses, and treatment of the injuries and affections which the surgeon is most frequently called upon to treat .... It has been my intention to keep in constant view the difference between the cellular processes, as we observe them in regeneration and inflammation, and

to connect the modern science of bacteriology more intimately with the etiology and pathology of surgical affections . . . . I have attempted to show the direct etiological relationship which exists between certain pathogenic micro-organisms and definite pathological processes . . . .

The twenty-four chapters discuss mostly inflammatory and infectious processes. Examples include "Suppuration"; "Necrosis"; "Erysipelas"; "Tetanus"; "Hydrophobia"; "Actinomycosis"; "Anthrax"; and "Glanders." It was initially available in cloth for $4.50 or sheepskin or half russia for $5.50. Further editions were published in 1895, 1901, and 1909. (See also GS138, GS139, GS140, GS162, GS168, OR49, and GU36.)

GS145. **CHRISTIAN BERRY STEMEN** (1836–1915). *Railway surgery, a practical work on the special department of railway surgery; for railway surgeons, and practitioners in the general practice of surgery.* 315pp. St. Louis: J. H. Chamber, 1890.

Stemen was professor of surgery at Fort Wayne College of Medicine. He writes in the preface:

> This book is the result of my experience in the practice of accidental or railway surgery, and my strong belief that a treatise on this special department was greatly demanded. While the volume is not what I had desired, being written while engaged in active practice, connected with the duties of teaching and other literary work, several chapters being written while traveling in other countries, thus rendering it impossible to give to it that constant and continuous thought and labor which it demanded, it is the hope of the author that the profession will find it of value, and that many practical suggestions may be found that will prove of special interest to the large and constantly increasing number of surgeons engaged in the practice of this special branch of surgery.

There were eighteen chapters, including "Shock in railway injuries"; "Fractures"; "Hemorrhage from railway injuries"; "Concussion of the brain"; "Burns and scalds"; and "Transfusion." The modern version of railway surgery is trauma care, and this volume is one of the earliest American surgical texts to deal specifically with this topic.

GS146. **JOHN B. HAMILTON** (1847–98). *Lectures on tumors from a clinical standpoint.* 143pp. Detroit: G. S. Davis, 1891.

Hamilton graduated from Rush Medical College in 1869. The early years of his career were spent as a surgeon in the United States Marine Hospital Service. He was on the surgical faculty of Georgetown University at the time his *Lectures* was written. The work is now little appreciated, although three editions were published, the last in 1898. The volume contains two plates and was part of Davis's Physicians' Leisure Library series. These short, practical treatises were published to supplement the large medical textbooks, which were considered to contain much irrelevant matter and to be difficult to read. They were bound in either durable paper covers at twenty-five cents or in cloth at fifty cents. Hamilton was eventually named professor of the principles of surgery and clinical surgery at Rush Medical College. He served as editor of the Journal of the American Medical Association from 1893 to 1898.

GS147. **EDWARD MARTIN** (1859–1938). *The surgical treatment of wounds and obstruction of the intestines.* 169pp. Philadelphia: W. B. Saunders, 1891.

An instructor in operative surgery at the University of Pennsylvania, Martin won the Fiske Fund Prize from the Rhode Island Medical Society in 1890 for this essay. The research was carried out over a period of two years and included extensive experiments on animals. A table and summary of over 130 gunshot wounds of the abdomen appear on pages 145–65. Some of the earliest kymographs in an American surgical textbook are found in chapter 11. (See also GS134, GS142, GU31, and GU38.)

GS148. **GEORGE McCLELLAN** (1849–1913). *Regional anatomy in its relation to medicine and surgery.* 2 vols., 436pp. and 414pp. Philadelphia: J. B. Lippincott, 1891–92.

The grandson of George McClellan (1796–1847), McClellan graduated from Jefferson Medical College in 1870. In 1881 he founded the Pennsylvania School of Anatomy and Surgery, where he taught until 1893. In 1906 he was named professor of applied anatomy at Jefferson. McClellan's *Anatomy* is his major work and was written when he was lecturer on descriptive and regional anatomy at the Pennsylvania School of Anatomy and professor of anatomy at the Pennsylvania Academy of Fine Arts. It went through further editions in 1894, 1896, 1898, and 1901, and was also translated into French. The book is of exceptional beauty. There are ninety-seven chromolithograph plates, the subjects of which were dissected, photographed and colored from nature by McClellan. McClellan writes in the preface:

> Accuracy has been the chief object, and I have relied upon the unfailing precision of the camera to present the true relations of the parts, which were in each case left in situ, only the adipose and connective tissues being removed, to give distinct impressions. Much thought, time, and expense have been given to the photographic details such as the arrangement of light to modify the shadows, the exposure and development of the negatives, and the subsequent printing and toning of the pictures to get the desired effect for the application of the watercolors. The coloring of the originals from which the plates were made on stone, under my personal supervision, was a study from nature, with perhaps some excess of tint or shade, as might be expected where the paints were mixed and applied with more enthusiasm than artistic skill. The dissections, in all about three hundred, were invariably the work of my own scalpel . . . .

McClellan's other important medical book is *Anatomy in its relation to art* (Philadelphia: W. B. Saunders, 1901).

GS149. **FRED BYRON ROBINSON** (1854–1910). *Practical intestinal surgery.* 2 vols. Detroit: G. S. Davis, 1891.

A graduate of Rush Medical College in 1882, Robinson taught anatomy and clinical surgery at the Medical College of Toledo. In 1891, he was named professor of gynecology at Chicago Postgraduate Medical School and later professor of gynecology and abdominal surgery at Illinois Medical College. His *Practical surgery* was written while he lived in Toledo. The work is part of Davis's Physicians' Leisure Library, and has twenty-four chapters and sixteen figures. It is dedicated to Nicholas Senn (1844–1908). The individual chapters deal with specific intestinal problems such as "Circular enterorrhaphy"; "Anastomosis"; "Gastro-enterostomy"; and "Gunshot wounds of intestines." The preface reads:

> The past six years I have devoted study and practice to gynaecology. The loss of a woman in abdominal section through intestinal perforation induced me to study, experimentally, how to avoid and repair such dangers. As the abdomen is the recognized field of the gynaecologist, I followed this experimental work with care and pleasure for three years, embracing about 200 operations. I thoroughly believe in specialists for the advancement of medicine, for new ideas; and that each man should practically cultivate from Nature his chosen department, as men do things well only when they do them automatically. This book is the result of original experimental work, and an attempt to add something to the field of gynaecology . . . .

Robinson's other medical works consist of *The peritoneum, part I, histology and physiology* (Chicago, W. T. Keener, 1897), *The abdominal brain and automatic visceral ganglia* (Chicago: Clinic Publications, 1899), *Arteria uterina ovarica; the utero-ovarian artery, or the genital vascular circle, anatomy and physiology, with their application in diagnosis and surgical intervention* (Chicago: E. H. Colegrove, 1903), and *The arteries of the gastrointestinal tract with inosculation circle, anatomy and physiology with application in treatment* (Chicago: E. H. Colegrove, 1908). (See also GY47.)

GS150. **HENRY REDWOOD WHARTON** (1853–1925). *Minor surgery and bandaging, including the treatment of fractures and dislocations, tracheotomy, intubation of the larynx, ligations of arteries and amputations.* 497pp. Philadelphia: Lea Brothers, 1891.

Wharton was demonstrator of surgery and lecturer on surgical diseases of children at the University of Pennsylvania. He attempted to present, in as concise a manner as possible, a description of the various bandages, surgical dressings, and minor surgical procedures that were employed in the practice of surgery. The preparation and application of antiseptic dressings were also discussed in detail. The volume has six parts: "Bandaging"; "Minor surgery"; "Fractures, dislocations"; "Ligation of arteries"; and "Amputations." There are 403 illustrations. Further editions were published in 1893, 1896, 1899, 1902, 1905, and 1909. (See also GS180.)

GS151. **DeFOREST WILLARD** (1846–1910) and **LEWIS H. ADLER** (?–?). *Artificial anaesthesia and anaesthetics.* 144pp. Detroit: G. S. Davis, 1891.

One of America's pioneer orthopedic surgeons, Willard graduated from the University of Pennsylvania Medical School in 1867. He was appointed lecturer in orthopedic surgery there in 1887 and served as clinical professor of orthopedic surgery from 1889 to 1903 and professor of orthopedic surgery after 1903. He was president of the American Surgical Association in 1901. At the time this volume was written, Adler was instructor in rectal diseases at the Philadelphia Polyclinic and College for Graduates in Medicine. The manual was intended to describe the uses, abuses, and dangers of multiple anesthetic agents. Among the topics discussed are "Ether"; "Chloroform"; "Nitrous oxide gas"; "Various anesthetic mixtures"; and "Local substances, including cocaine." Willard's other prominent medical book is *The surgery of childhood, including orthopaedic surgery* (Philadelphia: W. B. Saunders, 1910). (See also CR17.)

GS152. **FRED J. BROCKWAY** (1860–1901) and **A. O'MALLEY** (1858–1932). *Anatomy; a manual for students and practitioners.* 376pp. Philadelphia: Lea Brothers, 1892.

Brockway is an important but little-known figure in the history of American surgery. He was William Halsted's (1852–1922) first resident surgeon at Johns Hopkins Hospital. Brockway was born in New Hampshire and graduated from the College of Physicians and Surgeons in New York in 1887. He was then appointed an intern in the surgical division of Roosevelt Hospital in New York, where he served under Charles McBurney (1845–1913) from May 1887 to May 1889. When Halsted was organizing the surgical staff at Johns Hopkins, he wrote to McBurney asking him to suggest the name of a person who might serve as resident surgeon. Brockway was nominated and arrived in Baltimore on May 13, just in time to receive the first surgical patient to be admitted to the wards of the new hospital. Brockway left Johns Hopkins in October 1890 to become assistant demonstrator in anatomy at his alma mater. He never again performed surgical operations; his interests were in anatomy, and he worked for several summers at the Marine Biological Laboratory at Woods Hole, Massachusetts. In 1891 he married Marion L. Turner, who was the first pupil nurse to enter Johns Hopkins Hospital for training. O'Malley was an instructor in surgery in the New York Polyclinic. The *Anatomy* was part of Lea's Student Quiz Series; it cost $1.75 because it was considered a double number. The book contains six major sections: "Osteology"; "Arthrology"; "Myology"; "Angeiology"; "Neurology"; and "Splanchnology." A second edition, this one with plates, was published in 1893. Brockway wrote one other medical book, *Essentials of physics* (Philadelphia: W. B. Saunders, 1892).

GS153. **ROSWELL PARK** (1852–1914). *The Mütter Lectures on surgical pathology.* 293pp. St. Louis: J. H. Chambers, 1892.

An 1876 graduate of Northwestern University Medical School, Park was instrumental in the application of Listerian antiseptic techniques to American surgery. From 1884 to 1914 he was professor of surgery at the University of Buffalo. The Mütter Lectures were a series of ten presentations delivered at the College of Physicians of Philadelphia in 1890–91. They were initially reported in the volumes 13–15 of the *Annals of surgery*, but were later published as a textbook. Since Park had specialized in surgical pathology, the lectures reflected quite closely his own research and findings. Park's other medical books include *The physiology and hygiene of the house in which we live* (New York: Chautauqua, 1888), written in collaboration with Marcus Hatfield (1849–1909); *An epitome of the history of medicine* (Philadelphia: F. A. Davis, 1897); *The principles and practice of modern surgery* (Philadelphia: Lea Brothers, 1907); and *The evil eye: thanatology and other essays* (Boston: Richard G. Badger, 1912). A sample of Park's writings was collected in *Selected papers surgical and scientific from the writings of Roswell Park* (Buffalo: private printing, 1914). (See also GS173.)

GS154. **WILLIAM WILLIAMS KEEN** (1837–1924) and **JAMES WILLIAM WHITE** (1850–1916). *An American text-book of surgery.* 1,209pp. Philadelphia: W. B. Saunders, 1892.

An important textbook because of its strong advocacy of Listerian principles in surgery. The preface notes " . . . especial prominence has been given to surgical bacteriology, and to the most recent methods of treatment, particularly in relation to asepsis and antisepsis . . . . " The work fully discusses sutures and the various methods of disinfecting instruments, hands, and the field of operations. Some of the earliest color and halftone plates of bacterial infections are noted. The volume has additional importance because it was the first surgical textbook written by many authors in which only American surgeons were involved. Among the contributors were Charles H. Burnett (1842–1902), Phineas S. Conner (1839–1909), Frederic S. Dennis (1850–1934), Charles B. Nancrede (1847–1921), Roswell Park (1852–1914), Lewis S. Pilcher (1845–1934), Nicholas Senn (1844–1908), Francis J. Shepherd (1851–1924), Lewis A. Stimson (1844–1917), William Thomson (1833–1907), and John Collins Warren (1842–1927). However, no authors' names are assigned to any chapters. The preface notes:

> The entire book has been submitted in proof-sheets to all of the authors for mutual criticism and revision. As a whole, the book may therefore be said to express upon important surgical topics the consensus of opinion of the surgeons who have joined in its preparation, although it must be understood that, while it thus represents in general the views of all the authors, each individual author is free from absolute responsibility for any particular statement. Minor differences of opinion necessarily exist, and are recognized in the text.

The text is divided into four books: general surgery, special surgery, regional surgery, and operative surgery, totaling forty-seven chapters, 473 figures, and thirty-seven plates. Further editions were published in 1895, 1899, and 1903. The first edition was available in cloth for $7.00, sheepskin for $8.00, and half russia for $9.00.

Keen was professor of the principles of surgery and of clinical surgery at Jefferson Medical College. On pages 48–50 of an unpublished autobiography (Collection of the Brown University Library, 1912), Keen discusses the writing of this book:

> I found no Text-Book that was satisfactory; large enough to give a fairly thorough knowledge yet small enough to be practical for busy students in the then lamentably brief course, only two years. Especially were all the text-books deficient in that they taught nothing of surgical bacteriology, then a new but rapidly growing science. The name "bacteriology" was first used in 1884. As my colleague in the Chair of Pathology was a sceptic as to the role of these "bugs" as he disdainfully called the bacteria, I felt it to be of the utmost importance that this subject should

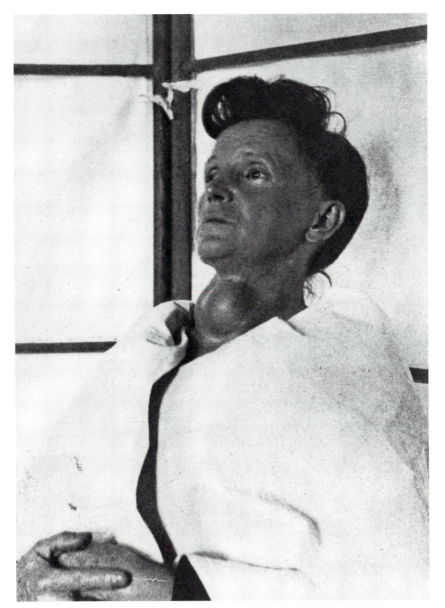

Fig. 45. (GS154) Keen and White's textbook was an outstanding summary of the state of American surgery. This plate, figure 18 on page 636, shows a patient with goiter or as it was called, bronchocele.

be the foundation of a new Text-Book of Surgery, which I at once planned. This was the genesis of the "American Text Book of Surgery" written by thirteen of the Professors of Surgery in our chief Medical Colleges which ensured both its financial and its professional success in spite of the accidental number of its authors. It was published in 1892 by W. B. Saunders & Co. in one volume of 1209 pages under the joint editorship of myself and Dr. J. William White, professor of surgery at the University of Pennsylvania. Its first chapter was upon "Surgical Bacteriology," and throughout the work bacteriology and anti- or a-septic surgery were expounded and enforced. The amount of labor that Dr. White and I gave to this book was, I may say, enormous. Not a line of it but was read by both of us in MS. and in proof and fully discussed wherever either of us questioned the statements made or advice given. Then we discussed each chapter with all the authors by letter and often at length. Moreover after we had completed our work the whole book

was read by Mr. McCreary, the most accomplished and exacting critic
as to English style I have ever known among many proof readers. The
galley proofs of the entire work were sent to each author with a request
to read, criticize and return to the editors. All serious criticisms or suggestions were then referred to the author of the chapter concerned. The
result was a homogeneous whole in careful English and representation
of the best surgical thought of the profession of the United States and
Canada. Its success was immediate and phenomenal. One of the peculiar features was that as all of the authors had revised all the chapters
and made various suggestions the book appeared with the thirteen
names on the title page but no chapter had any indication as to who
was the author of that particular chapter . . . .

Keen's other contributions to surgery were numerous and included a
description of linear craniotomy [G-M 4866] and the operative treatment of spastic torticollis by division of the spinal accessory nerve and
posterior roots of the first, second, and third spinal nerves [G-M 4867].
In addition, in 1874 he wrote a memorable sketch of the early history
of practical anatomy [G-M 442]. White was professor of clinical surgery
at the University of Pennsylvania. Keen's other books consisted of *The
bicentennial celebration of the founding of the First Baptist Church of the city
of Philadelphia, 1698–1898* (Philadelphia: American Baptist Publication
Society, 1899), *Addresses and other papers* (Philadelphia: W. B. Saunders,
1905), the eight-volume *Surgery, its principles and practice* (Philadelphia:
W. B. Saunders, 1906–21), *Animal experimentation and medical progress*
(Boston: Houghton Mifflin, 1914), *The surgical operation on President
Cleveland in 1893* (Philadelphia: George W. Jacobs, 1917), *The treatment
of war wounds* (Philadelphia: W. B. Saunders, 1917), *Medical research and
human welfare, a record of personal experience and observation during a
professional life of fifty-seven years* (Boston: Houghton Mifflin, 1917), *I
believe in God and evolution* (Philadelphia: J. B. Lippincott, 1922), *Selected
papers and addresses by William Williams Keen* (Philadelphia: George W.
Jacobs, 1923), *Everlasting life, a creed and a speculation* (Philadelphia: J. B.
Lippincott, 1924), and *The surgical operation on President Cleveland in
1893, together with six additional papers of reminiscences* (Philadelphia:
J. B. Lippincott, 1928). (See also GS58, GS178, and GU38.)

GS155. **HENRY ORLANDO MARCY** (1837–1924). *The anatomy and surgical treatment of hernia.* 521pp. New York: D. Appleton, 1892.
[G-M 3601]

Marcy's *Anatomy* is one of the most prominent and spectacular of
late nineteenth-century American surgical monographs. It is illustrated
with sixty-six full-page heliotype and lithographic plates, including
eight in full color, and thirty-seven woodcuts in text. Marcy dedicated
the work to Joseph Lister (1827–1912), of whom he wrote:

I would acknowledge his monumental labors, which have revolutionized the surgical art. Especially am I indebted for the faithful personal teachings which were rendered to me, his first American pupil.
Without the stimulus and profit received from his instructions, this
would never have been rendered possible.

Plates 64–66 and woodcuts 13, 14, 17–19, 25–30, and 33–37 are original
to Marcy. The others are from various European works. The twenty-seven
chapters provide comprehensive coverage of hernias, including high
ligation of the sac, transplantation of the cord, and careful reconstruc-
tion of the inguinal canal, but the major orientation of the text is
towards Marcy's "animal suture." Much of the credit for introducing the
Listerian doctrines to American surgeons and overcoming their stub-
born disbelief belongs to Marcy.
(See also GS137.)

GS156. **BERN BUDD GALLAUDET** (1860–1934) and **CHARLES N. DIXON-
JONES** (?–?). *Surgery, a manual for students and practitioners.* 301pp.
Philadelphia: Lea Brothers, 1893.

Gallaudet was a demonstrator of anatomy and clinical lecturer on
surgery at the College of Physicians and Surgeons in New York. His
coeditor Dixon-Jones was an assistant surgeon in the outpatient department of the Presbyterian Hospital in New York. This work was part of
the Students' Quiz Series published by Lea Brothers. The series covered
subjects considered part of a thorough medical education, arranged in
question-and-answer form. The authors were all teachers and examiners
from New York City. The volumes were usually priced at $1.00 except

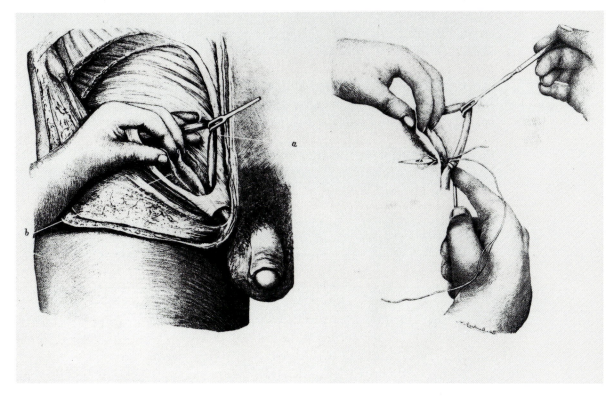

Fig. 46. (GS155) Marcy's book was beautifully illustrated, although most of the plates had been previously published
by other authors. However, this particular illustration, plate 64 on page 399, is original and shows dissection of the
deeper parts in an inguinal hernia and suturing of the posterior wall of the inguinal canal. The heliotype was drawn
by H. MacDonald.

for the double numbers *Anatomy* (GS152) and Gallaudet's *Surgery*, which were $1.75. Gallaudet, who was the series editor, writes in the preface:

> I became convinced that a book written not as a compend or digest of Surgery, but rather as one which would explain, would prove of advantage. Among the principles of Surgery, Inflammation is one the clear comprehension of which seems attended with peculiar difficulties. Therefore in writing this book one of the main purposes has been to elucidate this subject fully, and in doing so a method differing somewhat from that found in the regular textbooks has been pursued. In connection with this it will be observed that under Bacteriology neither the "specific" pathogenic bacteria nor the saprophytes are credited with any pyogenic functions. This course has been followed simply for the sake of making clearer the theory of the bacterial origin of inflammation, and with no intention whatever of controverting the latest discoveries, which seem to show that all bacteria whether pathogenic or saprogenic, are more or less capable of producing pus. Strictly speaking, therefore, the use of the terms "specific" and "non-specific" would be incorrect as applied to bacteria. But as it is a fact that the varieties of inflammation themselves are recognized as being either "specific" or "non-specific," and that putrefaction is a process distinct from inflammation, it was deemed best to avoid all discussion, and to classify the bacteria as causes in the same way in which their effects—i.e. inflammation and putrefaction—are classified.

The work consists of 22 chapters and has 149 figures.

GS157. **THOMAS HENRY MANLEY** (1851–1905). *Hernia; its palliative and radical treatment in adults, children, and infants.* 231pp. Philadelphia: Medical Press, 1893.

Manley received his M.D. in 1875 from the University of the City of New York. He later became visiting surgeon at Harlem Hospital and consulting surgeon at Fordham Hospital. The work was dedicated to Francis Charles Plunkett (1842–99), who was Manley's preceptor. The volume contains twenty-one chapters, but there is no table of contents and only a limited index, making the book difficult reading. There are sixty-four engravings and an extensive bibliography relative to hernia. Manley's preface explains his purpose in writing the book:

> My own reading and observations incline me to believe that there is a very wide-spread misconception with regard to what a hernia really is; its precise origin, and its morbid anatomy. Thousands of operations have recently been, and are being, performed for its radical cure; some operators claiming that intelligent surgical intervention will cure all, while on the contrary there are not a few, equally eminent, who deny that sanguineous methods ever effect a permanent cure. In this chaotic state it is but rational that we inquire just what surgery can do to relieve the infirmity, without danger to the patient's life . . . .

GS158. **DAVID WILLIAMS CHEEVER** (1831–1915). *Lectures on surgery.* 591pp. Boston: Damrell & Upham, 1894

Cheever was president of the American Surgical Association in 1889. He won the Boylston Prize for an essay in 1860 and was a dominant medical figure at Boston City Hospital. The *Lectures* is the only textbook he wrote. As professor of surgery at Harvard Medical School, Cheever wrote that "the reader who looks for a complete treatise on surgery in this volume may be disarmed when he learns that this is only a portion of a surgical course, which includes other teachers and varied departments . . . . These didactic lectures are meant to be only outlines of some surgical subjects." There are no illustrations or index, but among the thirty-three chapter headings are "Gunshot wounds"; "Special fractures"; "Frost-bite and burns"; and two chapters on "Hernia." A second edition was published in 1898. (See also GS69.)

GS159. **JOHN CHALMERS DACOSTA** (1863–1933). *A manual of modern surgery, general and operative.* 809pp. Philadelphia: W. B. Saunders, 1894.

DaCosta was named full professor of the principles and practice of surgery at Jefferson Medical College when he was thirty-seven. He was William W. Keen's (1837–1932) immediate successor. DaCosta's *Manual* went through ten editions, the last appearing in 1931. Encyclopedic in scope, it was for almost forty years one of the most used surgical texts and vied in popularity with William Osler's (1849–1919) *Principles and practice of medicine* (New York: D. Appleton, 1892) [G-M 2231]. DaCosta's clinical experience was enormous and it was reflected in the size of the book, which almost doubled by its sixth edition in 1910. Beginning with that sixth edition, DaCosta dedicated the book to William Halsted (1852–1922), about whom he wrote:

> This book is dedicated to the chief surgeon and inspiration of one of the greatest, most progressive, and most influential surgical clinics in the world. A clinic from which come important facts, real ideas, and brilliant men. To the operator, the teacher, the investigator, and the surgical philosopher. To Dr. William Stewart Halsted, the distinguished professor of surgery in Johns Hopkins University.

DaCosta's work was part of Saunders's New Aid Series of Manuals and originally sold for $2.50, available in cloth only. This new series was meant to complement Saunders's Question Compends. These volumes were intended to form a collection of advanced lectures, which would be valuable aids to students in reading and comprehending the contents of "recommended" works. Among DaCosta's other books are *Selection from the papers and speeches of John Chalmers DaCosta, M.D., LL.D.* (Philadelphia: W. B. Saunders, 1931) and two posthumous publications, *Poems of John Chalmers DaCosta* (Philadelphia: Dorrance, 1942) and *The trials and triumphs of the surgeon* (Philadelphia: Dorrance, 1944).

GS160. **GEORGE RYERSON FOWLER** (1848–1906). *A treatise on appendicitis.* 190pp. Philadelphia: J. B. Lippincott, 1894.

Fowler was examiner in surgery to the medical examining board of the regents of the University of the State of New York. His *Treatise* was the first American work to deal exclusively with appendicitis. It was a revised version of a series of articles by him that appeared in the *Annals of surgery*. At the time he wrote this work, Fowler had already completed over 200 laparotomies for appendicitis. There are four lithograph plates,

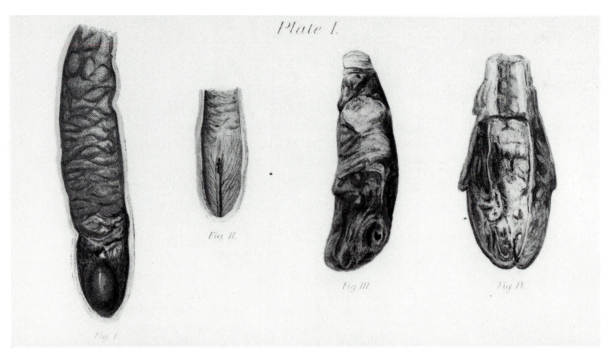

Fig. 47. (GS160) For the first American textbook on appendicitis, Fowler had F. A. Deck sketch specimens immediately after their removal. This lithographic plate, figure 1 on the frontispiece, depicts four differing stages of appendicitis.

two of which provide among the earliest representations of an infected appendix sketched in color. The twelve chapters and thirty-five figures supply a wealth of information about our initial understanding of appendicitis. A second edition was published in 1900. (See also GS128.)

GS161. **HUNTER ROBB** (1863–1940). *Aseptic surgical technique; with especial reference to gynaecological operations, together with notes on the technique employed in certain supplementary procedures.* 264pp. Philadelphia: J. B. Lippincott, 1894.

Robb was the first resident gynecologist to serve under Howard Kelly (1858–1943) at Johns Hopkins Hospital. He remained there until October 1894 as an associate in gynecology, then was appointed professor of gynecology at Western Reserve University in Cleveland. The techniques in the text were those practiced in the surgical and gynecological departments at Johns Hopkins. The twenty-five plates are of interest because they include several photographs of wards and other areas in the Johns Hopkins Hospital. The eighteen chapters cover such topics as "operating suits" to "operations in the country, in private houses, or in other places where the technique must necessarily be more or less imperfect." Later editions were published in 1902, 1904, and 1906.

GS162. **NICHOLAS SENN** (1844–1908). *Syllabus of lectures on the practice of surgery, arranged in conformity with the American text-book of surgery.* 221pp. Philadelphia: W. B. Saunders, 1894.

Senn was one of the prominent contributors to William W. Keen (1837–1932) and James W. White's (1850–1916) *American text-book of surgery* (GS154). The syllabus was meant to aid the advanced student in

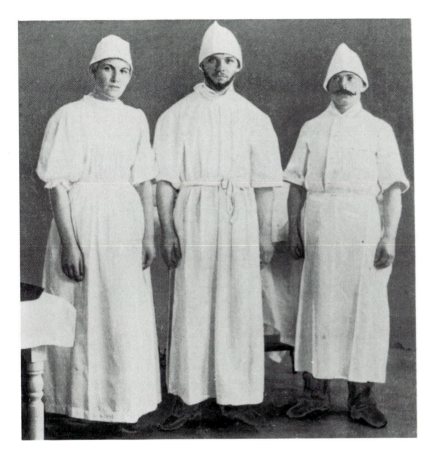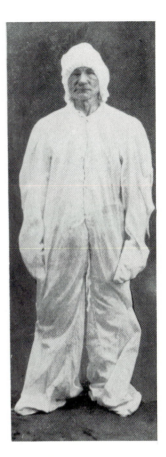

Fig. 48. (GS163) Beck introduced his own version of operating room attire. This plate shows a female nurse, surgeon, male nurse, and patient wearing their respective gowns (figure 8 on page 241).

surgery who adopted the *Text-book* as his major teaching source. Not only did the *Syllabus* provide a guide to its companion volume, but it also supplemented the larger work. Unlike the *Text-book*, which went through several editions, the *Syllabus* appeared in only one edition.

GS163. **CARL BECK** (1856–1911). *A manual of the modern theory and technique of surgical asepsis.* 306pp. Philadelphia: W. B. Saunders, 1895.

Beck graduated from the University of Jena in 1878. He emigrated to America in 1882 and settled in New York. He was eventually named professor of surgery at the New York Post-Graduate School of Medicine. At the time that his *Manual* was written, Beck was visiting surgeon at St. Mark's Hospital and at the German Poliklinik. Beck writes in the preface:

> An important feature of this book . . . is that a stricter line of demarcation than usual is drawn between wounds aseptically performed by surgeons and those otherwise inflicted or those dependent upon inflammatory processes. In the latter category antisepsis asserts its prerogatives, but only as subordinate to asepsis . . . . Among the antiseptic drugs, iodoform is assigned the most prominence . . . . An entire section is devoted to anesthesia, since, irrespective of its vital importance in most surgical procedures, its insufficient mastering is apt to impair seriously the aseptic condition of the patient.

Plates 1–3 provide early photomicrographs of bacteria. Plate 7 depicts a rather awkward-looking operating gown which Beck designed for his patients. The volume was originally available only in cloth for $1.25 and was part of Saunders's New Aid Series. Beck's other books are *Fractures* (Philadelphia: W. B. Saunders, 1900), *Röntgen ray diagnosis and therapy* (New York: D. Appleton, 1904), *Principles of surgical pathology* (Chicago: W. T. Keener, 1905), and *Surgical diseases of the chest* (Philadelphia: P. Blakiston's Son, 1907).

GS164. **CHARLES MILTON BUCHANAN** (1868–1920). *Antisepsis and antiseptics.* 352pp. Newark: Terhune, 1895.

Buchanan was professor of chemistry, toxicology and metallurgy at the National University in Washington, D.C. Although Buchanan was not a physician, his book was largely intended for a surgical audience. It is now relatively scarce. Among the eleven chapters are four on the history of antisepsis. Other topics of surgical interest include chapters 9 and 10 on the value and use of antiseptics in surgery and in obstetrics and gynecology. Among the most interesting aspects of this volume is a hand-written preface by Augustus Charles Bernays (1854–1907), professor of surgery from St. Louis:

> The material gathered for this work gives the views of the best living scientific biologists who have experimented in the field of pathogenic bacteriology. It also has compiled the practical rules followed by many of the best surgeons in the world in their daily work. These rules and recommendations are based on the results obtained in thousands of surgical cases .... Every surgeon must practice his art with all the safeguards afforded by antiseptics and asepsis. In modern surgery the life of the patient and the result of the operation depends as much upon the precautions against infection, as upon operative skill on the part of the surgeon ....

GS165. **FREDERICK SHEPARD DENNIS** (1850–1934). *System of surgery.* 4 vols., 880pp., 926pp., 919pp. and 970pp. Philadelphia: Lea Brothers, 1895–96. [G-M 5799]

An important work, this was the first multivolume American general surgical textbook in which the authors received credit for each individual chapter. The preface describes the authors:

> ... men of recognized authority in their respective branches have consented to contribute in order to present to the profession a complete review of the domain of modern surgery—a domain which has so wonderfully enlarged its boundaries through the achievements rendered possible by the systematic employment of antiseptic and aseptic methods of procedure .... The editor takes this occasion to acknowledge his obligations to the contributors, each one of whom is a teacher of surgery or a director in some large surgical clinic or hospital, and who, for this reason, is capable of speaking with clinical authority from an experience based on the study and observation of a large number of cases. Each department is thus treated by an acknowledged master of

the subject, who is able to present, the most modern and advanced views in the most cogent and demonstrative way.

Among the more important contents are Arpad G. Gerster (1848–1923) on the technique of antiseptic and aseptic surgery (volume 1), Roswell Park (1852–1914) on diseases and injuries of the head (volume 2), Charles McBurney (1845–1913) on the surgical treatment of appendicitis (volume 4), and William W. Keen (1837–1932) on the use of the roentgen or X rays in surgery (volume 4). The most prominent chapter is that by John S. Billings (1838–1913) on the history and literature of surgery (volume 1, pages 17–144) [G-M 5799]. Dennis was a graduate of Bellevue Hospital Medical College. He practiced in New York City and was elected professor of the principles and practice of surgery at his alma mater. Dennis served as president of the American Surgical Association in 1895. He was one of the earliest and most vociferous supporters of Listerism in America. This set was sold for $6.00 per volume in cloth, $7.00 in leather, and $8.50 in half morocco. A collection of Dennis's contributions to medical journals were published as the two-volume *Selected surgical papers (1876–1914)* (New York: private printing, 1934).

GS166. **JAMES GRANT GILCHRIST** (1842–1906). *The elements of surgical pathology with therapeutic hints.* 343pp. Minneapolis: Minneapolis Pharmacy, 1895.

Gilchrist was professor of surgery in the homeopathic medical department of the State University of Iowa. He notes:

> The following pages have been written to present . . . something systematic in the study of the etiology of morbid action, from the standpoint of one not in harmony with very much of the teaching of the day. The current literature, as well as the text-books, assume so much, and are apparently so oblivious of the fact that there is wide diversity of opinion on this question, that something seems necessary from the other side on this subject . . . . The attempt is here made to cover the ground somewhat systematically, commencing with an account of processes that are on the border line between physiology and pathology, and studying the development of morbid action as something due to perverted function, assuming that conditions leading to inflammation are common initiatives to all pathological states . . . .

The eighteen chapters are "Diagnosis"; "Prognosis"; "Therapeutics"; "Semi-pathological states"; "Anemia"; "Hyperemia"; "Surgical repair"; "Inflammation"; "Suppuration"; "Ulceration"; "Mortification"; "Surgical toxemia"; "Pathology of the lympathics"; "Pathology of the blood-vessels"; "Pathology of the nerves"; "Venereal contagion"; "Lithiasis"; and "Tumors." There was only one edition. (See also GS78, GS101, and GS117.)

GS167. **ROBERT TUTTLE MORRIS** (1857–1945). *Lectures on appendicitis and notes on other subjects.* 163pp. New York: G. P. Putnam's Sons, 1895.

Morris began private surgical practice in New York City in 1886. Although he never held a true academic post, he was a lecturer on surgery at New York Post-Graduate Medical School when this volume was written. Morris writes about this book:

> Eight years ago, when there was confusion in antiseptic methods of wound treatment, I presented a little book, which was accepted because it told of one way for accomplishing certain ends. At the present time, while there is confusion of ideas on the subject of appendicitis, it is perhaps a favorable time for blazing one clear trail through the subject in a similiar way. In the matter of operative procedures, I have due respect for methods which are different from my own, believing that in the art of surgery every surgeon is a law unto himself, and that he knows the factors of his own success. This collection of lectures includes the substance of my teaching on the subject of appendicitis at the Post-Graduate Medical School in New York, and I have added a series of notes on other subjects which have received little attention in literature, but which have interested my class.

The first four chapters deal with appendicitis. Chapter 5 is a compilation of twenty-eight short essays on various topics such as "Solvents on gallstones"; "On evolution trying to do away with the clitoris"; and "Ovarian transplantation." There are numerous illustrations, including photomicrographs, but no color plates. There was only one edition, which was reissued in 1896.
(See also GS125.)

GS168. **NICHOLAS SENN** (1844–1908). *The pathology and surgical treatment of tumors.* 700pp. Philadelphia: W. B. Saunders, 1895.

Senn was professor of the practice of surgery and clinical surgery at Rush Medical College. His *Tumors* was dedicated to Samuel D. Gross (1805–84). According to the preface:

> . . . the textbook should prove useful for the student, a work of reference for the busy practitioner, and a reliable, safe guide for the surgeon. For the purpose of simplifying diagnosis a special effort has been made to trace every tumor to its proper anatomical starting-point and histogenetic source, and to make a sharp histological and clinical distinction between true tumors, inflammatory swellings, and retention-cysts . . . . The increase in volume caused by a tumor is due entirely to erratic cell-growth from a matrix of embryonal cells of congenital or postnatal origin; the enlargement of a part or an organ caused by chronic inflammation which so often simulates a tumor is due to proliferation of pre-existing mature cells acted upon by pathogenic micro-organisms or their toxins, and to the vascular changes and cell-migration characteristic of inflammation; while a retention-cyst essentially consists of an accumulation of a physiological secretion in a pre-formed glandular space, the result of a mechanical obstruction. The classification of tumors in this work is in accord with this theory of the origin of tumors. The microbic origin of tumors is briefly disposed of, as it has not been established by any convincing experimental investigations or clinical observations. Should future research demonstrate a direct causative relationship between certain as yet unknown bacteria and the growth of some of the tumors, such tumors would have to be eliminated from this group of pathological products and be classified with the granulomata. The first part of this treatise is devoted to a general

consideration of tumors, and it is this part which is intended more especially for the use of students. Following the section on classification, each class of tumors is considered separately . . . .

There are numerous full-page color plates which depict staining patterns of bacteria. The thirty chapters are illustrated with 515 engravings that display microscopical pictures of tumors. (See also GS138, GS139, GS140, GS144, GS162, OR49, and GU36.)

GS169. **JOHN COLLINS WARREN** (1842–1927). *Surgical pathology and therapeutics.* 832pp. Philadelphia: W. B. Saunders, 1895.

Warren was professor of surgery at Harvard University. His *Pathology* was intended " . . . to associate pathological conditions as closely as possible with the symptoms and treatment of surgical diseases, and to impress upon the student the value of these lines of study as a firm foundation for good clinical work." The thirty-two chapters include such topics as "Inflammation"; "Shock"; "Tuberculosis"; "Carcinoma"; and "Aseptic and antiseptic surgery." Warren advises that "in cases of severe shock it is thought advisable by some to peform 'autotransfusion,' that is, to bandage the extremities so that the circulation may be limited to a confined area where the organs most essential to life are situated." There are 132 illustrations, 33 of which are chromolithographs. The four full-page color plates are remarkable, including one on page 223 that shows healing by first intention of an abdominal wound. When first published, the work was available in cloth for $6.00 or half morocco for $7.00. The second edition was issued in 1900. (See also GS77 and GS127.)

GS170. **JOHN BLAIR DEAVER** (1855–1931). *A treatise on appendicitis.* 168pp. Philadelphia: P. Blakiston & Son, 1896.

Deaver was an 1878 graduate of the University of Pennsylvania Medical School. He later was appointed professor of the practice of surgery at the school and eventually filled the John Rhea Barton Chair. Deaver served as president of the American College of Surgeons in 1921. Among the many operations he pioneered was that for appendicitis. He is particularly remembered for the Deaver incision, in which there was medial displacement of the rectus muscle following an incision in the right lower abdominal quadrant. Deaver's *Treatise*, his first full-length textbook, was written when he was surgeon at the German Hospital in Philadelphia. It reported his observations from over 500 cases, and he " . . . endeavored to emphasize the aetiology, symptomatology, and special technique in the operative treatment." The eleven chapters range from history to diagnosis, through complications and sequelae. There were thirty-two plates, most of which were chromolithographs. The book was available in cloth only for $3.50. Further editions were published in 1900 and 1905. Among Deaver's other medical books are *Surgical anatomy of the head and neck* (Philadelphia: P. Blakiston's Son, 1904); *Enlargement of the prostate, its history, anatomy, aetiology, pathology, clinical causes, symptoms, diagnosis, prognosis, treatment, technique of operations, and after-treatment* (Philadelphia: P. Blakiston's Son, 1905); the two-volume *Surgery of the upper abdomen* (Philadelphia: P. Blakiston's

Son, 1913), co-authored with Astley P. C. Ashhurst (1876–1932); and *The breast, its anomalies, its diseases, and their treatment* (Philadelphia: P. Blakiston's Son, 1917). (See also GS184.)

GS171. **CHARLES EDMUND FISHER** (1853–1932) and **T. L. MacDONALD** (?–?). *A homeopathic text-book of surgery.* 1,661pp. Chicago: Medical Century, 1896.

Fisher was professor of surgery at Hering Medical College in Chicago. MacDonald served as professor of surgery at Southern Homeopathic Medical College in Baltimore and as general and gynecologic surgeon at the National Homeopathic Hospital in Washington. The preface describes their intention in writing this text:

> . . . a new surgical literature has been made necessary, because of the exceedingly satisfactory development of surgical ambitions and successes among members of the homeopathic profession. While a number of text-books have lately been issued to meet the demand of the new order in the chirurgical art, in none has been outlined the application of remedial agents to surgical diseases and states according to the law of cure enunciated by Hahnemann—a law which a century of experience has amply demonstrated to be a most satisfactory principle of practice—and it is in part the function of this volume to remedy this defect . . . .

Many authors contributed, including William Helmuth (1833–1902) on tumors. With thirty-five chapters, fifty-two plates, and 1,102 illustrations, this work is monumental in scope. The chapters on surgical shock and antisepsis are of special value because of homeopathic disdain for allopathic claims. Fisher's other book is *A hand-book on the diseases of children and their homoeopathic treatment* (Chicago: Medical Century, 1895).

GS172. **WILLIAM J. MORTON** (1846–1920) and **EDWIN W. HAMMER** (?–?). *The X ray or photography of the invisible and its value in surgery.* 196pp. New York: American Technical Book, 1896.

A most important book, this was the first American medical text to describe and evaluate Wilhelm Roentgen's (1845–1923) momentous discovery. Morton was professor of diseases of the mind and nervous system and electro-therapeutics at New York Post-Graduate Medical School and Hospital. Hammer, his collaborator, was an electrical engineer. Morton is credited with producing the first dental radiographs in America in 1896 [G-M 3689], and two such radiographs appear in this textbook (figures 78 and 79). This work appeared less than one year after Roentgen's original paper of 1895. An interesting publisher's note states:

> The world-wide interest that has been taken in Prof. Roentgen's discovery of the marvellous properties of the X Ray prompted the publishers of this work to call on Dr. William J. Morton of New York, who had already been acknowledged the best X Ray expert in the United States, and urge him to write the result of his investigations with the X Ray for the benefit of the many who desired reliable information on

this scientific discovery . . . . All of the line illustrations contained in the work are from the dictation of the writers, and the half-toned plates are reproduced mechanically direct from the negatives of X Ray radiographs, taken by Dr. Morton. Much of the sharpness and delicacy of the original negatives has been lost in the reproduction, as it is impossible, to make exact copies of the negatives . . . . As many doctors, surgeons, dentists and others are contemplating the addition of the X Ray apparatus to their laboratories, Dr. Morton would be pleased to give any information gained by his experiments on the selection of the best material, and thus save them loss of time and money in experimenting with inferior apparatus.

The text has four sections: "Definitions"; "Apparatus"; "Operation"; and "Surgical value of the X ray." There is a colored frontispiece demonstrating a cathode ray tube and thirty-two halftone photographic plates of radiographs. In addition, the work has over fifty line drawings. In the appendix are an English translation of Roentgen's paper [G-M 2683], reports of a series of experiments with X rays by Thomas Alva Edison (1847–1931), and a paper by Oliver Lodge on X ray theory. Immediately following the index there is a list of radiographs available for sale from Morton. Morton's other book is *Cataphoresis; or, electric medicamental diffusion as applied in medicine, surgery and dentistry* (New York: American Technical Book, 1898).

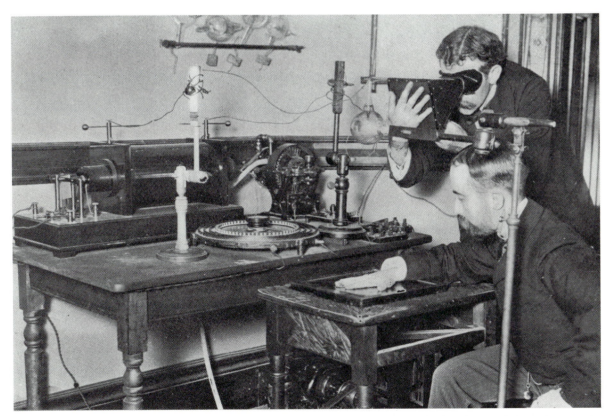

Fig. 49. (GS172) At the end of the nineteenth century it was not uncommon to find authors including photographs of themselves in their books. In this halftone photograph Morton and Hammer are shown in their laboratory conducting an experiment (figure 54 of the endplates).

GS173. **ROSWELL PARK** (1852–1914). *A treatise on surgery by American authors.* 2 vols., 799pp. and 804pp. Philadelphia: Lea Brothers, 1896.

Park was professor of the practice of surgery and of clinical surgery at the University of Buffalo Medical School and was president of the American Surgical Association in 1901. Park attended President William McKinley (1843–1901) after McKinley was shot. Park's *Treatise* was written with the expressed idea " . . . that the surest method of achieving success was to invoke the collaboration of those who unite the qualifications of teachers in our leading colleges with abundant experience in private practice and in hospital clinics." Among the authors were Frederick S. Dennis (1850–1934), Arpad G. Gerster (1848–1923), Charles Kelsey (1850–1917), Charles Nancrede (1847–1921), and Robert W. Lovett (1859–1924). The first volume contains mostly general subjects including "Pathology"; "General principles and theory of surgery"; and "Surgery of the tissues and tissue-systems." The second volume covers regional surgery and surgical procedures on particular organs. There are 356 engravings and twenty-one full-page color and monochrome plates in the first volume. Particularly striking is plate 4 of a microscopic view of an abscess in the kidney of a rabbit. The second volume contains 451 engravings and seventeen plates. The set was available for $4.50 per volume in cloth and $5.50 in leather. Further editions were published in 1896 and 1901. A one-volume condensed version (1,262 pages) was published in 1899. (See also GS153.)

GS174. **CHARLES THEODORE PARKES** (1842–91). *Clinical lectures on abdominal surgery and other subjects.* 477pp. Chicago: W. T. Keener, 1896.

Parkes graduated from Rush Medical College in 1868. In 1887, he was appointed to succeed Moses Gunn (1822–87) as professor of surgery at Rush. Parkes was a pioneer in abdominal surgery and was one of the first surgeons in America to engage in animal experimentation. For several years before his premature death, he compiled material for a textbook on general and abdominal surgery. His wife published the unfinished manuscript as his *Lectures*, and Albert John Ochsner (1858–1925) served as editor. Ochsner notes in the preface:

> Since Professor Parkes' early and unexpected death, many of his pupils and friends have expressed a wish to secure a collection of reports of his clinical lectures, and it is in response to these requests that this book has been compiled. These lectures were all delivered from stenographic notes . . . . Care has been taken to preserve almost entirely the language used by the lecturer, because in this, it would seem, by reason of its force and charm, lie the special value and fascination of this work for his pupils and his friends.

There is no table of contents, but an extensive index covers all the lectures.

GS175. **HERMAN MYNTER** (1845–1903). *Appendicitis and its surgical treatment, with a report of seventy-five operated cases.* 303pp. Philadelphia: J. B. Lippincott, 1897.

Mynter graduated from the University of Copenhagen in 1871. He practiced in Buffalo, where he was professor of operative and clinical surgery at Niagara University and surgeon at the Sisters of Charity Hospital in Buffalo. This monograph is somewhat unusual, as Mynter explains in the preface:

> The degree of Doctor of Medicine is not conferred in Denmark at graduation as in America. It requires the writing of a monograph showing special studies and individual experience, and is equivalent to Habilitations Schrifft in Germany, conferring the right to give lectures in the halls of the University as Private docent. Desiring to obtain the degree of Doctor of Medicine from his alma mater, the University of Copenhagen, twenty-six years after graduation, the author submitted this monograph to the University, and it was accepted in July, 1897 . . . . The author has attempted in this work to sift the evidence and weigh the testimony for and against the operative treatment of appendicitis. While in the United States this disease is considered an almost exclusively surgical lesion, the same is by no means the case in other countries. We find there men of undoubted authority, and whose opinions are entitled to respectful attention, in the ranks of the conservative physicians, who operate only in exceptional cases and advise against surgical interference as a standard treatment. The author has, however, after careful study of a large number of foreign and American authors and of numerous statistics, come to the same conclusions as most other surgeons, that appendicitis is a surgical lesion and ought to be treated by surgical means, and that medicine is unable to prophesy as to the result in a given case or to prevent gangrene and perforation with resulting fatal peritonitis. The surgical treatment, therefore, must be considered the conservative treatment, the quickly healing and least dangerous method, and it is radical in so far as a relapse is impossible. The medical treatment is a makeshift, uncertain in its results, unable to prevent the often fatal complications, and therefore dangerous.

The work contains no illustrations. Part 1 (pages 7–174) is divided into thirteen different sections dealing with varied topics, including "History"; "Anatomy"; "Histology"; "Function"; "Etiology"; "Pathology"; "Classification"; "Symptomatology"; "Complication and sequels"; "Diagnosis"; "Prognosis"; "Treatment"; and "Statistics." Part 2 (pages 175–291) consists of case descriptions. Further editions were published in 1898 and 1900.

GS176. **HOWARD CRUTCHER** (1865–?). *A practical treatise on appendicitis.* 134pp. Chicago: Hahnemann, 1897.

Crutcher was a homeopathic surgeon who was professor of surgical anatomy and the principles of surgery at Dunham Medical College, Chicago. The aim of this book was " . . . along practical lines, for the use of those whose bedside experience in appendicitis is limited. Much technical and theoretical matter has been purposely omitted as not coming properly within the scope of the work." There are eight chapters and thirty-one figures but no plates. Although Crutcher makes the point that appendicitis is a surgical disease, pages 61–62 give an interesting list of homeopathic remedies that can be used before surgical intervention.

GS177. **BLANTON L. HILLSMAN** (1872–1935). *Notes on principles of surgery from lectures by Stuart McGuire.* 224pp. Richmond: James E. Goode, 1897.

McGuire (1867–1948), the son of Hunter McGuire (1835–1900), was on the surgical faculty at the University of Richmond Medical School. He was later appointed professor of principles of surgery and clinical surgery at the University College of Medicine, Richmond. Hillsman was a member of the class of 1898 at the University College. McGuire offered a prize to his students for the best report of his lectures for the 1896–97 academic session. This volume presents the winning effort, and the lectures appear almost exactly as taken in the classroom. A total of forty-eight chapters cover a wide range of topics, among the major lectures are "Inflammation"; "Suppuration"; "Special wounds"; "Tuberculosis"; "Syphilis"; and "Tumors." There was just one edition, which is quite scarce due to a small printing and because it was available only to matriculating students at the university. McGuire later wrote his own text on surgery, *Lectures on principles of surgery* (Baltimore: Southern Medical Publishing, 1908).

GS178. **WILLIAM WILLIAMS KEEN** (1837–1932). *The surgical complications and sequels of typhoid fever.* 386pp. Philadelphia: W. B. Saunders, 1898.

In 1876, Keen delivered the fifth Toner Lecture on the surgical complications and sequels of continued fevers. The Toner Lectures were instituted in Washington by Joseph M. Toner (1825–96) who donated $3,000 to fund, " . . . two annual memoirs or essays relative to some branch of medical science and containing some new truths felt established by experiment or observation." The donation was administered by the Smithsonian Institution, and ten lectures were given from 1872 through 1889. Of these, Keen gave only one, which was published in 1877 as a 68 page monograph. In 1896, Keen delivered the Shattuck Lecture before the Massachusetts Medical Society, an updated version of his talk of twenty years before. These lectures served as the basis for his *Surgical complications*. He included in the volume the six complications and sequels discussed in his Toner Lecture and added a chapter on the surgical affections of typhoid fever and twelve chapters on complications of particular organs and regions. The surgical treatment of perforation of the bowel in typhoid fever did not exist in 1876. Nearly all of the cases in the second series are the surgical results of typhoid fever alone. In addition, there is a chapter by George E. de Schweinitz (1858–1938) on ocular complications of typhoid fever. There are five plates and four figures, none of which were original to Keen. Most books on complications of surgery were not written until the twentieth century. In this respect Keen's work is quite remarkable. It was originally available in cloth for $3.00. (See also GS58 and GS154.)

GS179. JOHN WILLIAM MacDONALD (1844–?). *A clinical textbook of surgical diagnosis and treatment for practitioners and students of surgery and medicine.* 798pp. Philadelphia: W. B. Saunders, 1898.

MacDonald was a graduate in medicine of the University of Edinburgh. He eventually settled in Minneapolis, where he became professor of the practice of surgery and of clinical surgery at Hamline University. The book is dedicated to Joseph Bell (1837–1911) and attempts to answer " . . . two questions which every surgeon must ask every time his professional advice or help is sought. The first question is, 'What is the disease or injury?' The second question is, 'What is the proper treatment? . . . '" Basic physiology and pathology are not discussed. The last of the seventeen chapters discusses X rays in surgical diagnosis, and includes five examples of early roentgenograms (figures 324–28).

GS180. HENRY REDWOOD WHARTON (1853–1925) and B. FARQUHAR CURTIS (1857–?). *The practice of surgery; a treatise on surgery for the use of practitioners and students.* 1,240pp. Philadelphia: J. B. Lippincott, 1898.

Wharton was demonstrator of surgery at the University of Pennsylvania and a fellow of the American Surgical Association. Curtis was professor of clinical surgery at the New York Post-Graduate Medical School and the Woman's Medical School of the New York Infirmary. The volume was written to be " . . . a useful guide to the student in the beginning of his work in the complicated science of surgery, and that it may also serve as a ready help in the solution of the surgical problems which confront the busy general practitioner." The work is mammoth in size and contains thirty-eight chapters and 923 illustrations. It provides little information about actual operative surgery, instead focusing on the practical aspects of surgical care. (See also GS150.)

GS181. WILLIAM WALLACE WINANS (?–?). *Quiz-compend on surgery.* 338pp. Philadelphia: Morris Press, 1898.

Winans was a student in the class of 1899 at Hahnemann Medical College when he wrote this volume. Other students who collaborated with him on it were Richard M. Haehl, who covered special and regional surgery, and Jarvis L. Thorpe, who discussed venereal diseases. This book is a compilation of all the quizzes given to the homeopathic students at Hahnemann for a period of several years. Winans notes:

> It is needless to say that such a work was not intended, nor does it presume in any way to usurp the place which any one of the valuable treatises on surgery now rightfully occupies in the student's course, the desire being merely that it should act as a substitute for the laborious though necessary task of note-taking . . . .

The work does not have a table of contents but does contain an extensive index.

GS182. GEORGE WASHINGTON CRILE (1864–1943). *An experimental research into surgical shock.* 160pp. Philadelphia: J. B. Lippincott, 1899. [G-M 5622]

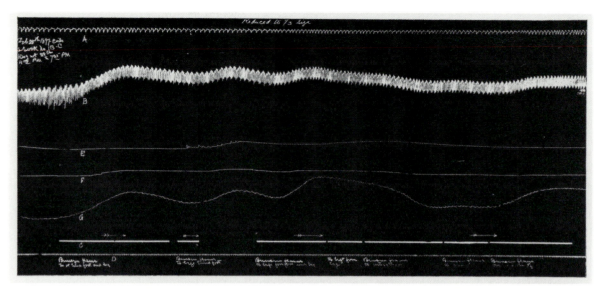

Fig. 50. (GS182) Some of the early experiments that Crile performed were completed in Victor Horsley's laboratory in London. This kymograph on page 97 demonstrates the effects of burning an extremity on: respiration, central blood pressure, peripheral venous pressure, and portal pressure.

Crile was an 1887 graduate of the Wooster Medical School (later the Western Reserve Medical School). His experiments in surgical shock and other related areas [G-M 5629] brought him worldwide fame. He was president of the American College of Surgeons in 1916 and of the American Surgical Association in 1924. This essay was awarded the Cartwright Prize for 1897. Crile describes the awarding of the prize in his autobiography (Philadelphia: J. B. Lippincott, 1947, volume 1, page 74–75):

> The chance reading of an announcement of the Cartwright Prize, awarded by Columbia University, reminded me sharply of my intention to publish my notes on shock. This prize of five hundred dollars was awarded every three years for the ablest article on medical or surgical research, but the time limit for the current award, said the announcement, would expire in two days. Immediately I engaged two public stenographers . . . . I started with the first sixteen experiments performed in Victor Horsley's laboratory. We began in the early afternoon and finished at two in the morning. I sent the manuscript to Columbia University by special registered mail. It arrived just in time to be considered—and won the prize! Meanwhile, in 1899, my Cartwright Prize manuscript was published by J. B. Lippincott Company and became my first book.

The work includes an extensive historical section reviewing previous research in the field. Crile advocated the use of saline solutions in cases of circulatory collapse but warned that it was possible to overload the body with too much saline, leading to an accumulation of fluid in the tissues. Crile's other books are *An experimental and clinical research into certain problems relating to surgical operations* (Philadelphia: J. B. Lippincott, 1901) [G-M 5624 and 5687], *Blood-pressure in surgery* (Philadelphia: J. B. Lippincott, 1903) [G-M 5627], *Hemorrhage and transfusion* (New York: D. Appleton, 1909) [G-M 5628], *Phylogenetic association in relation*

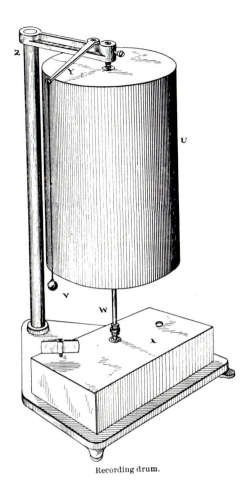

Recording drum.

Fig. 51. (GS182) This figure (page 17) demonstrates the recording drum which was used in making numerous kymographs. The machinery was constructed by Ulmer and Hoff under the supervision of Crile.

to certain medical problems (Cleveland: Barta, 1910), *Anemia and resuscitation* (New York: D. Appleton, 1914), *Anoci-association* (Philadelphia: W. B. Saunders, 1914), *The origin and nature of the emotions* (Philadelphia: W. B. Saunders, 1915), *A mechanistic view of war and peace* (New York: Macmillan, 1915), *Man—an adaptive mechanism* (New York: Macmillan, 1916), *The kinetic drive, its phenomena and control* (Philadelphia: W. B. Saunders, 1916), *The fallacy of the German state philosophy* (New York: Doubleday & Page, 1918), *Surgical shock and the shockless operation through anoci-association* (Philadelphia: W. B. Saunders, 1920), *A physical interpretation of shock, exhaustion, and restoration* (Oxford: Oxford University Press, 1921), *The thyroid gland* (Philadelphia: W. B. Saunders, 1922), *Notes on military surgery* (New York: William Feather, 1924), *The bipolar theory of living processes* (New York: Macmillan, 1926), *Problems in surgery* (Philadelphia: W. B. Saunders, 1927), *Diagnosis and treatment of diseases of the thyroid gland* (Philadelphia: W. B. Saunders, 1932), *Diseases peculiar to civilized man* (New York: Macmillan, 1934), *The phenomena of life, a radio-electric interpretation* (New York: W. W. Norton, 1936), *The surgical treatment of hypertension* (Philadelphia: W. B. Saunders, 1938), and *Intelligence, power and personality* (New York: Whittlesey House, 1941). (See also GS183.)

GS183. **GEORGE WASHINGTON CRILE** (1864–1943). *Experimental research into the surgery of the respiratory system.* 113pp. Philadelphia: J. B. Lippincott, 1899.

This work was a continuation of Crile's first book on surgical shock (GS182). Crile writes in his autobiography (volume 1, page 75):

> . . . I continued my researches on shock, investigating such special problems as drowning, and excessive variations of air pressure, as it is seen in deep-sea diving, in working in tunnels and in mountain sickness. An essay on this work was awarded the Nicholas Senn Prize of the American Medical Association in 1898 . . . .

Most of the experiments for this volume concentrated on wounds to the chest. He reinforced his conviction that the central phenomenon in shock was decreased blood pressure. Crile repeated earlier experiments showing the beneficial effects of cocaine and atropine in intubations of the larynx, and his ideas began to have considerable influence.

GS184. **JOHN BLAIR DEAVER** (1855–1931). *Surgical anatomy; a treatise on human anatomy in its application to the practice of medicine and surgery.* 3 vols., 632pp., 709pp., and 816pp. Philadelphia: P. Blakiston's Son, 1899–1903.

Deaver was surgeon-in-chief at German Hospital in Philadelphia. His treatise is a monument to his anatomical knowledge and tenacity of spirit. The book was twelve years in preparation, during which time he constantly expanded its original scope. Deaver wrote in the preface:

> My book has kept pace with change and growth. I have in no case cut down descriptions nor the teaching devoted to surgical anatomy, nor directions for and procedure in dissection, but I have added much relating to surgical work. I have endeavored to regard fully the necessities of undergraduates, and at the same time have had in mind constantly the requirements which they will meet as surgeons in their chosen fields, and have tried to make for them a sufficient work of reference for use in actual practice.

Volume 1 contains discussions of the "Upper extremities"; "Back of neck"; "Shoulder"; "Trunk"; "Cranium"; "Scalp"; and "Face." Volume 2 discuses the "Neck"; "Mouth"; "Pharynx"; "Larynx"; "Nose"; "Orbit"; "Eyeball"; "Organ of hearing"; "Brain"; "Female perineum"; and "Male perineum". The third volume discusses the "Abdominal wall"; "Abdominal cavity"; "Pelvic cavity"; "Chest"; and "Lower extremity." Almost all the 499 plates were drawn for this work from original dissections. (See also GS170.)

GS185. **CHARLES BEYLARD GUERARD** DE **NANCREDE** (1847–1921). *Lectures upon the principles of surgery.* 398pp. Philadelphia: W. B. Saunders, 1899.

Nancrede was named to the chair of surgery at the University of Michigan in 1889. Interestingly, at the same time he was professor of surgery at Dartmouth, taking care of his New Hampshire work during the summer months. Nancrede was president of the American Surgical Association in 1909. Dedicated to Phineas Sanborn Conner (1839–

1909), professor of surgery at the Medical College of Ohio and at Dartmouth Medical College, this volume was in essence the lectures which the Michigan students received during their medical school years. Nancrede was a vigorous Listerian, as is apparent in his use of drainage by tubes, capillary drains, and from his advocacy of chemical antiseptic dressings and irrigations. A large portion of the thirty-six lectures in the book are devoted to such topics as "Sapremia"; "Septicemia"; and "Hectic fever." Other noteworthy topics are shock and treatment of trauma (chapters 31–33) and various types of anesthesia (chapters 34–36). An appendix (pages 371–384) containing a resume of the principal views held concerning inflammation was written by William A. Spitzley, senior assistant in surgery at the University of Michigan. The book has thirty-seven illustrations in total, all of which are rudimentary in composition. There are no plates. A second edition was published in 1905. Nancrede's other book is *Surgical disease, certain abnormities [sic], and wounds of the face* (New York: William Wood, 1908). (See also GS126.)

GS186. **CLINTON B. HERRICK** (1859–?). *Railway surgery, a handbook of the management of injuries.* 265pp. New York: William Wood, 1899.

Herrick was lecturer in clinical surgery at Albany Medical College, New York. He also served as president of the New York State Association of Railway Surgeons. As the railway system grew in America, the number of railway-related injuries increased dramatically. Herrick describes his work in this manner:

> On account of the great increase in the number of injuries received on the railway, the peculiarities that many of them present, and the absence of any manual defining their distinctive features and their proper management, this volume is introduced to the profession . . . . There is no aim at scientific completeness, nor any attempt made to discuss theories or to settle dogmatic points . . . . The book will not be found to treat every variety of injuries, nor to go into detail in the consideration of any, but rather to give concise practical directions for handling the everyday cases that are met with.

There are eighty-six illustrations, including rather gruesome pictures of amputated extremities. The twenty-three chapters cover a wide range of topics, including jurisprudence in railway surgery.

GS187. **ALEXANDER JOHNSTON CHALMERS SKENE** (1837–1900). *Electro-haemostasis in operative surgery.* 173pp. New York: D. Appleton, 1899.

Born in Scotland, Skene graduated from the Long Island College Hospital in 1863. He advanced through the academic ranks, becoming dean and later president of his alma mater. This textbook was written when he was professor of gynecology at Long Island College Hospital, having served as president of the American Gynecological Society in 1887. The book was dedicated to John Byrne (1825–1902). The preface states:

> This contribution relating to electro-haemostasis and the electric cautery in general and special surgery, is issued to supplement the third edition of my work on diseases of women . . . . The interest manifested

by the profession in this subject, the employment of the new methods of operating in other than gynaecological surgery, a number of recent improvements in instruments and in the technique of operating, and a larger experience confirmatory of the value of the principles and practice advocated, both prompted the undertaking and raise the hope that the results will be acceptable to the profession. The part of the work devoted to electro-haemostasis may appear to be rather aggressive, not to say revolutionary, and therefore it might be judicious to give in this preface a statement explanatory of the principles involved and a preliminary argument in their favor; but past experiences remind me that it is unnecessary to do so.

The work consists of sixteen chapters detailing the use of electro-haemostasis in a number of pathologic conditions. The most interesting chapters (15 and 16) discuss asepsis and antisepsis specifically regarding architectural plans relative to sanitary hospital construction. There are eighty illustrations and two color plates. There was only one edition. (See also GY21, GY33, and GY51.)

GS188. JOHN EDWARDS SUMMERS (1858–1935). *The modern treatment of wounds.* 149pp. Omaha: Medical Publishing, 1899.

Summers was a graduate of the United States Military Academy at West Point. He attended the College of Physicians and Surgeons in New York and received an M.D. in 1885. Most of his professional life was spent in Omaha, where he was professor of surgery at Omaha Medical College and professor of clinical surgery at the University of Nebraska Medical School. Virtually all of his scientific writings appeared in medical journals. *Modern treatment* was his only textbook and is a compilation of cases from his large clinical practice. Summers notes in the preface:

> In the preparation of this little book I have tried to indicate means towards ends. An attempt has been made to keep within the subject title of the book, yet it has been thought necessary occasionally to discuss pathology and diagnosis in order to lead up to a rational practice. If at times some statements appear dogmatic, they will, I hope, be pardoned, because they have the merit at least of being based upon a liberal personal experience, both as a teacher and practitioner of surgery.

There are twenty chapters, including "Bacteria and wounds"; "Operations on infected tissues"; "Penetrating wounds of the chest"; "Treatment of septic blood poisoning"; and "Use of rubber gauntlets or gloves."

GS189. CHARLES TRUAX (1852–1918). *The mechanics of surgery, comprising detailed descriptions, illustrations, and lists of the instruments, appliances and furniture necessary in modern surgical art.* 1,024pp. Chicago: Privately Printed, 1899.

The most comprehensive and authoritative book ever published on 19th century American surgical instruments and their usage. A massive and unique work, with 2,381 illustrations in the text, *Mechanics of surgery* was dedicated " . . . to the medical profession, from the teachings and writings of which the information contained in this work has been almost exclusively gleaned . . . . " Truax was not a physician, but instead the owner of a surgical instrument company based in Chicago. One of the major suppliers and fabricators of surgical equipment, Truax, Greene & Company issued catalogues beginning in the early 1880s. The preface reveals Truax's conception of the work:

> In the . . . preparation of this work it is not assumed to offer advice as to when or how surgical operations should be performed. The pathology, etiology, prognosis and non-mechanical treatment of disease have been studiously avoided, save where necessary to completeness, the aim being to illustrate and describe such mechanical appliances as research and experience have proved to be suitable, or best adapted to the purposes for which they were designed. It has seemed fitting that the preparation of a book of this character should devolve upon one who has enjoyed abundant opportunities to acquire a knowledge of surgical appliances in their various and manifold forms and applications, and a practical knowledge not only of the different kinds of surgical instruments, and the several useful patterns of each, but also of their construction and mechanical differentiation. An almost daily intercourse with physicians and surgeons extending over a number of years, frequent attendance at clinics in many parts of the world, and extensive study of text-books and journals, together with a commercial knowledge of surgical instruments and appliances by no means inconsiderable, would seem to justify the attempt to fill what has appeared to be a hiatus in modern surgical literature . . . . Many generations have passed since a work in any way resembling this has been published. This is worthy of note, for it would seem that a book of this character, written by one competent to compile and arrange it, should find a place in the library of every practitioner of medicine or surgery . . . .

There are thirty-eight chapters covering almost every branch and specialty of surgery. Among the topics are the "History, construction, and care of instruments"; "Use of mechanical aids in diagnosis"; "Sterilization"; "Injection apparatus"; "Artificial respiration"; "Electro-therapeutics"; and "Minor operative surgery."

Surprisingly, Truax's work is still authoritative today because no equally comprehensive compilation of this sort has been attempted in recent times, and because many of the models and patterns of instruments in current usage actually date to the 1890's and earlier. The work has been reprinted by Norman Publishing with a definitive 45-page introduction on Truax and the development of the American surgical instrument industry by James M. Edmonson, Ph.D. This reprint is Number One in the Norman Surgery Series, published in 1988.

GS190. **LEWIS STEPHEN PILCHER** (1845–1934). *The treatment of wounds, its principles and practice, general and special.* 453pp. New York: William Wood, 1899.

Pilcher followed up his first book (GS114) with this massively revised and essentially new volume. He writes in the preface:

> In 1883 . . . the methods of Lister had reached their highest vogue and had begun to wane, although the spray and carbolized dressings were still much in use; the profuse use of iodoform, without exact

knowledge as to the real part it played as an antiseptic, was dominating many clinics . . . . During the period which has elapsed since the publication of my previous book the advances that have been made in the knowledge of the essential agents in most disturbances of wound-healing, and of the best methods of preventing or modifying the activity of these agents . . . have been such as to make it necessary for the author practically to write a new book in an effort to present the status of surgery in this most important department . . . .

The book consists of two parts. Section 1 in the first part deals with the principles of wound treatment, including an interesting chapter (chapter 3) on "The relations of micro-organisms to wound disturbances." Section 2 of part 1, on the practice of treating wounds, consists of eight chapters, most of which discuss the bandaging of wounds. Part 2, on special wounds, has three sections: "Varieties that may occur in any part of the body"; "Wounds of tissues common to all parts of the body"; and "Wounds of special regions." The latter deals specifically with the head, neck and thorax, abdomen and pelvis, and extremities, including amputations. At the time this volume was published, Pilcher was a surgeon on the staff of Methodist Episcopal Hospital in New York. This was the only edition, and it is relatively scarce. Pilcher does not even mention the book in his autobiography, nor is it found in any of the standard biographic references.

II. OPHTHALMOLOGY

OP1. **GEORGE FRICK** (1793–1870). *A treatise on the diseases of the eye; including the doctrines and practice of the most eminent modern surgeons and particularly those of Professor Beer.* 320pp. Baltimore: Fielding Lucas, 1823. [G-M 5844]

This is first American book on ophthalmology by the first American who is believed to have restricted his practice solely to diseases of the eye. Frick received his M.D. from the University of Pennsylvania in 1815 and spent several years in Vienna studying under George Beer (1763–1821). Frick later returned to Baltimore, where he became ophthalmic surgeon at Baltimore General Dispensary. In 1840, he abandoned the practice of medicine and spent most of the rest of his life in Europe, dying in Dresden in 1870. The *Treatise* is dedicated to Phillip Syng Physick (1768–1837), whom Frick considered among his most important mentors. Frick writes in the introduction:

> The volume which is here offered to the public is little more than the abstract of a course of lectures, which the author had prepared upon the diseases of the eye . . . It is a lamentable truth that the pathology of the eye has not kept progress with the advanced state of pathological science in general; and this is attributable no doubt to the circumstance, that this branch of the healing art has been confined for so long a time to exclusive oculists. In this country especially, the diseases of the eye have hitherto obtained but a small share of the attention of the profession, and a comprehensive work upon this highly important department of medicine, is a desideratum which still remains to be supplied . . . . Of all nations, the Germans have excelled in this particular department and we are indebted for most of the improvements in this branch of our art, to the industry and researches of this nation. Among the great and distinguished names consecrated to posterity . . . that of Professor Beer stands eminently conspicuous in his "Lehre von den Augenkrankheiten . . . . " It was the author's first intention to have presented to the public a translation of this work, but various considerations have induced him for the present to abandon the design . . . . The condensed manner in which the author has treated the subject, will he fears, occasion some disappointment to many of his readers; but he would remind them that the present work is intended simply as a manual for such as are but entering upon the study of these diseases, and claims no pretensions to an elaborate or systematic treatise . . . .

The work consists of four parts: "Ophthalmia" (five chapters); "Diseases which attack the individual textures of the eye" (six chapters); "Diseases of the appendages" (two chapters); and "Diseases which attack the eyeball" (one chapter). The book contains little that is original, although an excellent description of a cataract knife appears on page 175. There was one engraved plate but no other illustrations. The importance of this book is apparent from the fact that a second edition was published in 1826 in London by an English surgeon, Richard Welbank. He added numerous footnotes, rededicated the book to William Lawrence (1783–1867), but left the text essentially unchanged. Frick wrote no other books.

OP2. **JOHN MASON GIBSON** (?–?). *A condensation of matter upon the anatomy, surgical operations and treatment of diseases of the eye.* 203pp. Baltimore: W. R. Lucas, 1832.

Little is known of Gibson, who practiced in Baltimore, where he was a member of the Medical and Chirurgical Faculty of Maryland. He writes in the preface:

> In promulgating a work of this kind, an author labours under no little anxiety to foresee whether or not it will be viewed as a successful attempt at collecting the best matter upon diseases of the eye, it having

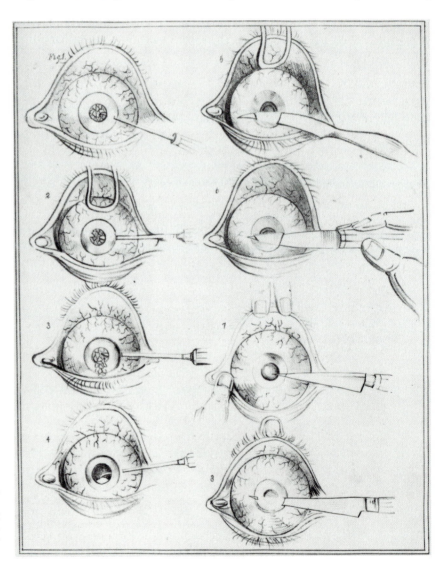

Fig. 52. (OP2). This black-and-white plate shows various types of operations for cataract extraction (figure 4 of the endplates). Gibson's work does not state who executed the drawings or performed the lithography.

been gotten up mostly with the intention of brightening the path of the more youthful practitioner ... that it may serve as a proficient helmsman to his barque when tossed upon the ocean of hypothesis, is devoutly to be wished for. It must be acknowledged that diseases casual to the organ of vision, are many, and frequently to be met with in this country; however, I believe upon the mind of the student, where and when the importance and great nicety of judgment are requisite in the treatment of them, and that by inadvertent and malpractice the victim may grope through his existence here in a valley of darkness. The work is one of compilation. It could have been more enlarged, but as the author has given insertion to what in his own judgment he deemed the best practice, he conceived it superfluous to add more. The author's claims to originality do not extend farther than to the construction of the plates ....

The contents include an opening section on "Anatomy" (pages 7–27); "Diseases of the eyeball" (pages 28–187); and "Diseases of the lachrymal apparatus" (pages 188–203). There are twelve lithographic plates which illustrate the anatomy, operations, and morbid appearance of the eye. There was only one edition. Because of its poor arrangement and lack of conciseness, the work had little affect on the direction of American ophthalmology.

OP3. **WILLIAM CLAY WALLACE** (?–?). *The structure of the eye with reference to natural theology.* 52pp. New York: Wiley & Long, 1836.

Wallace practiced in New York, where he was oculist at the New York Institution for the Blind and at the Orphan Asylum. He enjoyed considerable importance in ophthalmology due to his clinical skills and

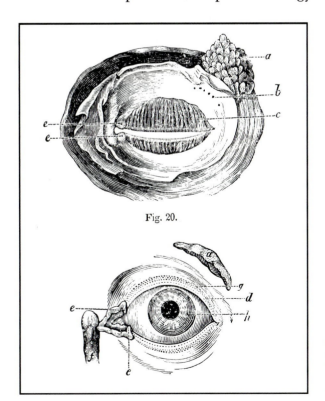

Fig. 20.

Fig. 53. (OP3) These two illustrations, figures 20 and 21 on page 44, show the lacrimal apparatus for tears in a human eye. Most of the other cuts from Wallace's work were of animal eyes.

to his writings on the comparative anatomy of the eye. Little biographical information is available, although it is known that early in his career Wallace served as a surgeon's assistant at the Glasgow Eye Infirmary under William MacKenzie (1791–1868). Wallace notes in the preface that

> the eye affords a wide and interesting field for observation. The ingenuity of the contrivance, and the adaptation of the means to the end that is to be accomplished, are exhibited in its structure, which is always varied to suit the wants of the possessor . . . . Owing to the difficulty of examining such a delicate structure, the nature and use of some of its parts are disputed. Independently of these, the evidences on which all are agreed are quite sufficient for the argument . . . .

There is no table of contents, but Wallace provides an interesting classification of structures of the eye by naming nine parts: "Refractors of light"; "Receiver"; "Reflector"; "Absorber"; "Regulator"; "Regulators to distances"; "Case"; "Movers"; and "Protectors and cleansers." There are twenty-two wood engravings, most of which are figures of various animal eyes. A greatly expanded second edition with eighty-eight pages was published in 1839 under a new title, *Treatise on the eye, containing discoveries of the causes of near and far sightedness, and of the affections of the retina, with remarks on the use of medicines as substitutes for spectacles.* Two forms of a third edition were printed in 1841, one with the same title as the second edition and the other with the title *Wonders of vision.* The latter contained ninety pages.

OP4. **SQUIRE LITTELL** (1803–66). *A manual of the diseases of the eye.* 255pp. Philadelphia: John S. Littell, 1837.

Littell was an 1824 medical graduate of the University of Pennsylvania. He immediately established himself in general practice in Philadelphia, and, except for the year 1825, when he lived in Buenos Aires, he remained in that city all his professional life. Littell did not regard himself as an ophthalmologic specialist, having edited the *Journal of foreign medicine* in 1828–29. When the Wills Hospital for the Blind and Lame was organized in 1834, he was elected one of the surgeons. Littell remained on the staff through 1863. The *Manual* was not a mere compilation but was rather based on the experience of Littell and his colleagues. The publisher was Littell's brother. The book's preface summarizes its purpose:

> The importance of the organ of vision, and the facilities afforded by its structure for the investigation of the various morbid affections to which it is exposed, have always rendered it a favourite object of regard; and the numerous publications which at different times have appeared, attest alike the skill and the research of those who have cultivated with especial attention this department of surgery . . . . the present volume has been composed . . . to present the points of chief importance in the symptoms, causes, and treatment of each disease, with as much brevity and perspicuity, and at the same time, with as much minuteness, as the nature of the plan would permit . . . .

The contents consist of "Diseases of the orbit"; "Wounds of the eye and its appendages"; "Diseases of the lachrymal organs"; "Palpebrae"; "Conjunctiva"; "Cornea"; "Sclerotica"; "Choroid"; "Retina"; "Iris"; "Crystal-line and capsule"; "Humours"; "Globe"; "Malignant diseases of the eye"; "Extirpation of the eye"; "Neuralgia"; and "Various states of defective vision." The book presents an interesting formula (page 221). It also contains an ophthalmologic vocabulary (page 235ff.). There are no plates. The work was so well received in England that a revised edition was edited by Hugh Houston and published by John Churchill in London in 1838. A second American edition was issued in 1846.

OP5. **JOHN HOMER DIX** (1813–84). *Treatise on strabismus, or squinting and the new mode of treatment.* 105pp. Boston: D. Clapp, 1841.

Born in Boston, Dix studied at Harvard and received his M.D. from Jefferson Medical College in 1836. He at once began the practice of medicine in Boston, giving special attention to diseases of the eye. In 1840 he became the first American to divide the internal rectus muscle for strabismus. The *Treatise* is an outgrowth of his interest in ophthalmology. It contains the following chapters: "Anatomy and function of the muscles of the globe"; "Strabismus"; "Division of the straight muscles of the globe for strabismus"; "Appendix of cases"; and "An analysis of 50 cases." There is one engraved plate. Dix never held an academic position but lists himself on the title page as a member of the Massachusetts Medical Society. (See also OP10.)

OP6. **ALFRED CHARLES POST** (1806–86). *Observations on the cure of strabismus; with an appendix on the new operation for the cure of stammering.* 67pp. New York: Charles S. Francis, 1841.

A nephew of Philip Wright Post (1766–1828), Post received his M.D. from New York's College of Physicians and Surgeons in 1827. He studied in Europe, returning to New York in 1829 to begin the practice of surgery. At the time this small volume was published, Post was a surgeon at New York Hospital, having formerly served on the staff of the New York Eye and Ear Infirmary. From 1851 to 1875, he held the chair of surgery at the University of the City of New York. Post notes in the preface:

> The branch of medical science, which relates to the rectification of deformities, may almost be said to have had its commencement within the last ten years. Before that period, it is true that some deformities existing in children were occasionally treated with success. But the true principles of the treatment were imperfectly understood, and the whole subject was overlooked or neglected by the great mass of the profession. And the treatment which was adopted, imperfect, as it was, was so entirely limited in its application to the period of childhood, as to have received the appellation of orthopaedia, which it still retains . . . . The operation for the cure of strabismus is one of the most recent applications of the principles which have previously been carried out in the treatment of other classes of deformities . . . . In the present essay, I propose to furnish a brief statement of the most important facts which are known with regard to the successful treatment of strabismus. It is not my intention to present an analysis of all that has been said or written on the subject, but to select from published records as well as from

Fig. 54. (OP6) This figure is the only uncolored plate from Post's work (figure 5 on page 50). Nathaniel Currier, of Currier and Ives fame, was lithographer for all seven plates, and Dr. Westmacott completed the drawing. The figure shows the initial stages of an operation to cure strabismus.

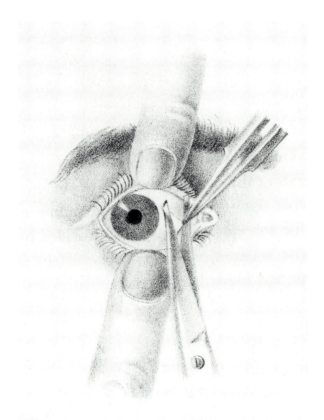

my own observation and experience, such facts as may appear to me to be useful in guiding the profession to correct practical views . . . .

The book has neither table of contents nor index, which makes it somewhat difficult to read. The seven plates are the most important part of the book; six of them are tinted in color. The lithographer was Nathaniel Currier (1813–88), and the engravings depict the anatomy of the muscles involved, the instruments used, and the methods of operation for strabismus. This book is the only one Post wrote. Among Post's eleven children was George Edward (1838–1909), a well-known medical missionary and author who spent most of his life working in Beirut.

OP7. **JAMES BOLTON** (1812–69). *A treatise on strabismus, with a description of new instruments designed to improve the operation for its cure, in simplicity, ease and safety.* 36pp. Richmond: P. D. Bernard, 1842. [G-M 5855]

Bolton was born in Savannah, but received most of his education in New York. He attended Columbia University and the College of Physicians and Surgeons, graduating in 1836. After graduation he immediately began study under John Kearney Rodgers (1793–1851), where he developed an interest in diseases of the eye and ear. Bolton established a practice in Richmond and eventually served in the Confederate forces as a surgeon. The *Treatise*, dedicated to Rodgers, treats strabismus much in the manner as other surgeons of the time. There is one engraved

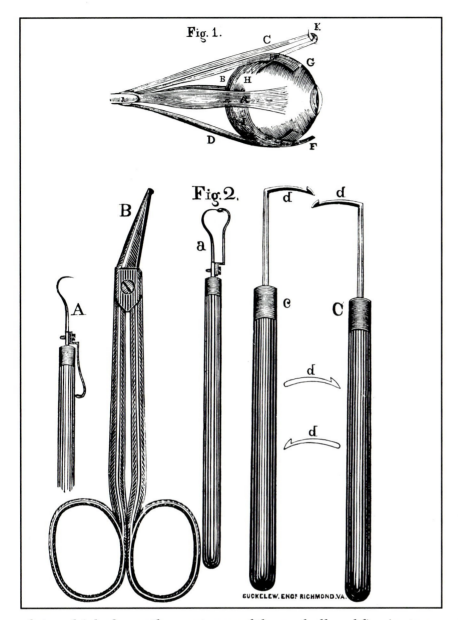

Fig. 1.

Fig. 2.

BUCKELEW. ENG? RICHMOND.VA.

Fig. 55. (OP7) In this engraved plate (frontispiece) Bolton shows the various instruments which he used in his operation for strabismus.

plate, which shows the anatomy of the eyeball and five instruments utilized in the operation. The book has no table of contents.

OP8. FRANK HASTINGS HAMILTON (1813–86). *Monograph on strabismus, with cases.* 69pp. Buffalo: Jewett & Thomas, 1845.

Hamilton was professor of surgery in Geneva Medical College at the time this small monograph was published. It was scarcely more than a bound pamphlet, the purpose of which he notes in the dedication: "To the students of Geneva Medical College, this brochure, prepared expressly for their use, is affectionately dedicated." Extremely scarce because of the limited number printed, this monograph provides a summary of the viewpoints Hamilton encountered while visiting Europe in 1843–44. It presents little in the way of original ideas, providing, for example, a fairly routine explanation of strabismus. The work is difficult to peruse because it lacks a table of contents. (See also GS50, GS70, GS75, OR7, and OR37.)

OP9. **JAMES WILLIAM POWELL** (?–?). *The eye: its imperfections and their prevention; comprising a familiar description of the anatomy and physiology, of the organ of vision: rules for the preservation, improvement, and restoration of sight, with remarks on near sight and aged sight; on optics, and the use and abuse of spectacles, with directions for their selection.* 139pp. New York: Privately printed, 1847.

Little is known about Powell. He lists himself on the title page as a member of the College of Surgeons, oculist, and aurist. This volume was probably written more for the purpose of advertising Powell than for enlightening the profession, since the book notes that his hours for appointments are from nine to four at his residence and office. He was a pupil of Arthur Jacob, professor of the diseases of the eye and ear at the Royal College of Surgeons in Dublin, attending his lectures from 1828 to 1833. Powell writes in the preface that

> . . . hitherto no work of a familiar nature, embracing the subjects specified in the title page, has appeared. I have attempted to fill up this hiatus in the popular literature of the day, by giving, in plain and concise language, which all can understand, a description of the human eye . . . . The disorders of the eye are indeed so numerous and diversified, and some of the operations for their relief require so nice a combination of skill and delicacy that they should be attempted only by the experienced oculist, and no one except the thorough surgeon can make the complete oculist . . . Shall we then trifle with this precious organ, or submit it to the rash treatment of the unskilled? How often is the oculist consulted, alas! when too late, where by neglect or mismanagement the sight is irretrievably destroyed? . . .

There are twenty-one chapters, including "Optics"; "Injuries and accidents"; "Artificial eyes"; "Exercise"; "Diet"; "Tobacco"; "Artificial light"; and "Spectacles." In an interesting "notice to persons at a distance" on page 141, Powell informs the reader that those residing at a distance may obtain his "opinion on various affections of the eye and ear by writing a description of their case and enclosing a fee of three dollars." A second edition was published in 1848 and a third in 1849. There is one plate, and a few wood engravings appear in the text.

OP10. **JOHN HOMER DIX** (1813–84). *Treatise upon the nature and treatment of morbid sensibility of the retina, or weakness of sight. Being the dissertation to which the Boylston medical prize for 1848 was awarded upon the following question: "What is the nature and best mode of treatment of that affection of the eyes, commonly called morbid sensibility of the retina?"* 146pp. Boston: W. D. Ticknor, 1849.

Dix was one of the founders of the American Ophthalmological Society and was among the preeminent ophthalmologic surgeons in Boston. He writes in the preface:

> The complaint to be treated of will perhaps be recognised by but few persons out of this region . . . . It is elsewhere most spoken of as weakness of sight, amblyopy or partial or incipient amaurosis. Admitting the

necessity of a distinctive scientific appelation for a disease which can with no propriety be classed under any other, and objecting to the term "morbid sensibility of the retina" as not expressing its true pathological condition, I would suggest the borrowing and appropriating to it the word "asthenopy," as being if not actually explanatory, at any rate not false in its signification. The remarkable frequency of this complaint here, where in fact it may be said to be among the intellectual classes of society the prevailing affection of the eyes, and the fact that medical literature furnishes no distinct treatise or chapter upon it, that its nature is hitherto unexplained, are considered to be sufficient reasons for the publication of these pages . . . .

There are four chapters: "Symptoms and diagnosis"; "Location and nature"; "Causes"; and "Treatment." (See also OP5.)

OP11. **FREDERICK A. CADWELL** (?–?). *Treatise on the eye and ear: rules for the preservation and restoration of sight: deafness, its causes and progress explained: new discoveries in treatment.* 279pp. Chicago: S. P. Rounds, 1853.

Cadwell lists himself in the book as an oculist and aurist and a graduate of Jefferson Medical College. He practiced in Chicago, but little biographical information is available about him. This work was essentially an advertisement for Cadwell's practice. He writes in the preface to the fifth edition in 1859:

If any apology were needed in offering a work to the public, treating on subjects of so much importance as sight and hearing, which is not in reality a work of practical advantage either to the medical practitioner or the student in medicine, it will be found in the greater advantage which a work of this description is intended to afford to those into whose hands it may chance to fall. And in order that it may be read alike by rich and poor, and its contents carefully perused and duly appreciated, the author has much pleasure in offering the fifth edition (20,000 copies) to the public gratuitously . . . .

Among the topics listed in the index under diseases of the eye are "No charge for an opinion and danger of wrong advice" (page 17); "Difference in cases, don't wait for your neighbors" (page 20); and "No opinion can be given without an examination" (page 74). In the section on deafness and diseases of the ear is a description of the author's miniature anatomical museum (page 110). The final section, "Miscellaneous," has extensive listings of references (pages 117–23), an advertisement for artificial eyes offering a "great reduction in prices" (page 128), letters from medical gentlemen and others (page 177ff.), and opinions of the press (page 181). There are numerous engravings, which Cadwell describes on page 279. The work went through seven editions, the last in 1869.

OP12. **JAMES HENRY CLARK** (1814–69). *Sight and hearing, how preserved, and how lost.* 351pp. New York: C. Scribner,1856.

An 1841 graduate of the College of Physicians and Surgeons in New York, Clark practiced in Newark. This volume is part of Scribner's Popular

Handbook series, and Clark explains the rationale behind its publication in the preface:

> The popular discussion of medical theories and methods of cure, in pamphlets and long conspicuous advertisements, does not tend to the real enlightenment of public opinion . . . . The healing art is too complicated for general appreciation, and is connected with too many collateral facts which must be first known, in order to the full comprehension of its essential truths. Though trite, it is on no other subject so eminently true, that "a little learning is a dangerous thing." A man may better be taught to become his own lawyer, because he deals in abstract truths. The physician, on the other hand, can only become truly competent by years of assiduous attention, and much accumulated experience. It is a life work . . . . The author does not seek to occupy a certain ill-defined middle position between the profession and the public; but this book is prepared with the full conviction that it fills an important place, and communicates truths which the public should know; the want of which is the cause of considerable suffering and loses the world much valuable service. The design of the work is to instruct the mother, the guardian, and the teacher, with regard to the dangers to which children and youth are exposed; to furnish hints to guide in the selection of trades; to advise the scholar when rest or change of employment is required; to point out methods which will tend to preserve the eye in its best condition to the latest period of life, and to induce the avoidance of those habits and practices which are calculated, in a great degree, to injure the important organs of sight and hearing . . . . It has been his endeavor to frame the language of this book to popular apprehension . . . .

There are twelve chapters under "Sight": "Functions and capabilities of the eye"; "Structure of the eye"; "Disorders incident to childhood"; "Disorders incident to youth"; "Near-sightedness"; "Middle-aged sight and accidents"; "Artificial light"; "Overwork and asthenopia"; "Aged sight"; "Glasses"; "Improper treatment of diseased condition of the eyes, popular notions and remedies, and quackery"; and "Artificial eyes." The contents of the section on hearing include "Structure of the ear and its functions"; "Curability of diseases of the ear, and popular opinions and practices"; "Diseases to which the ear is subject"; "Deaf-dumbness and ear trumpet"; "Comparative value of sight and hearing and revelations from the land of silence." This was the only edition. Clark also wrote *The medical men of New Jersey in Essex district from 1666 to 1866* (Newark: private printing, 1867).

OP13. **HENRY WILLARD WILLIAMS** (1821–95). *A practical guide to the study of the diseases of the eye; their medical and surgical treatment.* 317pp. Boston: Ticknor & Fields, 1862.

One of America's best known early ophthalmologists, Williams attended Harvard Medical School, where he graduated in 1849. He also studied in Europe, and it was there that he first became interested in the specialty of ophthalmology. Williams established a private practice in Boston in 1850 and worked in that city for his entire professional life. He was a founder of the American Ophthalmological Society (1864) and served as its president from 1868 to 1875. He is best remembered for his treatment of iritis without mercury [G-M 5878] and for a method of suturing the corneal flap after cataract extraction [G-M 5895]. He notes in the preface:

> . . . In offering this treatise to the profession, and to those who are about to enter it, the author does not assume to set forth all which is known in respect to diseases of the eye. He has endeavored to supply a want which his relations with junior practitioners and students have shown him to exist, and to prepare a work which shall afford, in a form as simple and concise as possible, a practical and serviceable knowledge of these diseases . . . . It has been the aim of the author to avoid encumbering his work, and confusing the reader, by the introduction of merely exceptional details . . . .

There are twenty-four chapters, including an early chapter on the ophthalmoscope (page 12ff.). There are no plates. Further editions were published in 1865, 1869, 1873 and 1886. (See also OP15, OP21, and OP34.)

OP14. **PETER DIRCK KEYSER** (1835–97). *Glaucoma, its symptoms, diagnosis, and treatment.* 88pp. Philadelphia: Lindsay & Blakiston, 1864.

Born in Philadelphia, Keyser received his medical degree from Jena University in Germany in 1864. He immediately returned to the United States and opened a practice in his native city. He soon founded the Philadelphia Eye and Ear Hospital, where he was surgeon-in-charge. For many years he also served on the staff of Wills Eye Hospital. In 1899, Keyser became professor of ophthalmology at the Medico-Chirurgical College of Philadelphia and dean of the institution. He notes in the preface to his *Glaucoma*:

> Should any apology be deemed necessary for obtruding on the medical public a new pamphlet on ophthalmic science, it may, perhaps, be furnished by the interest which that department of medicine and surgery has acquired in the last few years . . . . I have endeavored in these pages to lay before the reader, in an easy and practical form, the latest theories relating to glaucoma, so as to enable him at once to grasp the most salient and important points . . . . I have chiefly followed the views of Professor A. Von Graefe, of Berlin . . . from my notes taken while attending his clinical lectures, during the winter of 1863 and 1864 . . . .

There is no table of contents, nor does the book contain any plates.

OP15. **HENRY WILLARD WILLIAMS** (1821–95). *Recent advances in ophthalmic science. The Boylston Prize essay for 1865.* 166pp. Boston: Ticknor & Fields, 1866,

At the time this essay was written, Williams was ophthalmic surgeon at Boston City Hospital and university lecturer on ophthalmic surgery at Harvard University. He notes in the preface:

> . . . It is hoped that this essay may in a measure supply the demand, which becomes every day more urgent, for a work which, without being too elaborate, may assist the student and the general practitioner in ac-

quiring a knowledge of the principles of the ophthalmoscope and of its practical application,—and which may also elucidate, so far as is possible in a brief resume, other important points in regard to which immense progress has been made within a few years, leading to a more correct understanding of the optical powers and functions of the eye, and of the results of aberrations from the normal standard . . . .

Among the numerous chapter headings are "The ophthalmoscope"; "Lateral illumination"; "Optometers"; "Test letters"; "New therapeutic agents"; "Anesthetics"; "Tension of the eyeball"; "Paracentesis of the cornea"; "Iridectomy"; "Iridesis"; "Corelysis"; "Enucleation of the eyeball"; "Glaucoma"; "Apoplexy of the retina"; "Separation of the retina"; "Choroiditis"; "Posterior staphyloma"; "Cataract"; "The function of accommodation"; "Presbyopia"; "Paralysis of the ciliary muscle"; "Myopia"; "Hypermetropia"; "Asthenopia"; "Astigmatism"; and "Strabismus". On pages 90–91 is found a description of Williams's suture of a corneal wound, a procedure which met with great professional opposition. The few lithographic plates were drawn by John Green. There are also four charts, one of which is folding. The essay was also simultaneously published by James R. Osgood of Boston. Most of the important parts of this scarce work were incorporated into later editions of Williams's *Practical Guide* (OP13). (See also OP21 and OP34.)

OP15.1. **WALTER ALDEN** (?–?). *The human eye; its use and abuse: a popular treatise on far, near and impaired sight, and the methods of preservation by the proper use of spectacles, and other acknowledged aids of vision.* 138pp. Cincinnati: private printing, 1866.

Alden was an optician who practiced in Cincinnati. He often wrote in the lay press about problems related to the eyes. He explains in the preface that "This work is presented for the acceptance and approval of the public, touching a vital subject upon which little attention has hitherto been paid. The methods of preserving vision, the most precious and valuable of the senses, has been a subject too long neglected . . . . " The work contains thirteen chapters, but has no table of contents. A lengthy index is found on pages 133–38. An interesting rule for the selection of spectacles (page 129) notes that "never buy of an inexperienced person, peddler, jeweller, &c., but of an optician." The work contains twenty-nine engraved illustrations and two plates located as frontis-pieces. This was the only edition.

OP16. **ABRAM METZ** (1828–76). *The anatomy and histology of the human eye.* 184pp. Philadelphia: Office of the Medical and Surgical Reporter, 1868.

An 1848 graduate of Cleveland Medical College, Metz was professor of ophthalmology at Charity Hospital Medical College in Cleveland when this volume was published. The work was considered one of the more thorough American ophthalmologic texts of the mid-nineteenth century. Metz notes in the preface:

When, a few years ago, I commenced teaching ophthalmology, I seriously felt the want of a text-book on the anatomy and histology of the human eye. There does not exist, to my knowledge, a treatise on this subject that includes the results of the labors of the more recent histologists to be found in ophthalmological journals and in memoirs on special subjects. It has been my aim to collect this material into a connected form, and in such a manner as to adapt it alike to the requirements of the medical student and of the practicising physician . . . .

The contents include twenty-one chapters detailing various anatomical areas of the eyeball. The few engravings were made by Hugo Sebald of Philadelphia. Most of the titles cited in the bibliography were published in Germany after 1851, indicating that Metz was well abreast of the most recent developments in his field.

OP17. **JAKOB HERMANN KNAPP** (1832–1911). *A treatise on intraocular tumors, from original observations and anatomical investigations.* 323pp. New York: William Wood, 1869. [G-M 5902]

One of America's most renowned early ophthalmologists, Knapp was born in Dauborn, Germany. He received his M.D. from the University of Giessen in 1854 and within ten years became professor of ophthalmology at Heidelberg, where he founded that university's first ophthalmologic clinic. He emigrated to New York City in 1868, where he established the Ophthalmic and Aural Institute. From 1882 to 1888 Knapp was professor of ophthalmology at the University of the City of New York. He served in a similar position at the College of Physicians and Surgeons from 1888 to 1902. Among his major contributions was the founding of the monthly periodical *Archives of ophthalmology and otology* in 1869. Knapp trained many of America's early specialists in ophthalmology. He is best remembered for a valuable monograph on curvature of the cornea, *Die Krümmung der Hornhaut des menschlichen Auges* (Heidelberg: J. C. B. Mohr, 1859) [G-M 5884] and for a method of extraction of cataract with forceps [G-M 5964]. The *Treatise* is an English translation of his most important work, *Die intraocularen Geschwulste nach eigenen klinischen Beobachtungen und anatomischen Untersuchungen* (Carlsruhe: C. F. Muller, 1868). In the original German preface, Knapp writes:

> I have been induced by two reasons to study more minutely the subject of the present treatise: (1) Because the diseases here spoken of are perfectly harmless and masked in their earliest stages, but on further growth become so horrible and destructive to the patient and those about him, that they awaken, of themselves, the highest sympathy of the physician; and (2) because I am convinced that intraocular tumors especially are destined to throw light upon many general questions of fundamental significance for the theories and therapeutics of tumors in general . . . .

In a preface to the English edition, Knapp notes:

> The English translation of the present book has been made by my former pupil, Dr. S. Cole, of Chicago, who, at the time I was working at the subject, was a most industrious student of my clinical and didactic lectures at the Ophthalmic Hospital in Heidelberg. He not only saw most of my anatomical preparations, but observed some of the cases described even during life. He is therefore, thoroughly conversant with

the subject, a circumstance no less indispensable for a good translator than a perfect knowledge of both languages. I have availed myself of the very latest literature in making a few additions . . . . On my recent voyage through Germany, France, and England to America, I received

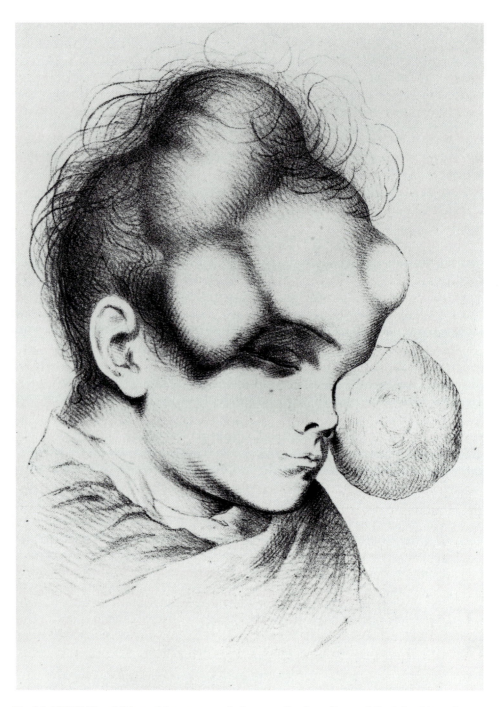

Fig. 56. (OP17) The child, aged two years and nine months, has glioma of the left orbit and metastases of glioma on the cranium, figure 4 of the end-plates. Knapp had extirpated the right eye when the infant was only three months old. The figure was drawn by C. P. Schmitt, and the lithography was produced by Chr. Fr. Muller of Carlsruhe.

the impression everywhere that great attention is now paid to the subject of intraocular tumors. Thus it is to be expected that many a question, actually beyond the reach of individual effort, will soon be settled by persistent and combined labor.

The book is divided into two parts: "Glioma (encephaloid) of the retina" and "Sarcoma of the choroid," with each part containing two sections. Seventeen cases are presented throughout the text. There is an extensive appendix which details other forms of tumors occurring in the eyeball. The book has one chromolithographic and fifty lithographic plates, which contain seventy figures. There were no further editions. (See also OT10.)

OP18. **JOHN PHILLIPS** (?–?). *Ophthalmic surgery and treatment: with advice on the use and abuse of spectacles.* 510pp. Chicago: W. B. Keen, 1869.

Little is known about Phillips, although he refers to himself in the book as an optician and oculist. He practiced in Illinois, where he was among the earliest to recognize the importance of the ophthalmoscope, and this work is among the first American textbooks to deal specifically with the instrument. The book contains one plate as a frontispiece and a few other rudimentary engravings. Phillips writes in the preface:

> So great an amount of talent and industry has of late years been devoted to the investigation of diseases of the eye, that a new volume on the subject appears to require a few words of introduction. Notwithstanding all the assistance the student may derive from systematic treatises and pictorial instructions, close personal examination of a large number of patients can alone enable him to recognize those delicate changes which the tissue of the eye presents under various morbid conditions. Specially to direct his attention to these changes, and to explain the best methods of observing them for himself, is the primary object of the following pages . . . . The matter contained in this book being, however, in great part derived from the labors of others, and adapted by myself to the requirements of men in general practice . . . . The ophthalmoscope, in its simplified form, has come into general use, and has proved indispensable to the oculist, as well as to the medical man . . . It not only enables us to view the retina, optic disk, etc., in health and disease, but often affords the earliest means of recognizing the presence of general morbid changes, such as albuminuria, syphilis, cerebral tumors, etc . . . .

Phillips also privately published the section on spectacles as a separate ninety-page monograph in 1869.

OP19. **HENRY CLAY ANGELL** (1829–1911). *A treatise on diseases of the eye; for the use of general practitioners.* 343pp. Boston: James Campbell, 1870.

Angell was an 1852 graduate of the Homeopathic Medical College of Pennsylvania. He studied in Vienna for one year after which he eventually established a general practice in Boston. In 1861, Angell again left for Europe, where he devoted three and a half years to studying diseases of the eye. On his return to Massachusetts, he devoted his practice solely to ophthalmology. Angell's *Treatise* was considered for many years the standard ophthalmologic text in schools of homeopathy and is quite important because it was the first comprehensive textbook to be published on ophthalmology by a non-allopathic physician. Angell describes himself in the book as an oculist and aurist and writes in the preface:

> My readers are requested to bear in mind that this work is written, not for specialists, but for homeopathic physicians in general practice—for those too busied with the whole, to devote a great amount of time to any one part of medicine and surgery. The endeavor has been, to treat the subjects embraced, clearly and concisely, in the hope of presenting a volume attractive enough, and small enough, to induce the busiest to give it some attention . . . . In the preparation of this work, I have had the advantage of copious notes taken during a somewhat prolonged attendance at the European clinics . . . .

There are twenty chapters, including a brief but interesting history of ophthalmic surgery in chapter 1. A discussion on the ophthalmoscope appears on pages 18–33, and homeopathic medications to treat ophthalmic affections are listed on page 311. The *Treatise* went through seven editions by 1891 because of its wide use in homeopathic schools. This was the only book Angell wrote.

OP20. **BENJAMIN JOY JEFFRIES** (1833–1915). *The eye in health and disease: being a series of articles on the anatomy and physiology of the human eye, and its surgical and medical treatment.* 119pp. Boston: A. Moore, 1871.

Jeffries was an 1857 graduate of Harvard Medical School. He spent two years in Europe, where he devoted himself to the study of ophthalmology and dermatology. On moving back to Boston, he established a practice devoted to these two specialties. He was serving as ophthalmic surgeon at the Massachusetts Charitable Eye and Ear Infirmary and at Carney Hospital at the time this volume was published. The work is a reprint of a number of articles that Jeffries had written over the course of several years. The articles were edited and substantial additions made to prepare them for publication in book form. The contents consist of "Anatomy of the eye"; "Physiology"; "Old sight and spectacles"; "Nearsightedness"; "Long-sightedness"; "Astigmatism"; "Cataract in children"; "Cataract"; "Artificial eyes"; "Squinting eyes"; "Artificial pupil"; "The ophthalmoscope"; "Injuries of the eye"; and "Type for testing vision." There was only one edition. Among his other books are *Diseases of the skin: the recent advances in their pathology and treatment* (Boston: A. Moore, 1871) and *Animal and vegetable parasites of the human skin and hair* (Boston: A. Moore, 1872) (See also OP28.)

OP21. **HENRY WILLARD WILLIAMS** (1821–95). *Our eyes and how to take care of them.* 103pp. Boston: James R. Osgood, 1871.

Williams was president of the American Ophthalmological Society at the time this small monograph was published. It consists of papers which had first been serially published in *The Atlantic monthly*. Williams states in the preface:

> The author's purpose . . . was to explain to parents, teachers, and all who have occasion to use their eyes, in the simplest language possible, some of the advances which have been recently made in our knowledge of the eye, its powers, and its proper uses; and to show what should be done and what avoided, that the sight, the most important of our senses, may be enjoyed and preserved . . .

The book has no table of contents nor index. The publisher, James R. Osgood & Co., was the successor to the important early Boston medical publishing firms of Ticknor & Fields and Fields, Osgood & Co. (See also OP13, OP15, and OP34.)

OP22. **ANDREW JACKSON HOWE** (1825–90). *Manual of eye surgery.* 204pp. Cincinnati: Wilstach & Baldwin, 1874.

Howe was professor of surgery at the Eclectic Medical Institute and one of the most prominent of American eclectic surgeons. He is the only American surgeon to have ever written books in four different specialties: general surgery, orthopedic surgery, eye surgery, and gynecologic sur-gery. Howe writes in the preface:

> In surveying the field occupied by ophthalmic writers I found the ground well covered with elaborate treatises; but, in most instances, the subject of eye surgery has been treated by "specialists" for the benefit of "specialists," and the general practitioner was left without a work adap-ted particularly to his wants. Recognizing the merits of the several hand-books already in existence on this subject, but thinking that in one feature or another they fail to meet the requirements of the ordi-nary physician, I have endeavored to supply this apparent need . . . . Although I have called this work a Manual, I have aimed at being thorough and systematic in the preparation and arrangement of what recent research has contributed to an eminently progressive branch of surgery. The physician of varied practice will find that degree of eluci-dation which will enable him to execute all the easier operations, and to comprehend what the expert oculist performs . . . .

There is no table of contents, but a detailed index appears on pages 199–204. No plates are included, and most of the illustrations are from other authors' works. Much to his discredit, Howe did not recognize the im-portance of the ophthalmoscope to all physicians because, as he writes in the preface:

> The ophthalmoscope has thrown so much light upon obscure diseases of the eye, that the instrument is indispensable to the proper diagnosis of certain morbid conditions; yet the beginner need not expect to gain much advantage from its use. It requires practice to become expert in making observations with any instrument of the kind . . . .

Based on this position, Howe did not include any discussion of the oph-thalmoscope in the text. There was only one edition. (See also GS84, OR25, and GY37.)

OP23. **CHRISTOPHER SMITH FENNER** (1823–79). *Vision; its optical de-fects, and the adaptation of spectacles. Embracing, first, physical op-tics; second, physiological optics; third, errors of refraction and defects of accommodation, or optical defects of the eye, with selections from*

the test types of Jaeger and Snellen. 299pp. Philadelphia: Lindsay &
Blakiston, 1875.

Fenner practiced ophthalmology in Louisville when he published
this volume. He writes in the preface:

> In preparing this work the endeavor has been made to give, in a con-
> cise and popular, yet comprehensive form, a resume of our present
> knowledge of physiological optics and of the defects of the eye as an
> optical instrument . . . . A brief elementary treatise on physical optics
> has been prefixed, as a knowledge of this subject is necessary in order
> to understand the explanation of many phenomena connected with
> the functions of vision. The manuscript was commenced during the
> past summer; but, owing to an affection of my eyes,—retinal hemor-
> rhage,—which came on suddenly before the writing of part first was
> finished, the work is not as complete as was intended. Having since that
> time been unable to make much use of my eyes in reading or writing,
> I was compelled to complete the manuscript by dictating to an aman-
> uensis, and to have my thoughts recorded, chiefly, as they were pre-
> viously arranged in my mind, or from notes before taken, but without
> regard to order, not being able to refresh my memory, as the book
> progressed, by more recent reading of authorities . . . .

There are three parts: "Physical optics (light)"; "Physiological optics
(visual sensations, visual perceptions)"; and "Errors of refraction and
defects of accommodation (hypermetropia, myopia, astigmatism, difference in refraction of the two eyes)." The illustrations consist of seventy-four engravings on wood. In addition, there are selections from the
test-types of Jaeger and Snellen. This was the only edition.

OP24. **TIMOTHY FIELD ALLEN** (1837–1902) and **GEORGE SALMON NOR-
TON** (1851–91). *Ophthalmic therapeutics.* 269pp. New York: Boericke
& Tafel, 1876.

Allen received his college education at Amherst and his M.D. from
the medical department of University of the City of New York in 1861.
Two years later, after having served in the Civil War, he entered private
practice in Brooklyn and soon converted to homeopathic medicine. In
1866, he became professor of chemistry at the New York Medical College for Women and in the following year, professor of anatomy at
New York Homeopathic College. At the time of this book's publication,
Allen was surgeon at New York Ophthalmic Hospital and professor of
materia medica and therapeutics at New York Homeopathic Medical
College. Quite well known as a homeopath, he served with William T.
Helmuth (1833–1902) as coeditor of the *New York journal of homeopathy*
in 1873–75. Allen was quite interested in botany and was one of the
founders of the New York Botanical Gardens. From 1888 to 1896 he
published in serial form a book called *The characeae of America,* which
was illustrated with magnificent plates by Evelyn Hunter Nordhoff.
Norton was surgeon at the New York Ophthalmic Hospital and ophthalmic and aural surgeon at the Homeopathic Hospital on Ward's Island in New York. The authors note in the preface:

> Material for this work has been accumulating for many years, especially
> since the adoption of the homeopathic method by the New York Oph-

thalmic Hospital . . . . It is proper to explain that the plan of this work is substantially the same as that projected by Dr. Allen a few years since, and prematurely announced; the material then in hand has been augmented by the observations of Dr. Norton, the whole work written out by him and revised by us jointly . . . .

The book consists of two parts: part 1 (pages 1–142) discusses an alphabetization of numerous homeopathic drug preparations related to ophthalmologic diseases. Part 2 (pages 145–269) presents eye pathology and is divided into various anatomical sections (i.e., orbit; lachrymal apparatus; and lids) and includes discussion of their homeopathic treatment. There are no illustrations. A second edition was issued under the direction of Norton in 1882. Among Allen's other books are the ten-volume *Encyclopedia of pure materia medica; a record of the positive effects of drugs upon the healthy human organism* (New York: Boericke & Tafel, 1874–79), an index to the preceding work titled *A general symptom register of the homoeopathic materia medica* (New York: Boericke & Tafel, 1880), and *A handbook of materia medica, and homoeopathic therapeutics* (Philadelphia: F. E. Boericke, 1889).

OP25. **EDWARD GREELY LORING** (1837–88). *Determination of the refraction of the eye by means of the ophthalmoscope.* 61pp. New York: William Wood, 1876.

Loring began his medical studies in Italy, but eventually returned to America and graduated from Harvard Medical School in 1864. He soon became associated with Cornelius Rea Agnew (1830–88) [G-M 5894] in New York, where he joined the staffs of the Brooklyn Eye and Ear Hospital and the New York Eye and Ear Infirmary. His writings on ophthalmoscopy were crucial in the development of this technique in the United States. This short work actually consisted of advance sheets from another study entitled *The ophthalmoscope,* which was never published separately: it was instead incorporated into one of Loring's textbooks (OP39). There is no table of contents and only a limited index. Among the chapters are "Directions for the use of the upright image"; "Description of suitable ophthalmoscopes"; "Determination of the optical condition of the eye with the ophthalmoscope"; "Astigmatism"; "Directions to be observed in case the observer is ametropic"; "Refraction by the mirror alone and by the inverted image"; "Determination of astigmatism with the mirror alone"; "Refraction by the inverted image"; "Determination of astigmatism with the inverted image"; and "The amount of enlargement produced by the upright image." There were no further editions.

OP26. **DANIEL BENNETT ST. JOHN ROOSA** (1838–1908) and **EDWARD T. ELY** (1850–85). *Ophthalmic and optic memoranda.* 264pp. New York: William Wood, 1876.

Roosa was professor of ophthalmology and otology at the University of the City of New York and surgeon at the Manhattan Eye and Ear Hospital. Ely, who attended University of Rochester as an undergraduate and received an M.D. from the College of Physicians and Surgeons in

New York in 1874, came under the postgraduate tutelage of Roosa. He is listed on the title page as an assistant to the chair of ophthalmology and otology, University of the City of New York, and attending surgeon to the class of eye and ear diseases, Eastern Dispensary. The authors explain their limited purpose in the preface:

> The little book that is herewith presented to students and practitioners of medicine has been prepared with great care. It aims to give a concise and correct outline of our present knowledge of ophthalmology and otology, and to serve as a kind of dictionary of these subjects. We shall be sorry if it is ever used to acquire a primary knowledge of either of these sciences, or if it is trusted for complete directions as to the diagnosis and treatment of ophthalmic and aural diseases . . . . We believe our book will prove especially useful to those who are attending lectures upon the subjects of which it treats, but who are too busy during the lecture-season to consult the larger treatises. We hope, also, that even experienced general practitioners and specialists will find it a trustworthy aid to the memory, in recalling facts which sometimes escape the minds of the most learned . . . .

The first part has three chapters: "Anatomy and physiology of the eye"; "Examination, therapeutics and surgery of the eye"; and "Diseases of the eye." The second part deals exclusively with the ear. The book has a minimal number of engravings but no plates. This volume was quite well received and further editions were published in 1880, 1885 and 1891. (See also OT14, OP43, OP60, and OP84.)

OP27. **CHARLES PORTER HART** (1827–?). *Homeopathic ophthalmic practice: a systematic treatise on diseases of the eye, for general practitioners and students.* 336pp. Detroit: E. A. Lodge, 1877.

Hart was a native of Norwich, Connecticut, and received his M.D. from New York University in 1854. The year before, he had attended a course of lectures given by Valentine Mott (1785–65). Most of his practice was devoted to the surgical specialties, although he was highly regarded as an adherent to the principles of homeopathy. At the time this volume was published, Hart was in practice in Wyoming, Ohio, having formerly served as chief surgeon in the eye department of Brown General Hospital in Louisville. The work is dedicated to T. Sterry Hunt. Hart writes in the preface:

> The present volume owes its origin to a desire on the part of some of the readers of the *American Homeopathic Observer*, that the series of articles on ophthalmology contributed by the writer to that journal, should, for the sake of convenience, be republished in book form. In complying with this request, the author has extended the series so as to embrace all the leading diseases of the eye, and in so doing has endeavored to exhibit, in a concise and practical form, a clear and exact account of the present state of ophthalmic science . . . . Unfortunately, the science of which we treat is still regarded by many as too abstruse, and the practice of it too difficult, for the general profession, and hence it has been relegated, for the most part, to a comparatively small number of practitioners. We say unfortunately, because the vast majority of ophthalmic diseases are still treated, and of necessity always will be

> treated, by the ordinary medical attendant. The important question, then, is, not whether diseases of the eye should be turned over to the specialist for more scientific investigation and treatment . . . but whether the general practitioner . . . shall be properly qualified to discharge a duty which, whether qualified or not, he is required to perform . . . .

The volume is divided into six major divisions: "Ophthalmic inflammation"; "Results of ophthalmic inflammation"; "Ophthalmic tumors"; "Cataract"; "Optical aids and tests"; and "Functional diseases." Among the more interesting and important discussions is an early description of the ophthalmoscope (page 272). There are numerous illustrations but no plates. This was the only edition. He also wrote *Repertory of the new remedies* (New York: Boericke & Tafel, 1876), *Homeopathic medical practice; a systematic treatise on diseases of the brain and eye* (Detroit: E. A. Lodge, 1878), *Diseases of the nervous system; being a treatise on spasmodic, paralytic, neuralgic and mental affections* (New York: Boericke & Tafel, 1881), *A treatise on the diseases of the respiratory passages* (Detroit: E. A. Lodge, 1882), *Treatise on intracranial diseases: inflammatory, organic and symptomatic* (Philadelphia: F. E. Boericke, 1884), and *Therapeutics of nervous diseases* (Philadelphia: F. E. Boericke, 1889).

OP28. **BENJAMIN JOY JEFFRIES** (1833–1915). *Color-blindness: its dangers and its detection.* 312pp. Boston: Houghton & Osgood, 1879.

Jeffries was one of the first American ophthalmologists to take an active interest in the study of color blindness. He was ophthalmic surgeon at Massachusetts Eye and Ear Infirmary, Carney Hospital, and the New England Hospital for Women and Children. This monograph was the first major contribution on the subject by an American and came at a time when European governments were already taking steps to guard against the occupational hazards of color blindness. Jeffries was the only authoritative American physician to research and call attention to the problems of color blindness among railway engineers, ships' captains, and other industrial workers. Jeffries discusses these problems in his preface:

> I have dedicated this volume to my friend Professor Holmgren, because I consider that to him above all others do we owe the present and future control of color-blindness on land and sea, by which life and property are safer, and the risks of travelling less. To his majesty, the King of Sweden, are due the thanks of all for his personal interest in the investigation of color-blindness, and his practical good sense in immediately putting into execution the plans and proposals of Professor Holmgren, by which the subject was so prominently brought forward as to command the attention and example of other nations. It is earnestly hoped that this country will follow rapid suit . . . . To bring before the community the dangers and the prevalence of color-blindness, I thought it best to prosecute my researches amongst the places of learning and teaching. Hence I chose our immediate universities, colleges, and public schools. Thus, whilst I was pursuing my own individual studies of color-blindness, I was at the same time gathering the necessary statistics in proof of the position I took, and disseminating a knowledge of the whole subject, very especially the important one of

its frequency. It is rather curious that this volume is only the third monograph in bookform on this subject . . . . I have not in this volume entered into the loss of time and money from color-blindness in the great industries where a perfect chromatic sense is needed; or the mortifications, &c., arising from constant mistakes of dress &c., in everyday life,—as all these bear no relation to the importance of the danger to life and property on land and sea from this curious visual defect. The railroads of England pay two million dollars a year for killed and injured travellers . . . . As this volume is intended to meet the wants of several quite different classes in the community, its contents are somewhat varied. Many of the chapters may be read by themselves, by those who are only interested in the subject from the point of view touched on in that special chapter. General readers will find the historical cases, and the curious mistakes caused by this chromatic defect, of most interest to them perhaps. Physicians will be interested in facts relating to color blindness from diseases, its heredity, and the supposed peculiarities heretofore connected with it, as also its incurability. Scientists and physiologists will naturally turn to the accounts of the precise condition of color-blindness and its relation to normal color-sense, as well as the additional methods of detection. The color-blind cannot but be interested in the palliatives of congenital color-blindness, since we can now do more for them than formerly . . . . Our national and state legislatures and railroad commissioners will naturally turn to the account of the present provisional European laws in reference to the control of color-blindness on land and sea . . . .

There are twenty-five chapters covering a wide range of topics. Among the more interesting ones are "Historical cases of color-blindness" (chapter 1); "Former classification of the color-blind" (chapter 3); "Dangers arising from color-blindness on railroads" (chapter 14) and "on the ocean" (chapter 15); "Methods of testing" (chapter 18); and "Efforts to conceal or to feign color-blindness" (chapter 21). There is an extensive bibliography on the subject (pages 291–308). The book has one chromolithographic plate. Interestingly, the volume is bound in linen with broad horizontal bands of red, green and blue. A second edition was published in 1883. (See also OP20.)

OP29. GEORGE CUVIER HARLAN (1835–1909). *Eyesight, and how to care for it.* 139pp. Philadelphia: Lindsay & Blakiston, 1880.

This monograph was the fourth of Lindsay and Blakiston's American Health Primers. It originally sold for fifty cents. Harlan, who received his M.D. from the University of Pennsylvania in 1858, was surgeon at Wills Eye Hospital. He held a number of other academic posts, including the first chair of ophthalmology at the Polyclinic and School for Graduates in Medicine in Philadelphia. Quite prominent politically, Harlan was president of the American Ophthalmological Society in 1893. The nine chapters consist of an "Introduction"; "Anatomy of the eye"; "Physiology of vision"; "Ophthalmoscope"; "Injuries and diseases of the eye"; "Optical defects"; "Spectacles"; "Practical suggestions for the care of the eyes"; and "Effects of school-life upon the sight." There are twenty-one rather rudimentary wood engravings. There was only one edition, and this was Harlan's only work in book form.

op30. **JOSEPH LeCONTE** (1823–1901). *Sight; an exposition of the principles of monocular and binocular vision.* 275pp. New York: D. Appleton, 1881.

LeConte was one of the more intriguing figures in nineteenth-century American medicine. At the time this book was written, he was professor of geology and natural history at the University of California. LeConte received his M.D. from the College of Physicians and Surgeons in New York in 1845, but practiced as a physician for only a few years. The reason for this change in career was his exceptional interest and ability in natural history, which led to his studying under the geologist and paleontologist, Louis Agassiz (1807–73). Although primarily known as a geologist, Le Conte continued to be interested in medicine, and *Sight* is a product of this concern. The book was well regarded by fellow ophthalmologists. It was issued as part of Appleton's International Scientific Series and was available for $1.50. LeConte states in the preface:

> In writing this treatise I have tried to make a book that would be intelligible and interesting to the thoughtful general reader, and at the same time profitable to even the most advanced specialist in this department. I find justification for the attempt in the fact that there is not, to my knowledge, any work covering the same ground in the English language . . . . As a means of scientific culture, the study of vision seems to me almost exceptional. It makes use of, and thus connects together, the sciences of physics, physiology, and even psychology. It makes the cultivation of the habit of observation and experiment possible to all; for the greatest variety of experiments may be made without expensive apparatus, or, indeed, apparatus of any kind. And, above all, it compels one to analyze the complex phenomena of sense in his own person, and is thus a truly admirable preparation for the more difficult task of analysis of those still higher and more complex phenomena which are embraced in the science of psychology.

Part 1, "Monocular vision," consists of "General structure of the human eye, and the formation of images"; "The eye as an optical instrument"; "Defects of the eye as an instrument"; and "Explanation of phenomena of monocular vision." "Binocular vision," part 2, includes "Single and double images"; "Superposition of external images"; "Binocular perspective"; "Theories of binocular perspective"; and "Judgment of distance, size, and form." Part 3, which discusses some disputed points in binocular vision, includes "Laws of ocular motion"; "The horopter"; "On some fundamental phenomena of binocular vision usually overlooked and on a new mode of diagrammatic representation based thereon"; "Visual phenomena in ocular divergence"; and "Comparative physiology of binocular vision." There are 130 illustrations, most of which are original to LeConte, but no plates. Among his other books are *Elements of geology* (New York: D. Appleton, 1878) and *Religion and science* (New York: D. Appleton, 1874). LeConte also wrote an autobiography which was edited by William D. Armes (New York: D. Appleton, 1903).

OP31. **WILLIAM F. MITTENDORF** (?–?). *A manual on diseases of the eye and ear, for the use of students and practitioners.* 445pp. New York: G. P. Putnam's Sons, 1881.

Mittendorf was a surgeon at the New York Eye and Ear Infirmary and ophthalmic surgeon at Bellevue Hospital's Out-Door Department. He received most of his post-graduate medical education serving as assistant to the chair of ophthalmology and otology at Bellevue Hospital Medical College. He notes in the preface:

> The importance of the study of the diseases of the eye and ear by every student of medicine is best shown by the fact that many of the medical colleges, especially those in England, have made the study of these diseases obligatory for graduation. The want of a short practical manual of the diseases of the eye and ear in the English language has long been felt by the medical student. I have, therefore, at the request of many members of my private classes, given in this little book my lectures upon these subjects, somewhat enlarged. It has been my aim to make this book as practical and brief as the great importance of the subject would permit . . . . The use of the more extensive text-books on the subject cannot be replaced by this little work, which is intended for the elementary study of the diseases of the eye and ear only . . . .

There are twenty chapters, seventeen of which concern the eye. The ten chromolithographic plates are copied from works by European authorities. (See also OP40.)

OP32. **HENRY DRURY NOYES** (1832–1900). *A treatise on diseases of the eye.* 360pp. New York: William Wood, 1881.

The *Treatise* was No. 75 in Wood's Library of Standard Medical Authors. Its author was professor of ophthalmology and otology at Bellevue Hospital Medical College and surgeon at the New York Eye and Ear Infirmary. He studied at New York University and received his M.D. from the College of Physicians and Surgeons in 1855. Noyes entered private ophthalmologic and otologic practice in 1859 and eventually wielded a great influence in American ophthalmology. He was one of the founders of the American Ophthalmolgical Society (in 1864) and served as president from 1878 to 1884. Noyes was among the earliest in this country to employ cocaine as a local anesthetic in eye operations, but he is best remembered as the first investigator to understand the relationship between retinitis and glycosuria [G-M 3938]. It was under his guiding hand that the New York Eye and Ear Infirmary achieved worldwide acclaim as one of the finest specialty hospitals in America. The *Treatise* served as the basis for Noyes's famous *Textbook* (OP46). He writes in the former's preface:

> In this treatise the writer has attempted to condense into the limits assigned to him the substance of modern ophthalmic knowledge. The standpoint is clinical and the purpose is practical; but, whatever is necessary to a correct understanding of a disease is presented, because sound treatment can only be attained by a proper knowledge of causes, connections, and processes. Brief statements of anatomy, including microscopic structure, have been introduced. In microscopic pathology, the writer has been obliged to depend upon the labors of others, and

has endeavored to present views which are most recent, in so far as he
has offered any . . . .

The book is divided into two parts: the first focuses on general disturbances of refraction and of muscular function, while the second part
discusses specific diseases of the eye in eighteen chapters, including
"Lachrymal apparatus"; "Eyelids"; "Conjunctiva"; "Cornea"; "Sclera";
"Iris"; "Ciliary body"; "Wounds and injuries"; "Sympathetic ophthalmia"; "Functional troubles of the iris"; "Crystalline lens"; "Vitreous

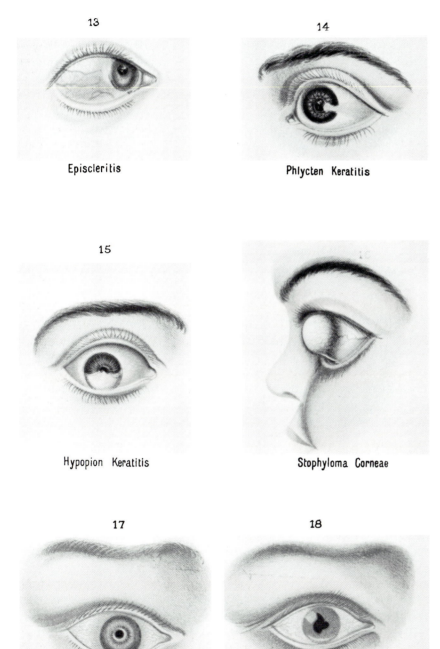

13

Episcleritis

14

Phlycten Keratitis

15

Hypopion Keratitis

Stophyloma Corneae

17

Iritis

18

Iritis, irregular pupil.

Fig. 57. (OP31) Mittendorf's
chromolithograph plate demonstrates various disease
states of the eye.

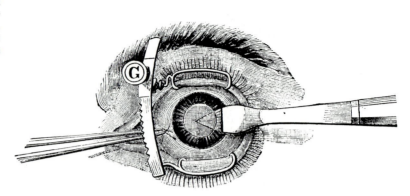

Fig. 58. (OP32) In 1866 Noyes invented a speculum for use in ophthalmic surgery. It is depicted in this wood engraving, figure 96 on page 242, as an adjunct to the extraction of a cataract.

body"; "Choroidea"; "Glaucoma"; "Retina and optic nerve"; "Diseases of the optic nerve"; "Orbit"; and "Optico-ciliary neurectomy." There are two color plates depicting various diseases of the retina and 111 wood engravings. This was the only edition. Among Noyes's other books is *Diagnosis of those diseases of the eye which can be seen without the ophthalmoscope* (New York: G. P. Putnam's Sons, 1876). This particular monograph was part of Edward C. Sequin's (1843–98) *Series of American clinical lectures*, which was issued in monthly numbers from January 1875 to December 1879 by Putnam.

OP33. **CHARLES HARRISON VILAS** (1846–?). *Spectacles; and how to choose them, an elementary monograph.* 160pp. Chicago: Duncan Brothers, 1881.

Vilas was a homeopath who served as professor of diseases of the eye and ear at Hahnemann Medical College and Hospital in Chicago. Well known in homeopathy, he was president of its Western Academy. The preface is quite succinct in its message:

> The aim of this little work is so plain as scarcely to need an explanation. It is the intention to make clear, by an agreeable compound of medical and common terms, the uses and modes of fitting spectacles. Such intercurrent facts only as may serve to elucidate these subjects will be incorporated. The medical treatment, often so essentially accompanying the correction of diseases due to the anomalies of refraction and accomodation, forms no part of the scope of the work. The attempt to render the whole as entertaining as possible, must be an apology for a certain lack of connection apparent throughout the book. A too close adherence to any one topic would render the subject somewhat tedious, and while undoubtedly scientific, might induce the less ardent student to throw away in the beginning that which, when led on by easy stages, he would gladly read to the end . . . .

There are thirteen chapters: "The uses of spectacles"; "Lenses"; "Selection of a proper frame"; "The old and new ways of numbering lenses"; "How to test the eyes"; "How the sight is measured"; "The adjustment of glasses for hypermetropia"; "The adjustment of lenses for myopia";

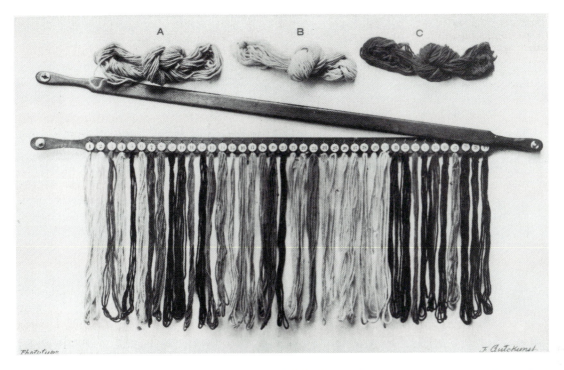

Fig. 59. (OP34) This photograph, on page 248, by noted Philadelphia photographer Frederick Gutekunst (1831–1917), shows one of the earliest tests for color blindness. Williams describes it as consisting of multiple strands of colored linens hung next to one another; the patient was asked to pick out certain shades.

"The adjustment of glasses for presbyopia"; "Spectacles for irregular-sight"; and "Other devices for aiding the accommodative effort." There are numerous interesting illustrations of various types of eyeglasses. The introduction provides a fascinating history of the use of spectacles (page 17). This was the only edition. (See also OP35, OP37, and OP49.)

OP34. **HENRY WILLARD WILLIAMS** (1821–95). *The diagnosis and treatment of the diseases of the eye.* 464pp. Boston: Houghton & Mifflin, 1882.

At the time this volume was published, Williams was professor of ophthalmology at Harvard University and ophthalmic surgeon at City Hospital. He was the first professor of ophthalmology at that institution. Williams writes in the preface:

> Several editions of a smaller work on diseases of the eye having been received with steadily increasing favor, the author ventures to offer to the profession another contribution to its literature, which he hopes may be acceptable and useful. In carefully preparing this new treatise, in which he has sought to embody that which his own observation and the recorded experience of others has proved to be of most value, the author has kept always in view his original purpose, and has endeavored to make his book a practical guide, serviceable to the general practitioner and to students . . . . Too elaborately scientific descriptions and statements of theories have been for the most part avoided . . . .

There are twenty-eight chapters covering a wide range of topics, including "Traumatic injuries" and "Artificial eyes." The book contains thirty-seven engraved illustrations and five plates, two of which are chromolithographs. The book also includes a folding eye chart plus five leaves of diagrams for eye examinations. The work was concurrently published in London. (See also OP13, OP15, and OP21.)

OP35. **CHARLES HARRISON VILAS** (1846–?). *The ophthalmoscope; its theory and practical uses.* 150pp. Chicago: Duncan Brothers, 1882.

This was the first book on ophthalmoscopy by a homeopath. The preface provides a rather apologetic introduction:

> This little volume is published to occupy a place hitherto vacant in medical literature, and supply a want which the author has felt as a teacher. Much labor has been expended to make a book of practical value. The author regrets that in his endeavor to be concise, omit all unnecessary diagrams, and abstain from rendering the volume hard to the novice, he is compelled to forego discussing the higher mathematics involved . . . . Inaccuracies in the details of some of the black-board diagrams are unavoidable. Mathematical precision must not be expected in rude sketches drawn to enable the reader to lay hold on points seemingly a little obscure . . . .

The fourteen chapters include "Reflection, refraction, and the formation of images"; "Theory of the ophthalmoscope"; "Description of different instruments"; "Practical application of the ophthalmoscope"; "The relative value of the direct and indirect methods"; "Examination of the healthy eye"; "Ophthalmoscopic appearances in disease and malformation"; "Refractive disorders"; "Fundus of the eye"; and "Ophthalmoscopic optometry." There was only one edition. (See also OP33, OP37, and OP49.)

OP36. **JOSEPH HOWARD BUFFUM** (1849–?). *The diseases of the eye: their medical and surgical treatment.* 428pp. Chicago: Gross & Delbridge, 1884.

Buffum was professor of ophthalmology and otology at Chicago Homeopathic Medical College. He dedicated his book to Timothy F. Allen (1837–1902), who had been his mentor at New York Homeopathic Medical College. Buffum received his post-medical school training at the New York Ophthalmic Hospital. He writes in the preface: "In the preparation of this work it has been the design of the author to state as concisely and briefly as possible the present views of ophthalmic science. The endeavor has been to make the work practical and at the same time as thorough as the importance of the subject demands . . . . " The twenty-one chapters consist of "General anatomy"; "Methods of examination"; "General treatment"; "Wounds and injuries"; "Errors of refraction"; "Affections of the muscles"; "Diseases of the orbit"; "Lachrymal apparatus"; "Lids"; "Conjunctiva"; "Cornea"; "Sclera"; "Iris"; "Ciliary body"; "Lens"; "Vitreous"; "Choroid"; "Retina"; "Optic nerve"; "Glaucoma"; and "Sympathetic ophthalmia." There are 150 wood engravings and twenty-five color lithographs. Most of the color plates were taken from Jules Sichel's (1802–68) *Iconographie ophthalmologique* (Paris: J. B. Baillière, 1852–59). In addition, the book contains a sheet of Snellen test-types. Buffum also wrote *Household physician* with Ira Warren (Boston: Physician's Publishing, 1905). (See also OT62 and OP59.)

OP37. **CHARLES HARRISON VILAS** (1846–?). *Therapeutics of the eye and ear.* 233pp. Chicago: W. A. Chatterton, 1883.

Vilas was quite prominent as an oculist and aurist. In 1883, Vilas was president of the American Ophthalmological and Otological Society. He writes in the preface:

> When the author began his teaching of diseases of the eye and ear . . . he found no text-book adapted to the wants of beginners. This volume is the outgrowth of some notes then made on the therapeutics of the eye and ear, and printed for the author's convenience as a teacher. Published for the use of his students they found favor to an extent beyond what he deemed their merits, and he allowed them to be sold to the profession. They were never designed as, or thought to be, complete, or necessarily original, but aids embracing that which the author considered ought to be understood by the pupils entrusted to his teaching . . . . Many of his old pupils have requested the publication of the notes in bookform; from which it is hoped that this volume will prove valuable to the general practitioner who, though he shun all operations, is compelled from the nature of the diseases to treat many of them until such time as the patients can be sent to a specialist in these diseases. No endeavor, therefore, has been made to get up a large volume, but one as practical as possible . . . .

Under "Ocular therapeutics" are found discussions of the "Cornea"; "Iris"; "Conjunctiva"; "Glaucoma"; "Local applications"; "Refraction and accomodation"; "Lids"; "Lachrymal apparatus"; "Injuries"; and "Tumors." "Aural therapeutics" includes the "External ear"; "Middle ear"; and "Internal ear." The most interesting aspect of the entire text is a massive homeopathic repertory of the eye (pages 147–230). (See also OP33, OP35, and OP49.)

OP38. **ADOLF ALT** (1851–1920). *A treatise on ophthalmology for the general practitioner.* 244pp. Chicago: J. H. Chambers, 1884.

Alt played a major role in the development of American ophthalmology. He received his medical education and training in Germany but settled in America in 1875, where he spent a few years in New York as an assistant to Hermann Knapp (1832–1911). In 1879, Alt moved to Toronto and permanently settled in St. Louis in the following year. In 1880 he published simultaneously in America and Germany a treatise on the normal and pathological histology of the human eye, *Lectures on the human eye in its normal and pathological conditions* (New York: G. P. Putnam's Sons, 1880). In Germany the book was published under the title, *Compendium der normalen und pathologischen histologie des auges* (Wiesbaden: J. F. Bergmann, 1880). The success of this book provided him worldwide recognition. In 1884 he established the *American journal of ophthalmology*, which was the first ophthalmological journal published in America west of New York. The *Treatise* is dedicated to John Green, about whom Alt writes:

> I have taken the liberty of dedicating this book to you, and I hope you will accept it as a token of my grateful esteem and friendship. You may, however, ask what motives prompted me to write this book, and thus to add one more to the long list of manuals on ophthalmology, which

the last few years have produced. Was there any need of another such manual? Or, can this book offer anything new? I confess that I would not have undertaken to write this book, had I not been asked to do it . . . . It appeared to me that, after all, there may be a want which previous works do not exactly supply, and which I might, perhaps, succeed in supplying. I mean that a book on ophthalmology, written solely for the general practitioner and his wants, was not among them. I mean a book, which the general practitioner would really peruse, and not lay aside because overburdened with details relating to subjects of little or no use to him; in short, a book which would give the general practitioner a clear idea of the principles of ophthalmology, together with so much only of its practice as he might be reasonably justified in attempting . . . . The present volume, then, is not intended for specialists, nor does it aim at making an oculist out of every general practitioner. It is, however, intended to serve as a guide for the general practitioner, as to when he may conscientiously take upon himself the responsibility of dealing with an eye affection, and when he had better not do so . . . .

This difficult-to-find work is divided into twenty-six chapters: "Anatomy"; "Examination"; "Diseases of the eye-lids"; "Lachrymal apparatus"; "Orbit"; "Minor manipulations in the treatment of eye-diseases"; "Conjunctiva"; "Cornea"; "Sclerotic"; "Iris"; "Ciliary body"; "Choroid"; "Retina"; "Optic nerve"; "Crystalline lens"; "Vitreous body"; "Injuries of the eye-ball and their consequences"; "Sympathetic ophthalmia"; "Errors of refraction and accommodation"; "External muscles"; "On the diagnostic value of eye-diseases in intra-cranial affections"; "Eye-affections caused by diseases of distant organs"; "On the detection of one-sided simulated blindness and congenital color-blindness"; "On the most important operations on the eye-ball and the eye-lids"; and "Drugs most commonly used in ophthalmic practice." The book contains one

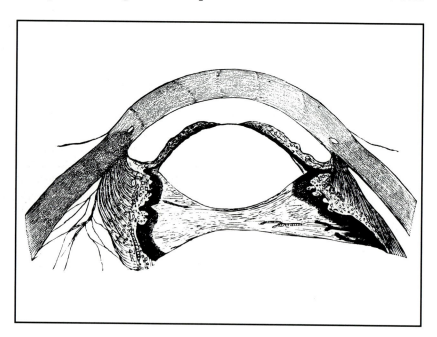

Fig. 60. (OP38) Alt describes a fibrino-plastic cyclitis as the most frequent form of inflammation of the ciliary body. This illustration, figure 47 on page 118, shows a cyclitic membrane which lies upon the posterior surface of the crystalline lens.

plate and eighty-two wood engravings. An extensive index is found at the end of the work.

OP39. **EDWARD GREELY LORING** (1837–88). *Textbook of ophthalmoscopy.* 2 vols., 259pp. and 253pp. New York: D. Appleton, 1886–91.

Loring's *Textbook* was issued in two volumes. Unfortunately, he died before finishing the second volume, and it was edited by Francis B. Loring, his brother, and published posthumously. This was Loring's most notable work. The first part focuses on the "Normal eye"; "Determination of refraction"; "Diseases of the media"; "Physiological optics"; and "The theory of the ophthalmoscope." It is the last topic which provides most of the contents of the six chapters. The editor's preface to the second volume describes how the work was finished:

> Dr. E. G. Loring, the author of this work, died suddenly on the 23rd of April, 1888, before its completion. It was my original intention, on assuming the charge of the manuscript that he left, to complete it, simply in order to present it in a finished state to the public. After a careful reading of it, however, I found that there was so much original matter in it, so much that from its very nature must provoke discussion and argument that I determined to publish it as it stood, without addition or correction . . . .

There are seven chapters in the first part, most of which concern "Diseases of the retina"; "Optic nerve"; and "Choroid." Four chromolithographic plates containing fourteen figures and 131 other illustrations are included in the first volume. Some of the plates in the second volume, unlike those in the first, are not original to Loring. Each volume was available in cloth for $5.00. There were no other editions. (See also OP25.)

OP40. **WILLIAM F. MITTENDORF** (?–?). *Granular lids and contagious diseases of the eye.* 110pp. Detroit: George S. Davis, 1886.

This work was issued as volume 10 in Series I of Davis's Physician's Leisure Library. At the time of its publication, Mittendorf was ophthalmic surgeon at the New York Eye and Ear Infirmary and Bellevue Hospital's Out-Door Department. He notes in the introduction:

> The importance of an early diagnosis of contagious diseases of the eye is so evident that it cannot be over estimated. The fact is, that thousands of children in our public institutions have been suffering from conjunctival affections when their existence was not known to the officers in charge, and in many instances not even to the attending physician. It is especially in the chronic forms of conjunctival troubles, the onset of which is often very insidious, that the disease is overlooked or not recognized until its ravages have crippled the patient for the remainder of his life . . . .

The eight chapters consist of "Methods of examination"; "Means of diagnosis"; "Anatomy of the conjunctiva"; "Symptoms and pathology"; "Causes"; "Treatment"; "Nature of granular lids"; and "Treatment of granular lids." There are no plates or illustrations. (See also OP31.)

OP41. SWAN MOSES BURNETT (1847–1906). *A theoretical and practical treatise on astigmatism.* 245pp. St. Louis: J. H. Chambers, 1887.

Burnett was an important figure in American ophthalmology. He served as professor of ophthalmology and otology at Georgetown University. He also served as surgeon at the Garfield Hospital and Central Dispensary and Emergency Hospital in Washington. Burnett received his M.D. in 1870 from Bellevue Hospital Medical College and soon established a practice in Knoxville. In 1875, he moved to the District of Columbia, where he gained prominence as a specialist in ophthalmology and otology. The *Treatise* is his best-known work and was one of the earliest such texts in the world. Burnett writes to the reader:

> The addition of one more medical book—even though it be a small one—to the scores that are annually issued from the press, carries with it a demand, on the part of the reading public, for its raison d'être. The cause of the existence of this little work has its foundation in my own needs as developed in my studies of refractive anomalies, and in my conception of the needs of others as manifested to me during the last eight years as a teacher of general and special students and general practitioners . . . fully aware that time and patience are two most important and indispensible factors, in unraveling the tangled threads of evidence, it cannot be doubted that nowhere in the whole range of medical practice, is accurate knowledge, based on positive science, of such avail as in the diagnosis of astigmatism. To lead to such accurate knowledge through the paths of positive science has been the chief incentive to my labor . . . . One word in regard to the bibliography. Without asking any undue indulgence for its imperfections and shortcomings, we would call to the mind of the captious critic the apothegm of an old and experienced bibliographer: "If a man have a pride of accuracy, and desires to be cured of it, let him make a bibliography." I trust that our labors in this regard may not be without value, particularly to the future writer on the subject, for we believe that, in that far away time, should the New Zealander, prowling among the ruins of the great medical library on the banks of the Potomac, stumble on a copy of this work, he will find recorded there the title of every important paper on the subject that has appeared up to the year of Grace 1886 . . . .

The thirteen chapters cover a wide array of topics related to astigmatism, with an interesting description of skiascopy (the shadow test) on pages 115–23. There are fifty-nine diagrams and illustrations. This is the only edition. Burnett's other book is *The principles of refraction in the human eye, based on the laws of conjugate foci* (Philadelphia: Keystone, 1904). Burnett's first wife, Frances E. Hodgson, wrote the famous children's classics *Little Lord Fauntleroy, The secret garden,* and *The little princess.*

OP42. LAWRENCE WEBSTER FOX (1853–1931) and **GEORGE MILBRY GOULD** (1848–1922). *A compend of the diseases of the eye, including refraction and surgical operations.* 148pp. Philadelphia: P. Blakiston, 1887.

This volume is the eighth in Blakiston's Quiz Compend Series. At the time of its publication, Fox was ophthalmic surgeon at Germantown Hospital and clinical assistant in the ophthalmological department of

FIG. 26.

Fig. 61. (OP42) Fox and Gould attributed this papillitis (number 26, page 102) to tobacco and called it tobacco amblyopia or chronic retro-bulbar neuritis.

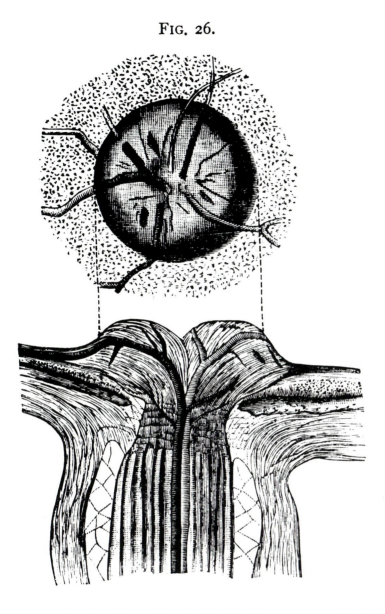

Jefferson Medical College Hospital. Gould was a student at Jefferson when he collaborated with Fox. Although he was older than the senior author, Gould did not receive his M.D. until 1888. He had previously served as a minister after graduating from Harvard Divinity School in 1874. Although Gould was well known as an ophthalmologist through his practice in Philadelphia and Ithaca, his primary reputation was based on his work as an author of medical dictionaries, editor, and writer. He served as editor of *Medical news* from 1891 to 1895, of the *Philadelphia medical journal* from 1898 to 1900, and of *American medicine* from 1901 to 1906. Fox and Gould write in the preface:

> It is needless to say the present little work aims at no exhaustive treatment of any branch of the subject, and is not designed for specialists. It has in view two definite and modest purposes: first, to supply the medical undergraduate with the most notable points concerning the

diagnosis and treatment of ocular disorders, whether pathological or refractive . . . . Our second object has been to give the busy general practitioner, who has never considered the importance of this knowledge to himself, or has relied upon his neighbor, the oculist, to do all such work for his patients, a few outlines of the science. Were he, even to a limited extent, master of such outlines, his patients would often be spared much suffering and himself much chagrin . . . .

There are four parts: "Refraction of the eye"; "Functional disorders affecting vision"; "Diseases of the eye"; and "Surgical operations, etc., instruments." There is one plate, which demonstrates a horizontal section of the right eye. A second edition was published in 1888. Gould issued a new edition without Fox in 1897. Walter L. Pyle (1871–1921) was coeditor of this work, which was itself revised in 1903.

Gould's other books consist of *A new medical dictionary; including all the words and phrases used in medicine; with their proper pronounciation and definitions* (Philadelphia: P. Blakiston & Son, 1890), *A pocket medical dictionary, giving the pronounciation and definition of about 11,000 of the principal words used in medicine and the collateral sciences* (Philadelphia: P. Blakiston & Son, 1892), *The meaning and the method of life; a search for religion in biology* (New York: G. P. Putnam's Sons, 1893), *An illustrated dictionary of medicine, biology and allied sciences* (Philadelphia: P. Blakiston & Son, 1894), and *Borderland studies; miscellaneous addresses and essays pertaining to medicine and the medical profession, and their relations to general sciences and thought* (Philadelphia: P. Blakiston & Son, 1896–1908). He was also editor of *An American year-book of medicine and surgery, being a yearly digest of scientific progress and authoritative opinion in all branches of medicine and surgery, drawn from the journals, monographs, and text-books of the leading American and foreign authors and investigators* (Philadelphia: W. B. Saunders, 1896); *Anomalies and curiosities of medicine; being an encyclopedic collection of rare and extraordinary cases, and of the most striking instances of abnormality in all branches of medicine and surgery, derived from an exhaustive research of medical literature from its origin to the present day* (Philadelphia: W. B. Saunders, 1897), with Walter L. Pyle; *Suggestion to medical writers* (Philadelphia: Philadelphia Medical Publishing, 1900); *A cyclopedia of practical medicine and surgery: a concise reference book, alphabetically arranged, of medicine, surgery, obstetrics, materia medica, therapeutics, and the various specialties, with particular reference to diagnosis and treatment* (Philadelphia: P. Blakiston's Sons, 1900); and the two-volume *Jefferson Medical College of Philadelphia, a history* (Chicago: Lewis Publishing, 1904). Gould's massive literary output has been chronicled in *Bibliography of the contributions of George M. Gould, M.D., to ophthalmology, general medicine, and literature* (Ithaca: Andrus & Church, 1909). Fox's other books are *Diseases of the eye* (New York: D. Appleton, 1904) and *A practical treatise on ophthalmology* (New York: D. Appleton, 1907).

OP43. **DANIEL BENNETT ST. JOHN ROOSA** (1838–1908). *The determination of the necessity for wearing glasses.* 73pp. Detroit: G. S. Davis, 1887.

Roosa was professor of diseases of the eye and ear at New York Post Graduate Medical School when this book was issued as part of Davis's Physician's Leisure Library (series I, volume 8). Roosa explains in the prefatory note:

> The object of this little book, is to serve as a guide to the general practitioner in determining whether a given patient does or does not require glasses, either to aid the vision or to relieve a symptom that may not be directly referred to the eye. It is by no means a complete manual of errors of refraction or failures in accommodation, but I believe that a careful study of these pages, will enable the practitioner to decide in a large proportion of cases, when the question comes up, whether or not glasses will probably be of service. I also hope, that the very busy man who is not inclined to seriously study the subject treated of in this little volume may get from the short time that he devotes to it, an accurate idea of how much has been accomplished in the last quarter of a century in adjusting glasses for the improvement of sight, and the mitigation and cure of distressing symptoms.

The five chapters consist of "History of test-types and the ophthalmoscope"; "Presbyopia"; "Myopia"; "Hypermetropia"; and "The value of prismatic glasses." (See also OT14, OP26, OP60, and OP84.)

OP44. **JOHN HERBERT CLAIBORNE** (1861–1922). *The theory and practice of the ophthalmoscope; a handbook for students.* 77pp. Detroit: G. S. Davis, 1888.

Claiborne received his M.D. from the University of Virginia in 1885. He established a practice in New York, where he eventually became professor of ophthalmology at New York Polyclinic and instructor at Columbia University. Claiborne makes no claim to originality in the preface:

> In presenting this brochure to the medical profession the author has not hoped to establish a claim for originality. The lines are cast in familiar places. His object has been to present in a clear and brief manner the main facts in ophthalmoscopy and the method of using the ophthalmoscope . . . .

The work was part of Davis's Physician's Leisure Library (series III, volume 4). The nine chapters cover a wide range of topics; a detailed selection of mydriatics appears on pages 74–77. There are no plates. Claiborne's other medical book is *Cataract extraction; being a series of papers with discussion and comments read before the ophthalmological section of the New York Academy of Medicine, 1907–1908* (New York: William Wood, 1908). (See also OP62.)

OP45. **CHARLES FREDERICK PRENTICE** (1854–?). *Dioptric formulae for combined cylindrical lenses applicable for all angular deviation of their axes.* 48pp. New York: J. Prentice & Son, 1888.

Prentice is an important person in the history of American ophthalmologic sciences. He is considered the father of modern day optometry, and, although not a medical doctor, nonetheless played a substantial role in the development of ophthalmology. He practiced in New York, where he was a partner with his father, James Prentice. This small monograph was dedicated to both Swan M. Burnett (1847–1906) and Richmond Lennox (1861–95). Prentice notes in the preface that

> . . . Dr. Swan M. Burnett . . . kindly suggested the execution of plastic models of combined cylindrical lenses, by placing a set of these, conceived and hastily prepared by himself, in my hands for further elaboration; with the request, if possible, also to produce two combinations in which the cylinders were to be united at angles other than right angles. As the result of my research, during the time devoted to the construction of the latter more especially, and with a view to establish confidence in the precision of these models, this mathematical demonstration is presented . . . . Suspecting my attempt to instruct, while in the capacity of an optician, may call forth unusual criticism, I trust the same will be mitigated when it is known that this effort is based upon the mere recollections of my earlier mathematical studies in Germany, which were prematurely terminated while in pursuit of a technical profession.

The contents include "Dioptric formulae for combined congeneric cylindrical lenses"; "Dioptric formulae for combined contra-generic cylindrical lenses"; "Dioptral formulae for combined cylindrical lenses"; "Sphero-cylindrical equivalence"; and "Verification of the formulae." There are four plates, and the frontispiece is an Albertype. Prentice also wrote *A treatise on simple and compound ophthalmic lenses, their refraction and dioptric formulae, including tables of crossed cylinders and their spherocylindrical equivalents* (New York: J. Prentice & Son, 1886), *Ophthalmic lenses, dioptric formulae for combined cylindrical lenses, the prism-dioptry & other optical papers* (Philadelphia: private printing, 1900), and *Legalized optometry and the memoirs of its founder* (Seattle: C. Fletcher, 1926).

OP46. **FRANCIS VALK** (1845–1919). *Lectures on the errors of refraction and their correction with glasses.* 241pp. New York: G. P. Putnam's Sons, 1889.

Valk practiced in New York City, where he was assistant to the chair of ophthalmology and otology and assistant demonstrator of anatomy at the University of the City of New York at the time the *Lectures* was published. He also lectured on diseases of the eye at New York Post-Graduate Medical School. These lectures, delivered in the years 1886 and 1887, were "received with many words of approval, and also with the request that I would publish them . . . . I know that many text-books treat this subject in perhaps a more scientific manner than it is here presented, but I have endeavored to make this work as simple and practical as possible . . . . " Most of the illustrations and diagrams are reproductions of blackboard drawings that Valk used in his lectures. The eleven lectures include "Anatomy"; "Refraction"; "Emmetropia"; "Hypermetropia"; "Myopia"; "Ophthalmoscopy"; "Muscular asthenopia"; "Astigmatism"; "Retinoscopy"; "Presbyopia"; and illustrative cases from Valk's practice. The first edition was reissued in 1890, and a complete revision was published in 1892. A third and final edition was printed in 1895. Valk also wrote *Strabismus, or squint, latent and fixed; a supplement to the errors of refraction* (New York: G. P. Putnam's Sons, 1904).

OP47. **EDWARD JACKSON** (1856–1942) and **E. BALDWIN GLEASON** (1854–1934). *Essentials of refraction and the diseases of the eye, and essentials of diseases of the nose and throat.* 276pp. Philadelphia: W. B. Saunders, 1890.

Number 14 in Saunders's Question-Compends, this widely read text, actually two volumes in one, was illustrated with 118 engravings. It was available in cloth for $1.00 or interleaved for notes for $1.25. Jackson was professor of diseases of the eye at Philadelphia Polyclinic and College for Graduates in Medicine at the time this volume was published. He was a graduate of Union College in New York and received his M.D. from the University of Pennsylvania in 1878. One of America's most prominent ophthalmologists, he resettled in Denver in 1898, and from 1905 to 1921 served as professor of ophthalmology at the University of Colorado. Gleason was surgeon-in-charge of the nose, throat and ear department of the Northern Dispensary of Philadelphia. The work includes two prefaces. Jackson writes in his preface:

> In deciding what to include, the writer has been guided by an acquaintance, gained in post-graduate teaching, with the needs and desires of the mass of medical graduates. For until the time of undergraduate study is extended, and ophthalmology made a compulsory branch of undergraduate instruction, but few will give it much attention during that period. A fair acquaintance with the general principles and facts of medicine and surgery is therefore presumed, and starting from this, the attempt is made to introduce the student to the essentials of this branch. It is also borne in mind that points of anatomy and physiology are given in other volumes of this series, which must be consulted, if their contents be not already stored for mental reference . . . . The student cannot be too strongly urged to combine with his reading a study of the laws of refraction, as they can be illustrated with a magnifying glass and piece of card-board; and of the appearance of his own normal eye, with a mirror. And if he can get a single normal fundus to study with the ophthalmoscope every day for a month, he has the best opportunity in the world for beginning the use of that instrument.

Part one on the eye (pages 17–148) contains ten chapters on essentials of refractions and nineteen chapters on diseases of the eye. Gleason notes in his preface:

> It is hoped that the following pages will be a sufficient excuse for themselves. It is admitted that, to the learned specialist, the information they contain will appear superficial; but superficial information has its value to a beginner as a foundation for that more profound knowledge which only comes slowly through years of extensive reading, thought, and actual work in the diagnosis and treatment of disease . . . . It is also thought that this little book may prove useful to the busy general practitioner who, from the force of circumstances, finds himself obliged to treat disease of the nose or throat, and can find quickly here, in a condensed form, the essentials of diagnosis and treatment in any given case . . . .

Part 2 contains sixteen major topic headings, including "Laryngoscope"; "Laryngoscopy"; "Laryngeal image"; "Rhinology"; "Rhinoscopy"; "Accessory instruments"; "Physiology and pathology of mucous membranes and 'catching cold'"; "Diseases of the nasal cavities"; "Septum"; "Pharynx"; "Tonsils"; "Larynx"; "Foreign bodies in the nose"; "Elongation of the uvula"; and "Post-nasal space or naso-pharynx." Further editions were published in 1894, 1901 and 1906. Among Jackson's other books are *A manual of the diagnosis and treatment of the diseases of the eye* (Philadelphia: W. B. Saunders, 1900). (See also OT60 and OP63.)

OP48. **HENRY DRURY NOYES** (1832–1900): *A textbook on diseases of the eye.* 733pp. New York: William Wood, 1890.

This is Noyes's major work and, although it was never published outside the United States, it commanded a significant amount of international attention. At the time it was written, he was professor of ophthalmology and otology at Bellevue Hospital Medical College and executive surgeon at the New York Eye and Ear Infirmary. It is illustrated by six chromolithographic plates, five black-and-white plates and 236 wood engravings. Noyes writes in the preface:

> This volume is an outgrowth from a treatise on diseases of the eye, published in December, 1881, in Wood's Library of Standard Medical Authors .... The spirit of the book is clinical, but an adequate preparation for clinical and practical work includes a wide range of preliminary knowledge .... This knowledge finds its chief application in unravelling functional disorders of sight, viz., such as concern the errors of refraction and accommodation, and motility .... In accordance with the practical intent of the book, mathematical formulae have been omitted .... the share which micro-organisms have in exciting diseases of the eye, has been fully recognized ....

The first part contains ten chapters: "General anatomy of the globe"; "General physiology of the eye"; "How to examine the eye"; "Ophthalmoscope"; "Glasses"; "Accommodation and its errors"; "Errors of refraction"; "Binocular vision"; "Strabismus"; and "Asthenopia." Part 2 presents twenty-two different topics, among which are specific anatomical areas of the eye and a final chapter (pages 698–703) of statistics on eye diseases. A second edition was published in 1894. (See also OP32.)

OP49. **CHARLES HARRISON VILAS** (1846–?): *Diseases of the eye and ear.* 117pp. Chicago: Boericke & Tafel, 1890.

This volume is actually a continuation of Vilas's previous work on the same subject, which he initially prepared for his students (OP36). He writes in the introductory notes that

> this volume is the outgrowth of some notes then prepared for the students and printed for the author's convenience as a teacher. They were never designed as, or thought to be, complete, or necessarily original, but were supplemented by clinical teaching, demonstrating the great majority of known diseases, and affording the opportunity to witness operations incidental to all branches of the art ....

There is no table of contents, but a brief index appears at the end of the work. There were no further editions. (See also OP33, OP35, and OP37.)

OP50. **CASEY ALBERT WOOD** (1856–1942). *Lessons in the diagnosis and treatment of eye diseases.* 154pp. Detroit: G. S. Davis, 1891.

Wood is remembered not only as an ophthalmologist, but also as an influential ornithologist and bibliophile. He was born in Wellington, Ontario, and received both a master of surgery and his M.D. from the University of Bishop's College, Montreal (now McGill University), the latter degree in 1877. After graduation, he practiced medicine, but his interest was eventually drawn to ophthalmology. In 1886, he trained at New York Eye and Ear Infirmary and shortly thereafter traveled to Europe for further study. He spent two years at the Royal London Ophthalmic Hospital (Moorfields) as a clinical assistant. On returning to America in 1890, he settled in Chicago, where he eventually became professor of clinical ophthalmology at Northwestern University. He lists himself on the title page of this work as microscopist and pathologist at the Illinois Eye and Ear Infirmary and oculist and aurist at Alexian Brothers Hospital. Among other positions he held within ophthalmology was the presidency of the American Academy of Ophthalmology and Otolaryngology. Wood also served as editor of the *Annals of ophthalmology* from 1896 to 1898 and of the *Ophthalmic record* from 1897 to 1918. The last twenty years of his life were devoted to ornithology and book collecting. In 1918 he was appointed to the editorial board of the *Annals of medical history*. The purpose of his *Lessons*, which was part of Davis's Physician's Leisure Library and available for twenty-five cents was

> ... to aid the physician to detect and treat, by means always at hand, those diseases of the eye which experience has shown are most frequently overlooked in the course of general practice .... Ocular diseases which are commonly and easily diagnosed by the nonspecialist are not so much dwelt upon as those that are more obscure .... Of course, this manual makes no pretension to being a complete treatise upon the subjects of its chapter headings ....

Among these ten headings are "The normal eye"; "The eye in disease"; "Diseases of the eyelids and conjunctiva"; "Lachrymal apparatus"; "Cornea and sclerotic"; "Iris and anomalies of the pupil"; "Cataract and other affections of the crystalline lens"; "Glaucoma"; "Ocular affections in general diseases"; and "Paralysis, squint, and other muscular troubles." There are no plates but numerous woodcuts. This was the only edition.

Wood's other books include *The eye, ear, nose and throat yearbook* (Chicago: Year Book Publishers, 1902), coedited on a biannual or triennial basis with Albert H. Andrews; *The common diseases of the eye; how to detect them and how to treat them* (Chicago: G. P. Englehard, 1904), cowritten with Thomas A. Woodruff; *A system of ophthalmic therapeutics; being a complete work on the non-operative treatment, including the prophylaxis of diseases of the eye* (Cleveland: Cleveland Press, 1909); the two-volume *A system of ophthalmic operations* (Chicago: Cleveland Press, 1911), the eighteen-volume *American encyclopedia and dictionary of ophthalmology* (Chicago: Year Book Publishers, 1913–1921), of which he was editor; and *The fundus oculi of birds, especially as viewed by the ophthalmoscope* (Chicago: Lakeside Press, 1917). As a bibliophile Wood compiled and edited *An introduction to the literature of vertebrate zoology based chiefly on the titles in ... libraries of McGill University* (Oxford: University Press, 1931).

OP51. **DAVID NEVENS SKINNER** (1841–92). *The care of the eyes in health and disease.* 116pp. Boston: J. G. Cupples, 1891.

Skinner practiced in Maine after receiving his M.D. from Bowdoin Medical College in 1867. He died a few months after publication of this volume. The nine chapters include "Anatomy and physiology of the eye"; "Physiology of vision"; "Defects of vision"; "Spectacles, their use and abuse"; "Diseases of the eyes of common occurrence"; "Injuries of the eyes"; "Suggestions pertaining to the care of the eyes"; and "Diseases of the eyes in infancy and childhood, with the results of school life upon the eyes." There are no plates and few illustrations.

OP52. **GEORGE EDMUND DE SCHWEINITZ** (1858–1938). *Diseases of the eye; a handbook of ophthalmic practice for students and practitioners.* 641pp. Philadelphia: W. B. Saunders, 1892.

Available by subscription only, this book was de Schweinitz's major contribution. At the time it was published, he was professor of diseases of the eye at Philadelphia Polyclinic and lecturer on medical ophthalmoscopy at the University of Pennsylvania. One of America's leading ophthalmologists, de Schweinitz received his M.D. from the University of Pennsylvania in 1881. In 1902, he was appointed professor of ophthalmology at his alma mater, where he served until 1924. Among his many honors were presidencies of the American Ophthalmological Society in 1916, the American Medical Association in 1922, and the International Congress of Ophthalmology in 1922. The *Diseases* was bound in either cloth for $4.00, sheepskin for $5.00 or half russia for $5.50. Illustrated with 216 woodcuts, the book also contains two chromolithographic plates. Among the most popular of ophthalmologic textbooks, it went through ten editions by 1924, and was one of the most respected works by an American ophthalmologist. De Schweinitz notes in the preface:

> This book has been written in the hope that it may prove of service to students and practitioners who desire to begin the study of ophthalmology. The methods of examining eyes, and the symptoms, diagnosis and treatment of ocular diseases have received the largest share of attention. The subject-matter has been given in greater detail than is customary in books written for students . . . .

James Wallace, chief of the eye dispensary at the University of Pennsylvania Hospital, wrote the sections on "General optical principles" and "Normal and abnormal refraction". Edward Jackson (1856–1942) wrote the section on "Retinoscopy." The twenty-two chapters include a detailed section (pages 92–138) on "Reflections"; "The ophthalmoscope and its theory"; "Ophthalmoscopy"; and "Retinoscopy." The final chapter (pages 572–624) presents various ophthalmologic operations. Among de Schweinitz's other books is *Pulsating exophthalmos, its etiology, symptomatology, pathogenesis, and treatment* (Philadelphia: W. B. Saunders, 1908), which he wrote with Thomas B. Holloway. (See also OT70 and OP67.)

OP53. **HOWARD FORDE HANSELL** (1855–?) and **JAMES H. BELL** (?–?). *A manual of clinical ophthalmology.* 231pp. Philadelphia: P. Blakiston & Son, 1892.

Hansell was lecturer on ophthalmology at Jefferson Medical College and Bell was demonstrator of anatomy and a member of the ophthalmological staff at Jefferson when this volume was published. It was their purpose

> . . . to place before the undergraduate and general practitioner of medi-cine, a brief review of the anatomy, physiology, refraction, and common diseases of the eye. No attempt has been made to treat the subjects exhaustively. Simplicity and brevity of statement have not been sacri-ficed to the mere attractiveness of literary finish. We have, in a word, endeavored in good faith, to make the volume conform to the purpose for which it was written, by giving it the character, directness, and practicability of clinical teaching and practice . . . .

None of the 120 illustrations or the few plates are original to the authors. The fifteen chapters include "General considerations"; "Physiological optics"; "Refraction"; "Ocular muscles"; "Diseases of the conjunctiva"; "Lids"; "Cornea and sclera"; "Crystalline lens and lens capsule"; "Uveal tract"; "Vitreous"; "Retina"; "Optic nerve"; "Orbital cavity"; "Glaucoma"; and "Operations." This was the only edition. Hansell's other books include *A text-book of diseases of the eye* (Philadelphia: P. Blakiston's Son, 1903), written with William M. Sweet; *Diseases of the eye; a treatise on the principles and practice of ophthalmic medicine and surgery* (Philadelphia: P. Blakiston's Son, 1906), also written with William M. Sweet; and *The ocular muscles; a practical handbook of the muscular anomalies of the eye* (Philadelphia: P. Blakiston's Son, 1910). (See also OP80.)

OP54. **J. MILTON JOHNSTON** (?–?). *Eye studies, a series of lessons on vision and visual tests.* 228pp. Chicago: J. M. Johnston, 1892.

Johnston was not a physician but an early optometrist. The book's dedication is quite interesting:

> To my mother whose spiritual face and spectacled visage have been before me since early childhood and still abide a living presence and inspiration,—to the growing thousands of students and practitioners in optics, whose high vocation is but just beginning to be appreciated,—to the many whose eyes have been correctly fitted, and the many more whose sight has been injured by inexcusable ignorance and misfits,—to all these this volume is dedicated, with the hope that their experience in the things of vision may prove an increasing delight till the dawn of an eternal morning, when we shall begin to see as we are seen.

Johnston notes in the preface:

> We first prepared and published our eye studies serially, in the *Johnston Eye Echo*, an optical journal edited by the author. With some exceptions . . . the contents of the series . . . appeared during the five years' continuance from 1885 to 1891 . . . . Those who read these lessons in serial form will notice a marked change in their character as now combined. Each topic, as here presented, is created in a single lesson . . . . We cannot forbear brief reference to encouraging progress in optical literature in the last few years. There was painful need of it . . . . To the best of the

writer's knowledge and belief he was the editor of the first journal of exclusively optical character. Its initial number appeared in Detroit 1886 . . . . The next purely optical journal of which we have knowledge was started in Chicago in the summer of 1886. Its career was brief. In 1891, optical journals were started respectively in London and New York, both called the *Optician* . . . . Now these journals, of which there are many of excellent quality, keep under pay a regular oculist or expert optician to conduct an optical department . . . .

The fourteen chapters include "Constituents of vision"; "Rays of light"; "Refracting media"; "Reflecting media"; "Emmetropia or normal sight"; "Ametropia or abnormal sight"; "Hypermetropia or far-sight"; "Myopia or near-sight"; "Astigmatism or asymmetrical sight"; "Strabismus"; "Asthenopia or weak sight"; "Color-blindness"; "Construction of test type"; and "How to fit the eye practically illustrated." This was the only edition.

OP55. **ARTHUR BRIGHAM NORTON** (1856–1919). *Ophthalmic diseases and therapeutics*. 552pp. Philadelphia: Boericke & Tafel, 1892.

A homeopathic ophthalmologist, Norton was professor of ophthalmology at the College of the New York Ophthalmic Hospital. He was also visiting oculist at Laura Franklin Free Hospital for Children. Well known for his writings, he edited the ophthalmologic section of the *North American journal of homeopathy* and from 1895–1906 was coeditor of the *Eye, ear and throat journal* in New York. This work was a continuation of previous contributions by Norton's brother George Salmon Norton (1851–91) (OP23). According to the preface,

> . . . this work has been completed in order to continue and carry out the plans of my brother, the late Dr. George S. Norton. For several years prior to his death it had been his desire to present to the profession a text-book upon ophthalmology, devoting especial attention to the homeopathic treatment of the diseases of the eye . . . . Finding, however, that the extensive demands upon his time from both college and hospital work, in addition to a large private practice, such a work would become too severe a tax upon his strength, he arranged with the writer to bring out such a book together . . . . As the object of the work has been to furnish the student and the general practitioner with a concise, practical manual, all useless verbiage has been discarded . . . . Special attention has been devoted to the homeopathic treatment of diseases; at the same time, knowing the importance of both local and operative measures, it has been our aim to omit nothing that may be of value in these methods . . . .

The 117 chapters comprising the first section of the book cover various disease states of the eye. The second part of the text (pages 377–538) provides a most interesting and detailed explanation of the homeopathic remedies for eye diseases. Arranged in alphabetic order (acetic acid to zincum), this section is a pharmacopeia of homeopathic medicines. There are two plates and numerous woodcuts. A second and third edition were both published in 1902. Norton's other book is *Essentials of diseases of the eye* (Philadelphia: Boericke & Tafel, 1904).

op56. **RICHARD JONES PHILLIPS** (1861–?). *Spectacles and eyeglasses, their forms, mounting, and proper adjustment.* 97pp. Philadelphia: P. Blakiston & Son, 1892.

A student of Edward Jackson (1856–1942), Phillips was instructor in diseases of the eye at Philadelphia Polyclinic and College for Graduates in Medicine. He also served as ophthalmic surgeon at Presbyterian Hospital in Philadelphia. This short work was an outgrowth of the lectures which he gave and was

> . . . intended to supplement studies in refraction, and to give the student that knowledge of the correct placing of the glasses before the eyes without which the most painstaking measurement of the refraction will frequently fail of practical result. With the popularization, as one may call it, of ophthalmology in the profession, many physicians who prescribe glasses are compelled, by the lack of skilled opticians in their neighborhood, to themselves furnish the spectacles to the patient. To these, it is believed, the knowledge which I have endeavored to impart in these pages will prove especially useful . . . .

The four chapters cover "General considerations"; "Principles of spectacle fitting"; "Prescription of frames"; and "Inspection and adjustment of spectacles and eyeglasses." There are forty-seven illustrations but no plates. Further editions were published in 1895, 1902 and 1908.

op57. **WILLIAM FISHER NORRIS** (1839–1901) and **CHARLES AUGUSTUS OLIVER** (1853–1911). *A textbook of ophthalmology.* 641pp. Philadelphia: Lea Brothers, 1893.

Norris was the son of George Washington Norris (1808–75) (GS79). He received his M.D. from the University of Pennsylvania in 1861 and studied ophthalmology in Vienna following service in the Civil War. In 1870 he returned to Philadelphia, where he eventually became professor of ophthalmology at his alma mater and one of the surgeons at Wills Eye Hospital. Norris served as president of the American Ophthalmological Society in 1884. His influence in ophthalmology was mostly the result of the large number of ophthalmologists who trained under him. Oliver also obtained his medical education at the University of Pennsylvania, finishing in 1876. Shortly thereafter he was appointed clinical clerk to Norris, the beginning of their lifelong association. At the time this textbook was published, Oliver had no academic position but was on the ophthalmological staff at Wills Eye Hospital and Presbyterian Hospital. The authors state in the preface that

> . . . the main purpose has been the presentation of such material as is necessary to convey a working knowledge of ophthalmology to students and practitioners. The work is not only representative of extensive research into the rich literature upon the subject, but is expressive of the result of careful clinical experience that has extended over many years of active practice . . . .

There are twenty-nine chapters, with Oliver having written the first ten (pages 19–282). Among the topics are "Optics"; "Ophthalmoscopy"; "Fundus-reflex test"; and the "Correction of errors of refraction and accommodation." Norris wrote the remainder of the book, which deals with various anatomical sections of the eye and their disease processes. Pages 622–27 contain different test-types. There are five chromo-lithograph plates and 356 engraved illustrations. There was only one American edition. An abridged Chinese translation by James B. Neal was published in 1894. (See also OP73.)

OP58. **GILES CHRISTOPHER SAVAGE** (1854–1930). *New truths in ophthalmology.* 152pp. Nashville: private printing, 1893.

Born in Tennessee, Savage attended two courses of lectures at Jefferson Medical College and graduated in 1878. He studied at the Royal

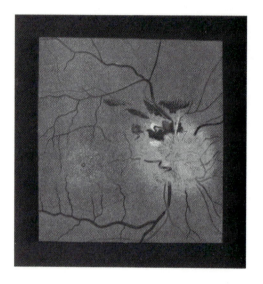

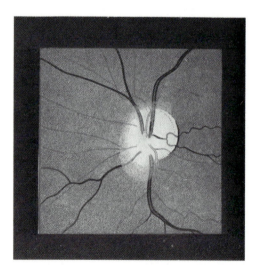

Fig. 62. (OP57) In this chromo-lithograph, figure 5 on page 474, Norris and Oliver demonstrate the ophthalmoscopic appearance of an early stage of papillitis and regressive neuritis.

Ophthalmic Hospital in London in 1884 and took ophthalmologic lectures at the General Hospital in Vienna from 1884 to 1885. In 1886 he settled in Nashville, where he practiced ophthalmology and otology for the remainder of his professional life. He founded the monthly journal *Ophthalmic record* in 1891 and served as professor of ophthalmology in the medical department of the University of Nashville and Vanderbilt University. *New truths* was dedicated to Samuel D. Gross (1804–85), who told Savage to "study a specialty." The volume consists of three parts: "New truths in ophthalmology"; "Contributions to old studies"; and "Operations." Many of the chapters are reprints of papers that Savage had published in medical periodicals. Savage makes little attempt to present the work of other ophthalmologists, and instead presents only his own views. There are thirty-two illustrations but no plates. A second printing of the work was issued in 1893, and a revised second edition was published in 1896. Among Savage's other books are *Ophthalmic myology, a systematic treatise on the ocular muscles* (Nashville: private printing, 1902), *Ophthalmic neuro-myology: a study of the normal and abnormal actions of the ocular muscles from the brain side of the question* (Nashville: private printing, 1905), and *The nervo-muscular mechanism of the eyes and routine in eye-work* (Nashville: private printing, 1916).

OP59. **JOSEPH H. BUFFUM** (1849–?). *Diseases of the eye and ear in children*. 80pp. Chicago: Gross & Delbridge, 1894.

Buffum was a well-known homeopathic aurist and oculist. He practiced in Chicago where he was one of the earliest members of the American Homoeopathic Ophthalmological and Otological Societies. This particular monograph is among the most difficult to find of American surgical texts. Even though it is listed in the Index catalogue of the library of the Surgeon-General's Office, neither the National Library of Medicine nor the Library of Congress has a copy. The book is important because it was one of the earliest full-length works devoted entirely to pediatric diseases. (See also OT62 and OP36.)

OP60. **DANIEL BENNETT ST. JOHN ROOSA** (1838–1908). *A clinical manual of diseases of the eye, including a sketch of its anatomy*. 621pp. New York: William Wood, 1894.

Roosa was professor of diseases of the eye and ear at New York Post-Graduate Medical School and Hospital and surgeon at the Manhattan Eye and Ear Hospital. He also served as president of the New York Academy of Medicine. This massive compendium was illustrated with 178 wood engravings and two chromolithographic plates. Roosa writes in the preface:

> This book has not been written because the author supposed, for an instant, that there were not already in the English tongue many excellent treatises on diseases of the eye. It is presented to the profession because I have not deemed that the debt I owe to it could be even approximately satisfied, nor my own reputation as a teacher, whatever

that may be, justly settled, unless I presented in a permanent and accessible form some of the results, with their personal coloring, of my long experience both in hospital and private practice, in ophthalmic

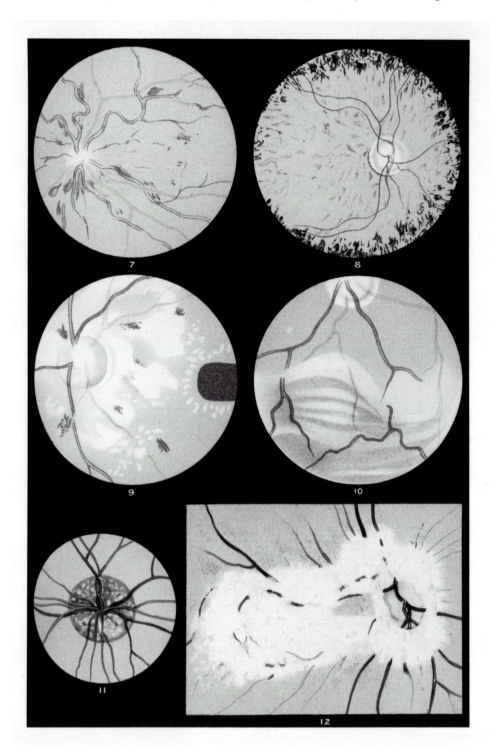

Fig. 63. (OP60) Various diseases of the retina and optic nerve are demonstrated in this chromolithographed plate. Roosa had Miss Elkins draw the bottom two figures from nature.

disease and therapeutics. To prepare a cyclopedic text-book of ophthalmology has not been my aim. The reader will not find in these pages a notice of all that has been described or suggested by the numerous writers upon diseases of the eye, but I trust that the book will be found a complete and safe guide to the practitioner . . . .

The work contains four parts: "Sketch of the anatomy and physiology of the various parts of the eye and its appendages"; "The relative frequency of different diseases of the eye, methods of examination, therapeutics and surgery of the eye"; "Diseases of the eyelids, the lachrymal apparatus, the conjunctiva, eyeball, and orbit"; and "Conditions of the eye requiring the use of glasses—errors of refraction and accomodation, strabismus, and affections of the ocular muscles." There was only one edition. (See also OT14, OP26, OP43, and OP84.)

OP61. **FLAVEL BENJAMIN TIFFANY** (1846–1918). *Anomalies of refraction and of the muscles of the eye.* 307pp. Kansas City: Hudson-Kimberly, 1894.

An 1874 graduate of the University of Michigan Medical School, Tiffany studied ophthalmology and otology in Europe from 1876 to 1877. After returning to the United States, he settled in Kansas City, where he eventually became professor of ophthalmology and otology at University Medical College of Kansas City. Quite fond of international travel, he wrote two interesting travel books, *Sojourn among the oculists of Europe* (Kansas City: Hudson-Kimberly, 1896) and *A trip around the world by an oculist* (Kansas City: Hudson-Kimberly, 1914). In the preface to *Anomalies* Tiffany writes:

> In no branch of medicine or surgery within the last decade has there been more attention given or more discoveries or advancements made than in the department of ophthalmology; particularly, the anomalies and affections of the ocular muscles and of refraction; and yet, these vast subjects of heterophoria and ametropia are still wrapped in a halo of uncertainties. That some anomaly of the ocular muscles, of refraction, or of both, is accountable for many of the pains, aches, and ills of the body and for many of the different forms of chorea and hysteria, is being more and more recognized by the profession in general . . . . It is said that the inmates of insane asylums, homes for the feeble-minded, and prisons are, with few exceptions, either ametropic or heterophoric. It would seem, then, that these anomalies may bear some intimate relation to man's moral nature . . . . In writing this little volume, it has been my purpose to present the subject in as clear, brief, and concise a manner as possible, embracing all essentials, besides collaborating recent advancements not to be found in the existing books . . . .

The comprehensiveness of the work is apparent from the very detailed nine-page index. Interestingly, Tiffany only devotes a few pages to the use of the ophthalmoscope. There are numerous illustrations, including several plates. Further editions were published in 1896, 1898 and 1900. Among his other books is *Anomalies and diseases of the eye* (Kansas City, Hudson-Kimberly, 1902).

OP62. **JOHN HERBERT CLAIBORNE** (1861–1922). *The functional examination of the eye.* 96pp. Philadelphia: Edwards & Docker, 1895.

Claiborne had received most of his ophthalmologic training under Emil Gruening (1842–1914) in New York. He was serving as adjunct professor of ophthalmology at New York Polyclinic and instructor of ophthalmology at the College of Physicians and Surgeon when this volume was published. The work was a result of a course of lectures which Claiborne had delivered for a number of years at both institutions. There are nine chapters: "Faculty of vision"; "Method of conducting the examination"; "Description of prisms, lenses and the trial case"; "Refraction of the eye"; "Application of the test card to the errors of refraction"; "Astigmatism"; "Cases of astigmatism"; "Presbyopia"; and "Mydriatics." Both Jaeger's and Snellen's test-types are located at the conclusion of the text. There are twenty-one illustrations. (See also OP44.)

OP63. **EDWARD JACKSON** (1856–1942). *Skiascopy and its practical application to the study of refraction.* 112pp. Philadelphia: Edwards & Docker, 1895.

Jackson held many important positions in American medical organizations. He was chairman from 1894 to 1895 of the American Medical Association's section on ophthalmology. In addition, he served as president of the American Academy of Ophthalmology and Otolaryngology in 1903 and of the American Ophthalmological Society in 1912. Jackson was chairman of the American Board of Ophthalmology for the first five years of its existence, from 1914 to 1919. Among the most prestigious posts he held was editor of the *American journal of ophthalmology* from 1918 to 1928. *Skiascopy* is considered among the more important of nineteenth-century American ophthalmologic contributions (the title reflects an obsolete term for both "retinoscopy" and "fluoroscopy"). Jackson was professor of diseases of the eye at the Philadelphia Polyclinic and College for Graduates in Medicine when the volume was published. He writes in the preface:

> This little book was written to bring about the more general adoption of skiascopy as an essential part of the examination for ametropia. It is not supposed that any ophthalmologist is quite ignorant of the test; but many do not know its full practical value, or how best to apply it. The demonstrations and descriptions here given assume a general knowledge of the eye and of physiological optics. And the writer, having observed that students of this subject do not generally think in the terms of algebraic formulas, but more readily grasp the graphic or geometric presentation of a fact, has governed himself accordingly . . . .

Among the eight chapters are "History, name, difficulties and study"; "General optical principles"; "Conditions of accuracy"; "Regular astigmatism"; "Aberration and irregular astigmatism"; "Practical application with plane mirror"; "Practical application with concave mirror"; and "General considerations." There are twenty-six illustrations but no plates. It was in this work that Jackson championed the use of the plane mirror and made five claims for its use: (1) skiascopy is an objective test, independent of the patient's intelligence or visual acuteness; (2) it is the most accurate objective test and the limits of its accuracy depend on details of its execution and the skill and patience of the observer; (3) it requires little more time than the use of the refraction ophthalmoscope or the ophthalmometer; (4) it requires no costly, complex or cumbersome apparatus; and (5) it reveals the refraction in each particular part of the pupil better than any other test. Further editions were published in 1896, 1898 and 1905. (See also OP47.)

OP64. **CHARLES N. McCORMICK** (1858–?). *Practical optics for beginners.* 101pp. Chicago: A. L. Swift, 1895.

McCormick taught at his family's Optical College in Chicago, where he was clinical instructor in ophthalmology. He notes in the preface:

> An expressed desire for elementary information, with reference to refraction and its application in optics, is the source of inspiration of this little work . . . . It is not our purpose to tell anything particularly new, but to use the simplest language and illustrations in telling an old story, so that those who, through a lack of time or opportunity, have failed to secure an optical education, may fit themselves at home sufficiently to treat successfully a very large per cent of the cases of defective vision which cannot be benefited by using the ordinary spectacles carried in stock by retail merchants . . . . Seventy-five per cent of the good optical service rendered the general public is performed by men and women who, without any claims of special prominence as "professor" or "doctor," conscientiously use their common sense and a set of trial lenses. Practical information on the use of the trial set and other instruments is herein given, with the hope that it may stimulate a more general desire for thorough education. We are all students. The field is broad, and we should endeavor to help one another for the common good to humanity.

There is neither a table of contents nor an index, which makes the volume difficult to peruse. This was the only edition. Among McCormick's other books are the two-volume *A system of mature medicine as taught in the McCormick Medical College* (Chicago: McCormick Medical College, 1916–22), and *Food composition and human ills, mental and physiological* (Chicago: McCormick Medical College, 1919). (See also OP78.)

OP65. **CHALMERS PRENTICE** (?–?). *The eye in its relation to health.* 214pp. Chicago: A. C. McClurg, 1895.

Prentice was a general physician who practiced in the Chicago area. Although not a specialist in ophthalmology, he firmly believed that nervous dysfunction and consequent diseases of the eye had a direct relationship to an individual's overall health. This work has no table of contents, but a detailed index (pages 211–14) lists his hypotheses. Among the topics are atrophy of the optic nerves and general debility (page 113) and the theory that latent eyestrain causes nervous derangement (page 43). Prentice also wrote *Eye, mind, energy, and matter* (Chicago: private printing, 1905).

OP66. **GERTRUDE ANNIE WALKER** (1863–?). *Students' aid in ophthalmology.* 183pp. Philadelphia: P. Blakiston & Son, 1895.

This volume is unique because it is the only book written by a female surgeon in nineteenth-century America. Walker was clinical instructor in diseases of the eye at the Woman's Medical College of Pennsylvania. She writes in the preface:

> Students entering upon a course of study of ophthalmology are confronted by many technicalities, and for this reason are often unable to profit by their observation of clinical cases. This book is intended for study preliminary to a course of clinical lectures upon the eye, or for reference during attendance upon such a course. Its preparation was suggested by experience in teaching and by observation of the difficulties felt by students of this branch of medicine. It is hoped that the book may prove useful to practitioners who desire to obtain sufficient knowledge of the specialty to enable them to diagnosticate and treat cases of ocular disease . . . .

The twelve chapters include "Method of examining the eyes"; "Lenses"; "Errors of refraction"; "Correction of errors of refraction"; "Optical instruments and their use"; "Ocular muscles"; "Diseases of the conjunctiva, lids, and lacrymal apparatus"; "Cornea, iris, and ciliary body"; "Choroid, sclera, and vitreous"; "Optic nerve, retina and glaucoma"; "Lens and orbit"; and "Brief descriptions of important operations." The book contains one chromolithographic plate of the normal fundus and forty other engravings. There were no further editions.

OP67. **GEORGE EDMUND** DE **SCHWEINITZ** (1858–1938). *The toxic amblyopias: their classification, history, symptoms, pathology, and treatment.* 238pp. Philadelphia: Lea Brothers, 1896.

De Schweinitz's essay was awarded the Alvarenga Prize of the College of Physicians of Philadelphia in October 1894. At the time he was professor of ophthalmology at the Philadelphia Polyclinic and clinical professor at Jefferson Medical College. This work and other writings by de Schweinitz in periodicals greatly advanced knowledge of toxic amblyopias, which were not then fully understood. He writes in the preface:

> Although the demonstration of axial neuritis has done much to clear away the fog which prevented the penetration of knowledge into the exact nature of the most important visual distrubances which arise under the influence of certain toxic substances, there are still many facts to be learned in regard to the etiology and pathology of a number of drug-amblyopias, and they furnish an inviting field for study and research. Therefore, a collection of our information with reference to them is desirable. To this end the present essay has been written . . . .

The book was printed in a deluxe binding as a limited edition and was available for $4.00. There were forty-six engravings and nine chromolithographic plates. Among the ten sections are "Drugs in class I with reference to alcohol, tobacco, bisulphide of carbon, iodoform, nitrobenzol, the coal-tar products, arsenic, and lead"; "Class II drugs especially anesthetics, opium, choral, bromide of potassium, and cannabis indica"; "Drugs in class III—caffein and thein"; "Class IV, quinine and salicylic acid"; "Classes V, VI, and VII, including mydriatics and myotics"; "Visual effects of filix mas in class VIII"; "Unclassified drugs"; "Ptomaines, toxal-bumins, meat-, fish-, and sausage-poisoning and serpent-virus"; and "Relation of hysteria to certain varieties of toxic amblyopia." This was the only edition. (See also OT70 and OP52.)

OP68. **JOHN ELLIS JENNINGS** (?–?). *Color-vision and color-blindness; a practical manual for railroad surgeons.* 115pp. Philadelphia: F. A. Davis, 1896.

Jennings practiced in St Louis, where he was lecturer on ophthalmoscopy and chief of the eye clinic at Beaumont Hospital Medical College. He graduated from the University of Pennsylvania and received most of his ophthalmologic training at the Royal London Ophthalmic Hospital in Moorfields. In the preface Jennings explains the importance of detecting color blindness:

> For a long time the theoretical problem of color-blindness has engaged the attention of the scientific world. The practical side lay dormant for many years until it was proved that this curious defect was the cause of disastrous accidents by rail and sea. Public attention became aroused, new and simpler methods of investigation were invented, and, as a result of much agitation, many railroad and steam-ship companies now require their employees to submit to an examination as to their color-sense . . . . The methods now employed have proved practical and efficient, and there is every reason to believe that all the railroads in this country would take measures to weed out the color-blind from the service if the frequency and dangers of this affection were brought to their notice. It is with the hope of stimulating further effort in this direction that this manual has been written. The author does not aim to be original, but has endeavored to produce a practical work on color-blindness which shall contain all that is essential to a perfect understanding of the subject, and to refer the reader to the proper authorities for many of the facts stated . . . .

Among the ten chapters are "An interesting historical sketch"; "Physiological anatomy of the retina"; "Physics of light and color-sensations"; "Theories of color-perception and color-blindness"; "Color-blindness"; "Methods for detecting color-blindness and selection tests"; "Pseudo-isochromatic tests, contrast tests, special tests"; "Acquired color-blindness"; "Pennsylvania Railroad Company's instruction for examination of employees as to vision, color-blindness, and hearing"; and "Descriptions of Oliver's series of tests for the detection and determination of subnormal color-perception (color-blindness), designed for use in railway service." The book has one plate and numerous engravings. A second edition was published in 1905. Jenning's other book is *A manual of ophthalmoscopy for students and general practitioners* (Philadelphia: P. Blakiston & Son, 1902).

OP69. **CLARENCE ARCHIBALD VEASEY** (1869–?). *Ophthalmic operations as practiced on animal's eyes.* 99pp. Philadelphia: Edwards & Docker, 1896.

This book is most unusual. Its author was adjunct professor of diseases of the eye at the Philadelphia Polyclinic and chief clinical assistant to the ophthalmological department of Jefferson Medical College Hospital. Veasey notes in the preface:

> This little work has been prepared in the hope that it may prove of assistance to those beginning the study of ophthalmology by enabling them to become acquainted with the technique of the various operative procedures through practice on animal's eyes, thus removing a certain amount of timidity and affording a larger experience and more confidence when attempting the operations on the human eye . . . .

The six chapters include "General considerations"; "Operations upon the cornea"; "Iris"; "Crystalline lens and capsule"; "Sclera"; and "Ocular muscles." There are fifty-six illustrations but no plates. Most of the engravings relate to various ophthalmologic instruments. The animal eyes described are those of a pig, sheep, and bullock. Veasey's other book is *A manual of diseases of the eye* (Philadelphia: Lea Brothers, 1903).

OP70. **CHARLES D'A. WRIGHT** (1863–?). *A handbook of the refraction of the eye, its anomalies and their correction.* 128pp. Ann Arbor: Sheehan, 1896.

Wright was a demonstrator of ophthalmology and otology at the University of Michigan when he dedicated this work to Flemming Carrow, who was his professor at the university. According to the preface

> the object of this little volume is to present, in a plain and practical form, an explanation of the anomalies of refraction and their correction. It substantially embodies the instruction given to the demonstration classes in the University of Michigan, and while it is intended, primarily, to facilitate the work of junior students in preparing the subject, the perusal of its pages may prove of benefit to other readers . . . .

The twelve chapters include "Lenses"; "Emmetropic eye"; "Visual acuity"; "Hyperopia"; "Myopia"; "Astigmatism"; "Presbyopia"; "Skiascopy"; "The ophthalmoscope"; "Eye muscle"; "Fitting of frames"; and "General remarks." This was the only edition.

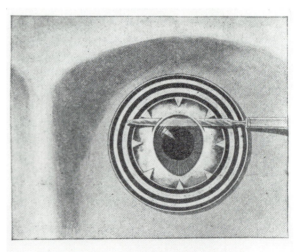

Fig. 64. (OP69) Veasey demonstrates an anterior sclerotomy in this engraving (number 43, page 72). He notes that it is "usually performed in certain cases of glaucoma—mostly of the chronic type, or in those cases in which an iridectomy had previously been performed, in spite of which an increase of the intra-ocular tension had returned."

Fig. 43. Anterior sclerotomy.

OP71. **JOHN WESTLEY WRIGHT** (1842–1935). *A textbook of ophthalmology.* 405pp. Columbus: J. L. Trauger, 1896.

Wright practiced in Columbus, Ohio, where he was professor of ophthalmology and clinical ophthalmology at Ohio Medical University. The object of his treatise was

> . . . to provide the medical student with a systematic text in the primary principles of ophthalmology, such as will be a reliable assistance to him in his pursuits of knowledge as a student of medicine. No apology can be necessary for the issuance of a work of this kind, when it is known that there is not a treatise that is particularly designed for the student in his class work in college, most works being intended for the skilled oculist . . . . While this treatise is especially intended for the student in his class work at college, it is no less adaptable for him as a general practitioner, for what is necessary for the student to know and understand thoroughly . . . .

The twenty-three chapters include a wide range of topics. Among the more interesting areas are "Therapeutics of the eye" (chapter 20); "Retinoscopy" (chapter 21); and "The perimeter-Placido's disc-ophthalmometry" (chapter 23). There are four pages (360–64) of illustrations of instruments and a detailed glossary of terms related to the eye (pages 365–98). The book has 101 illustrations. Second and third editions were published in 1900 and 1909, respectively.

OP72. **ALEXANDER DUANE** (1858–1926). *A new classification of the motor anomalies of the eye based upon physiological principles, together with their symptoms, diagnosis, and treatment.* 100pp. New York: J. H. Vail, 1897.

Duane graduated as valedictorian of his class from Union College in New York in 1878. After receiving his M.D. from the College of Physicians and Surgeons in New York, he practiced general medicine until 1887. He became associated with Hermann Knapp (1832–1911), and his interest turned toward ophthalmology. At the time the *Classification* was written, Duane was assistant surgeon at the Ophthalmic and Aural Institute of New York, and for this work he was awarded the Alumni Association Prize of his medical alma mater. Duane became quite prominent in American ophthalmology and served as president of the section on ophthalmology of the American Medical Association from 1917 to 1918 and of the American Ophthalmological Society in 1923. In 1919 he received an honorary doctorate from Union College and became a trustee of that college in 1923. The book has no table of contents nor index, but, as Duane writes in the preface:

> The following brochure represents the result of some ten years' labor and study expended upon the subject of muscular anomalies. Whatever merit it may have is due to the fact that it stands for original investigation in a field still full of difficulties and obscurities . . . . Many of these principles and methods have been enunciated in lectures given to successive classes of practitioners, and have been demonstrated in their practical applications upon patients before the same gentlemen . . . .

Duane also wrote the *Student's dictionary of medicine and the allied sciences* (Philadelphia: Lea Brothers, 1893) and *Rules for signalling on land and sea* (1899).

OP73. **WILLIAM FISHER NORRIS** (1839–1901) and **CHARLES AUGUSTUS OLIVER** (1853–1911). *System of diseases of the eye; by American, British, Dutch, French, German, and Spanish authors.* 4 vols., 672pp., 556pp., 962pp. and 949pp. Philadelphia: J. B. Lippincott, 1897–1900.

A massive compendium, this four volume set was the first such "system" to be published in the English language. According to the editors, the *System*

> . . . embraces the most advanced theoretical and practical views on the subject that could be systematically grouped in a single publication. The editors believe that, by a careful selection of material and by the aid of many and able collaborators, a work has been produced which will take a place in the English language similar to that occupied by the "Handbuch" of Graefe and Saemisch in German and by the "Traité complet" of de Wecker and Landolt in French, and which will be of service not only to ophthalmologists and special students, but also to the medical profession at large.

The four volumes contain 137 full-page plates and 973 text illustrations. Many of the plates have historical importance, since Norris was one of the early proponents of using actual photographs of the retina. He was probably the first to make photomicrographs with the wet-plate process in high powers. Both Norris and Oliver practiced in Philadelphia, where the latter was attending surgeon at Wills Eye Hospital. Oliver was later appointed associate clinical professor of ophthalmology at the Woman's Medical College in 1897 and full clinical professor in 1906. Oliver's association with Norris began in 1877 when, after receiving his M.D. from the University of Pennsylvania, he was appointed clinical clerk to Norris, who was then professor of ophthalmology at the university. Volume 1 deals with "Embryology"; "Anatomy"; and "Physiology" of the eye. Volume 2 covers "Examinations of the eye"; "School hygiene"; "Statistics of blindness"; and "Antisepsis". Volume 3 discusses "Local diseases"; "Glaucoma"; "Wounds and injuries"; and "Operations". The fourth volume includes "Motor apparatus"; "Cornea"; "Lens"; "Refraction"; and "Medical ophthalmology".

Among the American physicians who contributed to the *System* were Edward Jackson (1856–1942) (volume 1, pages 459ff., "Dioptrics of the eye" and volume 2, pages 89ff., "Skiascopy"); William Thomson (volume 1, pages 581ff., "Normal color-perception" and volume 2, pages 315ff., "Detection of color-blindness"); George M. Gould (1848–1922) (volume 2, pages 63ff., "The ophthalmoscope"); Samuel D. Risley (1845–1920) (volume 2, pages 353ff., "School hygiene"); Joseph A. Andrews (volume 2, pages 463ff., "Antisepsis"); Charles S. Bull (1844–1911) (volume 3, pages 3ff., "Diseases of the orbit"); George C. Harlan (1835–1909) (volume 3, pages 63ff., "Diseases of the eyelids" and pages 89ff., "Operations performed upon the eyelids"); Samuel Theobald (1846–1930) (volume 3, pages 133ff., "Diseases of the lacrymal apparatus");

Swan M. Burnett (1847–1906) (volume 3, pages 173ff., "Diseases of the conjunctiva and sclera"); Emil Gruening (1842–1914) (volume 3, pages 685ff., "Wounds and injuries of the eyeball and its appendages"); Robert L. Randolph (1860–1919) (volume 3, pages 721ff., "Sympathetic ophthalmia"); Hermann Knapp (1832–1911) (volume 3, pages 777ff., "Operations usually performed in eye-surgery"); Myles Standish (1851–?) (volume 4, pages 781ff., "Motor changes in the ocular apparatus associated with functional neuroses"); and George E. de Schweinitz (1858–1938) (volume 4, pages 797ff., "The toxic amblyopias"). Many of the foreign authors wrote their chapters in a language other than English. In these instances, American ophthalmologists provided the translation. There was only one edition. (See also OP57.)

OP74. **FRANK LARAMORE HENDERSON** (1865–?). *Notes on the eye, for the use of students.* 103pp. St. Louis: Shultz, 1897.

Henderson was professor of ophthalmology at Barnes Medical College in St. Louis. He also served as ophthalmic surgeon at St. Mary's Infirmary. The preface to this book, which was intended only for the use of his students, states:

> The object of this little handbook is to help students by giving them the elements of ophthalmology in a condensed form. It is not my desire to minimize medical education but to increase the knowledge of the graduate by simplifying the method of his instruction. The short time allotted to the eye in our medical schools and the large size of the text books on the subject are so disproportioned as to cause confusion and despair to the student. The result is abandonment of the textbook and reliance upon the notes taken in the lecture room. This little book, which contains nothing original, but has been compiled from standard works, is not intended to take the place of the large size text book, at least one of which every student and practitioner should have, but is designed to supplant the inaccurate notes taken by the student in the lecture room and to suppress a practice so disagreeable to the teacher and injurious to the pupil . . . .

Much to his discredit, Henderson comments on the utility of the ophthalmoscope in the preface: " . . . I have also slighted those diseases which have to be diagnosed with the ophthalmoscope as I doubt the diagnostic value of an ophthalmoscope in the hands of the average general practitioner . . . . " Further editions were published in 1900, 1903 and 1910.

OP74.1 **E. H. LINNELL** (?–?): *The eye as an aid in general diagnosis.* 248pp. Philadelphia: Edwards & Docker, 1897.

Linnell was at first a general practitioner but later devoted most of his time to the treatment of ophthalmologic conditions. He practiced in Norwich, Connecticut. Linnell dedicated this handbook to his father, J. E. Linnell, who was also a physician. He writes in the introduction:

> Examination of the eyes affords valuable aid not only in the diagnosis of diseases of the central nervous system, but also of constitutional affections and diseases of other organs. It has long seemed to the writer that this subject was too much neglected by the general practitioner . . . . It

has not been my purpose to enumerate all the eye symptoms . . . but rather to emphasize such as are of direct importance in the way of diagnosis, and to present such data so as to be of ready reference and practical value. The book has been written from the standpoint of the specialist for the student and general practitioner . . . .

There are three major sections with twelve chapters in all. The book contains four color plates, and a small number of engravings are scattered throughout the text.

OP75. **NATHANIEL L. MACBRIDE** (?–?). *Diseases of the eye.* 310pp. New York: Boericke, Runyon & Ernesty, 1897.

MacBride was dean of the College of the New York Ophthalmic Hospital and professor of ophthalmology at the same institution. He was a homeopathic physician. This volume was dedicated to Carl Theodore Liebold (1831–86), who had been one of MacBride's mentors. The rather succinct preface states:

> In preparing the following pages, the author has endeavored to set forth the results of his experience and study in a form that will prove most useful to the busy general practitioner. With this aim in view words have been used very sparingly, and only such remedies, operations, and means of diagnosis recommended as the writer believes will be found

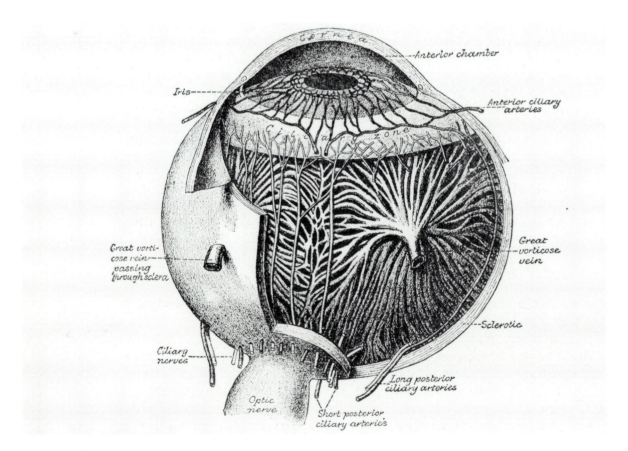

Fig. 65. (OP75) MacBride diagrams the principal nerves and blood vessels of the eyeball in this black-and-white engraving on page 92.

to be most useful in our present state of knowledge to the practical physician . . . .

There are sixteen chapters, including "Anatomy"; "Diseases of the conjunctiva"; "Cornea"; "Sclera"; "Iris and ciliary body"; "Retina"; "Principles governing vision"; "Refraction and accomodation"; "Glaucoma"; and "Operations." There is one chromolithographic plate, but diagrams and eyecharts are scattered throughout the text. Pages 267–68 contain engravings of various instruments used in ophthalmic surgery. On pages 11 and 12 is a list of remedies relating to eye pathology. Interestingly, the text notes only a few homeopathic preparations. This is the only edition.

OP76. **AMBROSE LOOMIS RANNEY** (1848–1905). *Eye-strain in health and disease; with special reference to the amelioration or cure of chronic nervous derangements without the aid of drugs.* 321pp. Philadelphia: F. A. Davis, 1897.

Ranney began to do research on a causal connection between eyestrain and functional nervous disease relatively early in his career, although he was already well known in New York, having served as president of the New York Academy of Medicine. His views were considered quite controversial. He was no longer affiliated with any academic institution when this volume was published. He notes in the preface:

> This volume comprises the substance of several monographs that the author has published from time to time during the past ten years in medical journals, with the addition of considerable new matter. He has added, also, the histories of many typical cases in detail with the view of illustrating some remarkable results of eye-treatment alone upon various forms of nervous disturbances that have persisted for years and failed to yield to any other form of treatment . . . . To the critics the author would say that three facts should not be lost sight of in this volume,—viz., that none of the cases here reported took any drugs while under his care, that they were chronic cases which had received no benefits from medical men under skillful hands, and that many of them were made absolutely well by eye-treatment alone . . . . While the author does not expect that his critics will accept all of his conclusions, he has a right to ask that the work be read without prejudice prior to criticism and that the reviews be dispassionate. The time has passed when violent antagonism or ridicule can have much weight in opposing the progress of any method of treatment of diseases that is scientific and positive rather than speculative or empirical . . . .

The ten chapters encompass "The bearings of eye-strain upon the duration of human life"; "Tests of vision and ocular movements"; "Eye-strain as a cause of headache and neuralgia"; "The eye-treatment of St. Vitus's Dance (chorea)"; "Sleeplessness"; "Eye-strain as a cause of chronic gastric and digestive disturbances"; "Eye-treatment of epileptics"; "Eye-treatment of nervous prostration and insanity"; "The surgical treatment of anomalies of the ocular muscles"; and "Eye-strain as a cause of abnormal eye-conditions." There are numerous text illustrations but no plates. This was the only edition. (See also GS94 and GS109.)

OP77. **JAMES THORINGTON** (1858–?). *Retinoscopy (or shadow test) in the determination of refraction at one meter distance, with the plane mirror.* 66pp. Philadelphia: P. Blakiston & Son, 1897.

Thorington practiced in Philadelphia, where he served as adjunct professor of diseases of the eye at the Philadelphia Polyclinic and College for Graduates in Medicine. Following graduation from medical school, he lived in Panama from 1882 to 1889, where he was a physician and surgeon with the Panama Railroad Company. Thorington writes in the preface:

> At the earnest solicitation of many students and friends, this book is presented as an abstract of the author's previous writings and lectures on retinoscopy . . . . While intended for college students and postgraduates, yet there is ample material given whereby the ophthalmologist at a distance may acquire a working knowledge of the method, by study and practice in his own office. For three reasons retinoscopy, in preference to skiascopy, has been chosen as the title; namely, that it may not be confounded with skiagraphy, as it is the name by which the test is universally known, and as it is the retina in its relative position to the refractive media, which we study.

There are six rather short chapters, the last two dealing with retinoscopy in irregular and regular ametropia. The book is illustrated with twenty-four engravings. The volume was quite well received and by 1911 had gone through six editions. Thorington also wrote *Refraction and how to refract; including sections on optics, retinoscopy, the fitting of spectacles and eye-glasses* (Philadelphia: P. Blakiston, 1900), *The ophthalmoscope and how to use it* (Philadelphia: P. Blakiston, 1906), and *Refractions of the human eye and methods of estimating the refraction* (Philadelphia: P. Blakiston, 1916).

OP78. **CHARLES C. BOYLE** (?–?). *Therapeutics of the eye.* 404pp. New York: Boericke, Runyon & Ernesty, 1898.

Boyle was a homeopathic physician who was professor of ophthalmic and aural therapeutics at the College of the New York Ophthalmic Hospital. The book was designed as a reference work and was available in cloth for $3.50 or half morocco for $4.50. Although there is no table of contents, the book is divided for convenience of consultation into three parts: "(I) A materia medica alphabetically arranged of symptoms pertaining to the eye"; "(II) Affections of the eye, under which are given different remedies with their applied therapeutics according to anatomical sections"; and "(III) A repertorial index, which serves either as a repertory or general index to the first two parts." This was the only edition.

OP79. **LAWRENCE J. DAILEY** (?–?). *Refractive and ophthalmic catechism, for the use of general practitioners, opticians, and students.* 218pp. Gloversville: Collins, 1898.

Dailey practiced in Gloversville, New York, where he was ophthalmologist and otologist at Nathan Littauer Hospital. He received his M.D. from the University of the City of New York in 1882 and later studied under Francis Valk (1845–1919) from 1891 to 1892. Dailey writes in the preface:

> In offering this little book to those who are interested in refractive work, it is in the hope that the author has succeeded in producing a work that will be, first of all, practical and accurate in its methods of determining and correcting the different refractive conditions. It makes no pretensions beyond being a concise and ready hand-book on the subject of refractive errors, and the instruments used in the work . . . . From the standpoint of the general practitioner, in which field the author labored for nine years previous to taking up special work, he hopes he has succeeded in presenting this subject to others in such a manner as to enable them to learn something about refractive errors and glasses without the necessity of reading several tomes . . . . To those who make a specialty of prescribing correcting glasses, and especially to the large number of opticians engaged in this work does the author recommend this book as embodying the most practical and latest methods of determining refractive errors . . . .

The fourteen chapters are "Anatomy of the eye"; "Refraction and lenses"; "Accommodation of the eye"; "Emmetropia and hypermetropia"; "Myopia"; "Astigmatism"; "Ophthalmoscopy"; "Ophthalmometry"; "Skiascopy"; "Presbyopia"; "Muscular asthenopia"; "Perimetry"; "Illustrative cases from note book"; and "Diseases and therapeutics of the eye." On page 199 there is an interesting glossary of ophthalmologic terms.

OP80. **CHARLES N. McCORMICK** (1858–?). *Optical truths, illustrated.* 152pp. Chicago: McCormick Optical College, 1898.

McCormick was president of McCormick Optical College in Chicago. As he did his previous work (OP64), he used this book as a diatribe against the influence of ophthalmologists in American medicine. The volume contains two parts, each with six chapters. The first six are "Laws of refraction stripped of complications"; "Measurement of lenses and prescription writing"; "Refraction of the dioptric system of the eye"; "The 'fogging' method of measuring errors of refraction"; "Machine test-objective and subjective methods compared"; and "The clinical value of perfectly adjusted frames and lenses." McCormick makes his accusations against ophthalmologists in the second part: "Exposing ophthalmological charlatans and their practices"; "Operations, medicines and prisms, three great ophthalmological blunders"; "Affection of the eyes"; "Anatomy and physiology of the eye"; "Mydriatics and myotics"; and "Color-blindness, and a comparison of the tests therefor." There is a fourteen-page appendix containing a quiz compend and embracing the principal points of practice. A glossary comprising a list of optical terms appears on page 147. A second edition was published in 1906.

OP81. **ALEXANDER W. STIRLING** (?–?). *Glaucoma; its symptoms, varieties, pathology and treatment.* 177pp. St. Louis: J. H. Parker, 1898.

Stirling was a native of England but was practicing in Atlanta when he published this volume. He received most of his ophthalmologic training at the Royal Westminster Ophthalmic Hospital in London. He eventually emigrated to America and became an assistant surgeon at the Manhattan Eye, Ear and Throat Hospital. This work consists of lectures that Stirling gave at the Post-Graduate Medical School and Hospital in New York. They were originally published serially in the *Annals of ophthalmology* and, on the urging of friends and professional acquaintances, he reproduced them in book form. There are fifteen chapters covering a wide range of topics. Chapters 4–7 are of particular interest because they present detailed discussions of various theories of the etiology of glau-coma. Sterling's work is important for two reasons: it is the first book by an American ophthalmologist to deal exclusively with glaucoma and it contains some of the earliest photomicrographs of the eye to appear in an ophthalmologic text. There were no further editions.

OP82. **HOWARD FORDE HANSELL** (1855–?) and **WENDALL REBER** (?–?). *A practical handbook on the muscular anomalies of the eye.* 182pp. Philadelphia: P. Blakiston & Son, 1899.

Hansell was a prominent ophthalmologist in Philadelphia, where he was clinical professor of ophthalmology at Jefferson Medical College and professor of diseases of the eye at Philadelphia Polyclinic and College for Graduates in Medicine. Reber was a recent medical school graduate and served as instructor in ophthalmology at the Polyclinic. The aim of the authors was

> ... to present to beginners in ophthalmic work, the principal facts in the diagnosis and treatment of abnormal states of the eye-muscles. The subject matter is an elaboration of a short series of lectures, delivered in successive winter courses at the Philadelphia Polyclinic. Stimulated by the interest displayed by the classes, and their constant inquiries for a practical text-book on the subject, the authors have endeavored to give book-form to their ideas about the muscular anomalies of the eye . . . .

The four parts include "An introduction to anatomy and physiology"; "Structural anomalies"; "Functional anomalies"; and "Operations on the eye muscles." There was one chromolithographic plate and twenty-eight illustrations. A second edition was published in 1912. (See also OP53.)

OP83. **CLIFFORD ELMORE HENRY** (1873–?): *A manual of osteopathic treatment of diseases of the eye.* 51pp. Minneapolis: private printing, 1899.

This book was one of the earliest books written by an American osteopath. It covers little in the way of operative treatment. Henry was professor of anatomy and osteopathic therapeutics at the Northern Institute of Osteopathy in Minneapolis. He states in the preface:

> This book is intended to deal with only those diseases of the eye that are amenable to osteopathic treatment, proven to be so by clinical results; where glasses or other treatment is necessary I have designated such treatment. The majority of the diseases of the eye are reflex, and the osteopath acting on this theory correcting the constitutional derangements, meets with a surprisingly large percentage of cures . . . .

The eleven chapters include "Method of examination"; "General consideration of treatment"; "Accommodation"; "Refraction"; "Abnormal conditions of the ocular muscles"; "Diseases of the lids"; "Lacrymal apparatus"; "Cornea and sclera"; "Iris, ciliary, body and choroid"; "Lens"; and "Optic nerve and retina." There are few illustrations and no plates. No further editions were issued. Henry's other book is *A manual of osteopathic therapeutics* (Minneapolis: private printing, 1898).

OP84. **DANIEL BENNETT ST. JOHN ROOSA** (1838–1908): *Defective eyesight; the principles of its relief by glasses.* 193pp. New York: Macmillan, 1899.

Roosa was professor emeritus of diseases of the eye in the New York Post-Graduate Medical School and Hospital and surgeon to the Manhattan Eye and Ear Hospital. He writes in a prefatory note:

> In 1888 the author of this volume published a little book entitled *The Determination of the Necessity for Wearing Glasses*. It was one of a series, by various authors, upon different subjects in medicine and surgery. It had a very favorable reception and large sale. The publisher, however, has lately retired from business, and transferred the copyright to the author with the suggestion that the book be republished, since it was still constantly asked for. On undertaking to revise this volume I found that it required a complete rewriting, so great has been the advance in our knowledge of the proper prescription of glasses, especially in the matter of simplicity in method. I have, therefore, carefully rewritten the book, introduced illustrations, and very much enlarged it. I have also ventured to change the title, as I think the present one explains its object a little better than the former. I hope this manual may be found a reliable guide to the student and practitioner in ophthalmology, and that it may also be of interest to those educated people and general practitioners who, without having a special interest in the subject, wish to know the principles upon which the prescription of glasses is based.

The seven chapters consist of "Measurement of visual power"; "Presbyopia"; "Myopia—short-sightedness"; "Hypermetropia"; "Corneal astigmatism"; "Asthenopia"; and "General remarks as to lenses." There are thirty-six illustrations but no plates. Pages 187–89 contain reading charts to measure effective vision. A foldout leaf appears at the end. (See also OT14, OP26, OP43, and OP60.)

III. OTORHINOLARYNGOLOGY

OT1. **HORACE GREEN** (1802–66). *A treatise on diseases of the air passages: comprising an inquiry into the history, pathology, causes, and treatment of those affections of the throat called bronchitis, chronic laryngitis, clergyman's sore throat.* 276pp. New York: Wiley & Putnam, 1846. [G-M 3261]

Considered the father of American laryngology, Green was the first specialist in the United States to devote his practice exclusively to diseases of the throat. He received his M.D. from Castleton Medical College in Vermont in 1824.

In the *Treatise* Green startled the medical profession by claiming to be able to pass a probang, a curved instrument of whalebone ten inches long tipped with a tiny sponge, through the larynx into the trachea and apply medication directly to the mucosa. His abilities were the subject of bitter controversy both in the United States and Europe. The book was reviewed adversely, and he was accused of plagiarizing from Armand Troussaeau (1801-67) and Hipployte Belloc's *Traité pratique de la phthisie laryngée, de la laryngite chronique, et des maladies de la voix* (Paris: J. B. Baillière, 1837) [G-M 3258]. These allegations were investigated by members of the New York Academy of Medicine but no definitive conclusions were reached. However, the controversy gave impetus to the study of laryngeal diseases in this country. At the time of the *Treatise*'s publication, Green was practicing in New York City, where he was instrumental in founding the New York Medical College. Green is described on the title page as formerly president and professor of the theory and practice of medicine at Castleton Medical College. He writes in the preface:

> I am fully aware, that views of the pathology of disease, and of its treatment, differing, in any degree, from those generally admitted, by the profession, are received by its members, with distrust and hesitation. But, so far from complaining of this, I am, and ever have been, among those, who have condemned the disposition, manifested by a part of the profession, in America, to receive, unquestioned, the observations and conclusions of certain pathologists; and to adopt such views, as established truths in medicine. In the following pages, I have presented a series of observations and facts, with regard to the phenomena of disease, and the effect of remedies, upon that disease, which, it may be in the power of every practical man, to verify, or disprove. Let the inquiry, then, be fairly made, and if it shall be found, that the conclusions which have been adopted; as to the nature of disease, and the effect of the treatment upon it; are unphilosophical and untenable—let them be discarded. As an apology, however, for what may be deemed by some, an obtrusion upon the profession, of individual views, of the nature

and treatment, of disease, I will take the liberty of stating, that I have been urged, in such a manner, by many distinguished medical gentlemen, of different parts of the Union, to publish these views, that I have not felt myself at liberty to refuse . . . .

There are ten chapters, including "Anatomy of the larynx, trachea, and bronchi"; "Physiology of the mucous follicles"; "Pathology of the throat, larynx, and bronchi"; "Follicular inflammation of the throat and air-passages"; "Malignant follicular disease of the esophageal tube"; and "Pathology of follicular disease of the air-passages." Descriptions of the plates are found on page 269. Subsequent editions were published in 1849 and 1852. Among Green's other books is *Selections from favorite prescriptions of living American practitioners* (New York: Wiley & Halsted, 1858). The New York Academy of Medicine has an unpublished autobiography in its collection that Green wrote in 1865. (See also OT2, OT4, and OT5.)

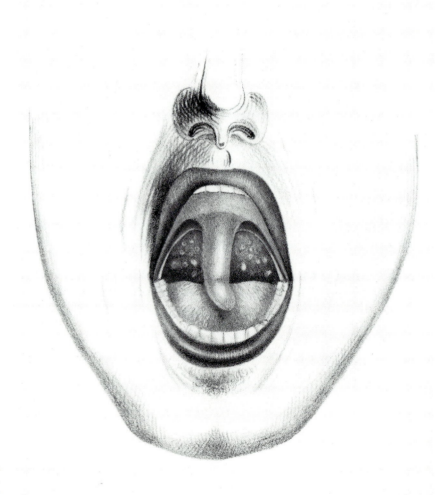

Fig. 66. (OT1) Green drew this color plate from life. G. and W. Endicott were the lithographers. The figure demonstrates tonsillar pathology and an enlarged uvula which interfered with the patient's breathing.

OT2. **HORACE GREEN** (1802–66). *Observations on the pathology of croup: with remarks on its treatment by topical medications.* 115pp. New York: J. Wiley, 1849.

In spite of the controversy which surrounded his claims of being able to pass an instrument through the glottis into the larynx, Green's practice in New York City grew quite rapidly. This volume was his first monograph to publically defend his findings. The preface is most important because in it Green provides his understanding of the entire controversy:

> When, about eighteen months ago, the author brought before the medical public, in a work on Diseases of the Air-Passages, the subject of the treatment of disease of the larynx and trachea, in the adult, by means of the direct application of therapeutical agents to the lining membrane of those cavities, the proposition was received with distrust by a large proportion of the profession; whilst another part publicly and peremptorily declared that it is practically impossible to convey medicinal agents, in the manner proposed, below the epiglottis. Less than two years have passed, and that practice which, as the *British and Foreign Medical Review* has remarked, was received by "some of the author's countrymen with a sneering incredulity," and was by them declared to be an "unwarrantable innovation," and "anatomical impossibility, as well as, physiologically impracticable," has been adopted, not only by distinguished medical men in almost every part of this country, but by the highest medical authority of Europe; and by the latter has been commended as a method of treatment which is not only the most effectual and certain in some forms of pulmonary disease, but as one that "will lead to important changes in the prophylaxis and cure of pulmonary phthisis." Less reluctantly, therefore, does the author now advocate—as he has done in the following pages—the practice of making topical application of medicinal agents into the larynges of young children, for the treatment of membranous croup. Nor does he hesitate to declare, although the proposition may be received by many with allowance, that it is a plan entirely practicable, safe, and, when judiciously employed, in the highest degree efficacious . . . . In conclusion, this little work, and the practice herein advocated, are commended to the candor of that portion of the profession who have the liberality to admit that improvements in the practice of our art can be made; and the energy and honesty to test such proposed improvements before condemning them.

The seven chapters include "Nature and pathology of croup"; "Laryngeal and tracheal croup"; "Membranous croup complicated with bronchial inflammation"; "Membranous croup complicated with spasmodic and bronchial symptoms"; "The treatment of croup"; and "Diphtherite, or the croup of adults." A greatly expanded edition was published in 1859. (See also OT1, OT4, and OT5.)

OT3. **JAMES BRYAN** (1810–81). *A treatise on the anatomy, physiology and diseases of the human ear.* 124pp. Philadelphia: Privately printed, 1851.

Bryan was professor of surgery at Geneva Medical College and professor of the institutes of medicine and medical jurisprudence at the

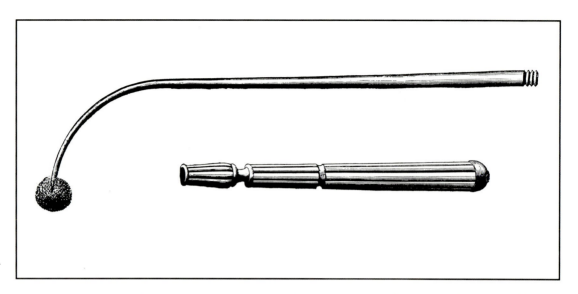

Fig. 67. (OT2) Green employed the probang for making direct medicinal applications to the fauces and larynx. This plate (frontispiece) portrays the instrument, which was made of a piece of whalebone about ten inches long. It was slightly curved at one end, and at this end was attached a small round piece of fine sponge.

Philadelphia College of Medicine. He dedicated this work to Valentine Mott (1785–1865) "whose pre-eminence among living surgeons, is universally acknowledged." It was Mott who had performed one of the earliest operations on the nose for removal of a fibrous growth by division of the nasal and maxillary bones [G-M 3259]. Bryan's monograph consists of two books; the first has three chapters on "Anatomy"; "Physiology"; and "Cophosis", while the second contains seven chapters dealing with specific diseases of the ear. The basis for the work was a series of lectures which Bryan delivered in the autumn of 1850 at the Philadelphia College of Medicine. He admits in the preface that

> the universal dearth of American literature on this subject, was another pretty strong incentive to the rash act of printing and publishing a book on a new subject . . . . The character of our people, like that of the Anglo-Saxons generally, is decidedly practical; the author has, therefore, avoided long dissertations, or theoretical speculations, on subjects purely speculative. Diseases whose existence has not been proved by post-obit or well attested clinical observations, are excluded. He has attempted to present as nearly as possible what is really known, and valuable, and avoided stating several operations which have not as yet received the sanction of the profession. The itch for publishing novelties has not to his knowledge swayed the course of his pen or thoughts; and he has preferred being a safe guide, to being more brilliant and striking, but less safe.

This was the only book Bryan wrote and it appeared in only one edition.

OT4. **HORACE GREEN** (1802–66). *On the surgical treatment of polypi of the larynx, and oedema of the glottis.* 124pp. New York: G. P. Putnam, 1852. [G-M 3262]

Green was one of the few to remove a laryngeal tumor before the invention of the laryngoscope: when the patient opened his mouth widely and coughed, a round white fibrous-looking tumor, about the

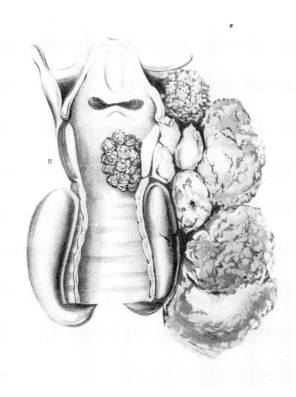

Fig. 68. (OT4) This plate, shows a fungating tumor of the larynx which Green removed at the time of death.

size of a cherry, could be seen arising from the larynx. Green succeeded in seizing the tumor with a tonsil forceps and dividing it with a long slender knife. This important work describes this surgical procedure. Written when Green was president of the faculty and professor of the theory and practice of medicine at New York Medical College, it consists of seven chapters. Among these are "Polypi of the larynx"; "History of polypi of the larynx"; "Morbid growths in the larynx"; "Diagnosis"; "Treatment of polypus of the larynx"; and "Oedema glottidis and its treatment." There are four plates. Green states in the preface:

> Happily, polypus of the larynx and oedema glottidis are diseases of very rare occurrence: so, at least, it has ever been considered; and yet the author does not hesitate to express the opinion, and to leave it for future experience to confirm or invalidate, that foreign growths have occurred in the opening of the air-passages, in many instances, where their presence was neither suspected nor discovered; and that, if the attention of the profession should by any means be directed to this subject, it will be found that the existence of polypus and other excrescences in these passages is an occurrence taking place much more frequently than has been supposed by medical practitioners . . . . In the forty cases of this disease to which allusion is made in the following pages, the result was fatal in every instance, with three exceptions . . . . The happy result which, in some many instances, has followed the employment of topical applications in the treatment of oedema glottidis, has encouraged the author to commend, with much confidence, to his professional brethren, this method of treating one of the most formidable, and hitherto one of the most fatal, of all the diseases of the larynx.

(See also OT1, OT2, and OT5.)

OT5. **HORACE GREEN** (1802–66). *A practical treatise on pulmonary tuberculosis, embracing its history, pathology, and treatment.* 355pp. New York: J. Wiley, 1864.

This book was written at the end of Green's career while he was past president and emeritus professor of the theory and practice of medicine at New York Medical College. Although not strictly related to the growth of otorhinolaryngologic surgery in America, the *Treatise* is important to the subject because of Green's overall influence on the specialty. He comments in the preface:

> I am quite aware of the charge of presumption which, very properly perhaps, may be brought against me for venturing to give my own views on the subject of tuberculous disease, when our country is so full of mature and learned works on this subject. But I have no apology or excuse to offer. I am not ambitious of thrusting forward new or peculiar opinions on any medical subject. I have only embodied views which twenty-five years of constant and extensive experience in the treatment of this class of diseases have given me, and do not ask my professional brethren to accept them, only so far as they are convinced of their truth . . . . These views are submitted to the profession with entire confidence in their willingness to carry out the injunction, prove all things; hold fast that which is good.

The work is divided into three parts: the first is a historical sketch of the views of ancient and modern authors concerning tuberculosis; the second consists of Green's opinions of the pathology of the disease; and the third discusses treatment. An interesting formulae of remedies for tuberculosis is found on pages 336–43. This was the only edition. (See also OT1, OT2, and OT4.)

OT6. **LOUIS ELSBERG** (1836–85). *Laryngoscopal surgery illustrated in the treatment of morbid growths within the larynx, being the prize essay to which the American Medical Association awarded the gold medal for MDCCCLXV.* 56pp. Philadelphia: Collins, 1866.

Elsberg was one of the preeminent figures in American laryngology. He graduated from Jefferson Medical College in 1857 and later founded the American Laryngological Association, of which he was the first president. He was the first in the United States to demonstrate in public the laryngoscope for diagnosis and treatment. The short-lived *American archives of laryngology* was issued under his editorial guidance from 1880 to 1884. Elsberg taught laryngosocopy at the University of New York, where he was lecturer on the diseases of the larynx. This rather scarce volume contains twelve woodcuts and two black-and-white and two color lithograph plates. The plates are especially impressive because of their representation of laryngeal pathology as seen through a laryngoscope. The book consists of four sections: "Introduction"; "Operations heretofore practised"; "Surgical treatment of today"; and "Report of eleven cases, occurring in the writer's practice, with portraits as reflected by the laryncoscope." There was only one printing.

OT7. **EDWARD HAMMOND CLARKE** (1820–77). *Observations on the nature and treatment of polypus of the ear.* 71pp. Boston: Ticknor & Fields, 1867.

Clarke graduated from the University of Pennsylvania in 1846 and immediately left to travel through Europe. It was there that he began the study of otology, a specialty to which he devoted himself in the early years of practice. He eventually settled in Boston, where he was chosen professor of materia medica at Harvard University. Clarke is also remembered as the editor of *A century of American medicine, 1776–1876* (Philadelphia: Henry C. Lea, 1876) [G-M 6586]. His *Observations* is difficult to read because it has no table of contents or index. The book does contain two plates with line drawings of microscopic structures. He notes in the preface:

> The observations on polypus of the ear contained in this essay were made a few years ago. Owing to the engrossing labors of general practice, and the still more engrossing duties of collegiate instruction they were laid aside. The interest which diseases of the ear have recently excited, both in this country and in Europe, especially in Germany, recalled my attention to these observations, and have induced me to collate them, and give to them their present form . . . .

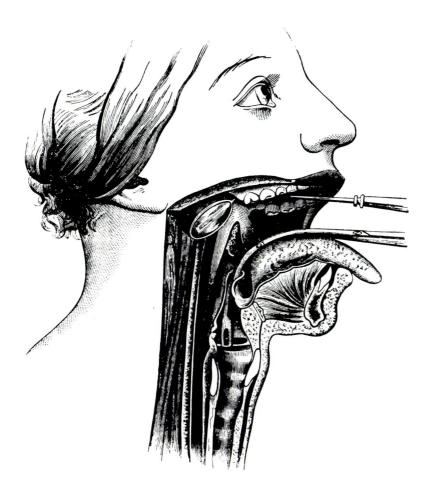

Fig. 69. (OT6) This woodcut, figure 2 on page 30, demonstrates Elsberg's technique of examining the larynx and pharynx by mirror.

Clarke's other medical books consist of *The physiological and therapeutical action of the bromide of potassium and bromide of ammonium* (Boston: J. Campbell, 1872), *Sex in education; or, a fair chance for the girls* (Boston: J. R. Osgood, 1873), *The building of a brain* (Boston: J. R. Osgood, 1874), and *Visions: a study of false sight (pseudopia)* (Boston: Houghton & Osgood, 1878).

OT8. **JACOB DASILVA SOLIS COHEN** (1838–1927). *Inhalation: its therapeutics and practice; a treatise on the inhalation of gases, vapors, nebulized fluids, and powders, including a description of the apparatus employed.* 305pp. Philadelphia: Lindsay & Blakiston, 1867.

Solis Cohen helped establish laryngology as a surgical specialty in the United States. He graduated from the University of Pennsylvania in 1860. In 1867 he removed a fibrous polyp from the inferior surface of the right vocal cord with the aid of a laryngoscope. This was the first successful operation for cancer of the larynx [G-M 3274]. He was a founder of the American Laryngological Association and served as its president from 1880 to 1882. This volume is the first American work to describe inhalation and its benefits. In the preface, Solis Cohen explains the reason for the publication of *Inhalation*:

> Inhalation, especially by the method of nebulization, is at present attracting favorable attention from the profession. At the annual meeting of the American Medical Association, in 1866, a committee, of which the writer was chairman, was appointed to prepare for the meeting of 1867 a report on the Therapeutics of Inhalation. In the preparation of this report, the writer accumulated a quantity of material much too voluminous for that purpose, and determined to incorporate the most valuable portions in book-form, presenting in some detail the historical record of experiments, pathological studies, &c., from which conclusions were drawn for the report. The principal literature on the subject is foreign . . . .

The book consists of three parts: "Inhalation of nebulized fluids"; "Inhalation of medicated airs, gases, and vapors"; and "Inhalation of powders." There are twelve engraved figures but no plates. A second edition was published in 1876 with many more illustrations. (See also OT11, OT15, and OT20.)

OT9. **ANTOINE RUPPANER** (1825–92). *The principles and practice of laryngoscopy and rhinoscopy in diseases of the throat and nasal passages.* 153pp. New York: A. Simpson, 1868.

Ruppaner completed his medical degree at Harvard in 1858. He soon began to specialize in laryngology and eventually settled in New York. He notes in the preface:

> The value of the Laryngoscope and Rhinoscope in the diagnosis and treatment of disease is beginning to be daily more appreciated by the profession, it is desirable that the principles and application of the same should come as speedily as possible into general use. To advance this purpose, to enable the busy practitioner and the inexperienced student to overcome, by a moderate amount of practice and perseverance, that which is most essential to the successful application of this art, this

treatise has been prepared, omitting nothing, as is hoped, which may be considered essential, but eschewing everything that has no immediate practical bearing upon the subject, tending only to confuse the student, and to increase the size and expense of the volume . . . . Having been commissioned during a visit to Vienna in 1865 by Prof. Turck, to translate and edit an English edition of his work *Die Krankheiten des Kehlkopfes und der Luftrohre*, the preparation and execution of which English edition has been necessarily delayed on account of the great expense involved in the publication of such an extensive work with atlas, and its naturally limited sale, I have liberally availed myself of Prof. Turck's work, and especially of his admirably well-executed drawings, regarding this as an excellent opportunity to introduce an author of such high merit and reputation to an American medical public, hoping thereby to awaken an interest for the study of the original work among students in this department of practical science.

Ruppaner's *Principles* contains fifty-nine engravings on wood. There are seven chapters in the first part, including "Auto-laryngoscopy"; "Recipro-laryngoscopy"; and "Infra-glottic laryngoscopy or tracheoscopy"; and eight chapters in part 2. The two appendices (pages 145–53) are of interest because they contain illustrations concerning laryngologic mirrors. Ruppaner's other medical book is *Hypodermic injections in the treatment of neuralgia, rheumatism, gout, and other diseases* (Boston: T. O. H. P. Burnham, 1865).

OT10. **JAKOB HERMANN KNAPP** (1832–1911). *A clinical analysis of the inflammatory affections of the inner ear.* 80pp. New York: William Wood, 1871.

Best known as an ophthalmologist, Knapp was born in Germany and became professor of ophthalmology at Heidelberg. For various reasons he emigrated to New York City in 1868. He immediately established the Ophthalmic and Aural Institute. Its reputation soon spread, and it became the largest such institution in the United States. Most of his written work was on ophthalmology, and the *Analysis* was his only book devoted to diseases of the ear. It remains exceedingly scarce due to its small press run. There was only one edition. (See also OP17)

OT11. **JACOB DASILVA SOLIS COHEN** (1838–1927). *Diseases of the throat: a guide to the diagnosis and treatment of affections of the pharynx, aesophagus, trachea, larynx, and nares.* 582pp. New York: William Wood, 1872. [G-M 3280]

Solis Cohen was lecturer on laryngoscopy and diseases of the throat and chest at Jefferson Medical College. He is credited with having performed the first laryngectomy in this country. His *Diseases* is considered the first systematic textbook on the subject to be published in the United States. It was a widely distributed volume that for many years was the only comprehensive English-language work in its field. There are fifteen chapters covering a multitude of topics. This edition contains 133 illustrations on wood. It was a tremendous undertaking, as Solis Cohen notes in the preface:

Fig. 70. (OT11) Cohen shows
glandular tissue at the vault of
the pharynx in a case of cleft
palate in this wood engraving
on page 185.

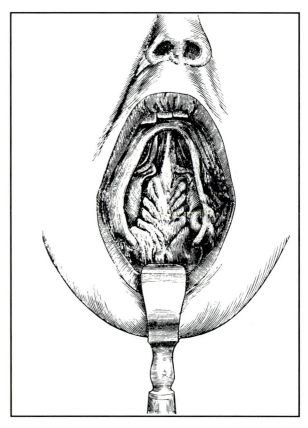

The preparation of the following pages has been no holiday task on the
part of the author. Only such irregular intervals as could be snatched
from the requirements of an unusually arduous practice could be
devoted to the purpose . . . . With the exception of a few hospital and
dispensary patients, seen from time to time at the request of his professional friends, the author's entire experience has been confined to his
own private and consultation practice. This has debarred him from
much opportunity for personal pathological research; but it has faci-
litated the description of morbid processes as they are met with in the
ordinary routine of practice . . . .

A second edition was published in 1879. (See also OT8, OT15, and
OT20.)

OT12. **LAURENCE TURNBULL** (1821–1900). *A clinical manual of the diseases of the ear.* 486pp. Philadelphia: J. B. Lippincott,1872.

Turnbull was born in Scotland and graduated from Jefferson Medical College in 1845. He spent the year 1859 in Europe, where he devoted
himself to the study of diseases of the eye and ear. He returned to the
United States and settled in Philadelphia, where he became a physician
in the department of diseases of the eye and ear of Howard Hospital.
Turnbull is best remembered as having performed the first mastoid
operation in the United States. In the preface, Turnbull states:

The author's object has been to present the subject of diseases of the
ear in such a manner that every well educated physician may approach
their treatment with as much confidence as he would the diseases of
the heart, lungs, brain, etc. The day has passed for medical men, as a

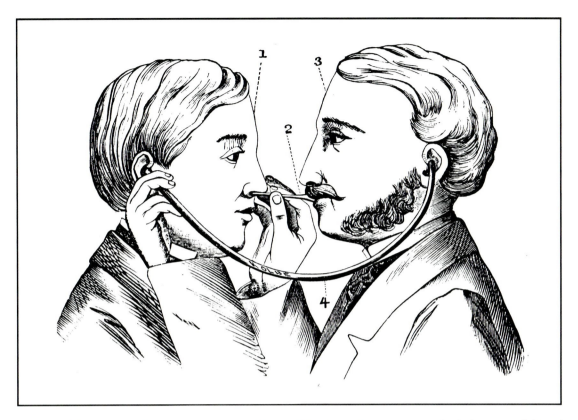

Fig. 71. (OT12) This wood engraving (number 89, page 270) shows the manner in which the permeability of the Eustachian tube could be diagnosed by a Eustachian catheter.

rule, to affirm that they "know but little of the anatomy and physiology of the ear, and nothing about its diseases." A scientific reformation has taken place on the subject of otology, and some of the best men in the profession are devoting their time and talents to its study, in the extended field of the phsyiological and pathological connection between the organs of sight and hearing . . . .

The work contains 107 illustrations on wood and a single color lithographic plate. There are twenty chapters dealing with a wide range of topics. The most interesting section of the work is an extensive chronologic bibliography (pages 453–76) listing important articles on the ear and its diseases published from 1683 to 1871. A second edition appeared in 1887. (See also GS93, GS124, and OT30.)

OT13. **A. D. WILLIAMS** (?–?). *Diseases of the ear including the necessary anatomy of the different parts of the organ immediately preceding the consideration of the diseases of those parts.* 209pp. Cincinnati: Robert Clarke, 1873.

Williams practiced in St. Louis, although he had earlier been lecturer on otology at Miami Medical College. This book does not have a table of contents, and is only notable for a superb color plate of the tympanic membrane and acute myringitis. Williams explains in the preface why he wrote the work:

The author presents this little book to the profession of the great Mississippi Valley, in the hope that it will be of interest to those who do him the honor to peruse its pages. The growing importance of Otological Science is his only excuse for its production. In composing the matter, he has endeavored to condense everything as much as the nature and extent of the subject would allow . . . . It appeared to him that the necessary anatomy of each individual part should precede the consideration of the diseases of that part, as the most convenient arrangement of a work of the kind. The author has confined himself mainly to his own experience, but has endeavored to state correctly the opinions of others, particularly when they differed from his own. So far as the author knows, this is the first work of the kind ever written in the West, so that it may be said to represent particularly western ideas.

OT14. **DANIEL BENNETT ST. JOHN ROOSA** (1838–1908). *A practical treatise on the diseases of the ear, including the anatomy of the organ.* 535pp. New York: William Wood, 1873.

Roosa graduated in 1860 from the University of the City of New York. Immediately after the Civil War, he began to devote his practice exclusively to diseases of the eye and ear. He practiced in New York City and became professor of the disease of the eye and ear at his alma mater. One of the earliest members of the American Otological Society, he eventually served as its president. His *Treatise* was

> . . . intended to be a guide to those who wish to treat the diseases of the ear. The portion that is devoted to a description of these diseases, and the means for their relief and cure, is founded upon my own experience in the observation and treatment of more than thirty-eight hundred cases, in public and private practice. I have, however, taken pains to give the experience of other practitioners, both at home and abroad . . . . Considerable space has been given to illustrative cases, with a view of showing the actual symptoms of aural diseases and the results of treatment. I have also added historical sketches upon all points of practice that are new or still under discussion, in order that the successive steps by which our present position has been reached might be distinctly traced . . . . The practice of Otology in this country was, a few years since, almost exclusively confined to charlatans; but it is now cultivated by a class of men who are the equals of any in the profession. Ten years ago, in most parts of the country, those who wished advice upon a disease of the ear were forced to seek aid outside of the profession . . . . The day will soon arrive—if indeed it be not already upon us—when Otology will take equal rank with Ophthalmology, to which department it has so long been a mere appendage, and when some knowledge of the diseases and treatment of the ear, will be required of every practitioner.

Part 1 contains eight chapters on the external ear. Part 2 deals with the middle ear and has nine chapters. The two chapters on the internal ear are in part 4. Part 4 also has a single chapter on deaf-muteness with an interesting description of ear trumpets. The book contains numerous wood engravings and chromolithographs. This volume was well received and went through further editions in 1874, 1876, 1880, 1881, 1885, and 1891. Among Roosa's other books are *A vest-pocket medical lexicon; being a dictionary of the words, terms, and symbols of medical science* (New York: William Wood, 1865), *A doctor's suggestion to the community; being a series of papers upon various subjects from a physician's standpoint*

(New York: G. P. Putnam's Sons, 1880), *Handbook of the anatomy and diseases of the eye and ear* (Philadelphia: F. A. Davis, 1904,), and *A textbook of the diseases of the ear, nose and pharynx* (New York: Macmillan, 1905). (See also OP26, OP43, OP60, and OP84.)

OT15. **JACOB DASILVA SOLIS COHEN** (1838–1927). *Croup, in its relation to tracheotomy.* 78pp. Philadelphia: Lindsay & Blakiston, 1874.

Solis Cohen was lecturer on laryngoscopy and diseases of the throat and chest at Jefferson Medical college when this monograph was written. The volume has neither a table of contents nor an index, which makes it difficult to peruse. Solis Cohen presents the following conclusions on page 78:

> . . . there are no insuperable contra-indications to tracheotomy in croup; 2. That the administration of an anesthetic for the purpose of controlling the child's movements is admissible in performing the operation; . . . 3. That a careful dissection should be made down to the windpipe, and hemorrhage be arrested before incising it; . . . 4. that the incision should be made into the trachea as near the cricoid cartilage as possible, to avoid excessive hemorrhage, and subsequent accidents which might occasion emphysema; 5. That a dilator should be used; . . . 6. That the tube should be dispensed with as soon as possible; . . . 7. and that a skilled attendant should be within a moment's call for the first twenty-four or forty-eight hours immediately following the operation.

This was the only edition. (See also OT8, OT11, and OT20.)

OT16. **LUCIUS D. MORSE** (?–?). *On nasal catarrh; its symptoms, causes, complications, prevention, treatment, etc., with illustrative cases.* 72pp. Memphis: A. F. Dod, 1876.

Morse was a homeopathic physician who practiced in Memphis. This was his only major work. He notes in the preface that

> nasal catarrh, in its various forms, afflicts a large number of people, and it cannot be denied that the results of medical treatment are, often, far from satisfactory, both to physician and patient. Anything positive, on the score of its Therapeutics, we feel certain, will not come amiss. While no pretentions are made, as elsewhere stated, to an exhaustive consideration of the subject, the clinical department of this little work will be found tolerably full . . . .

The book comprises four parts: the first part discusses the symptoms, complications, causes, prevention, and treatment of catarrh; the second part consists of cases from practice and observations on the use of remedies; the third part focuses on acute catarrh-coryza; and the fourth part lists numerous homeopathic remedies (pages 54–72). There was only one edition.

OT17. **CHARLES HENRY BURNETT** (1842–1902). *The ear; its anatomy, physiology, and diseases.* 615pp. Philadelphia: Henry C. Lea, 1877.

Burnett received his M.D. from the University of Pennsylvania in 1867. He was always interested in the study of hearing and set up practice in Philadelphia in 1872, devoting his work to diseases of the ear.

Published as an octavo volume with eighty-seven illustrations, the book was available in cloth for $4.50, in leather for $5.50, and in half-russia for $6.00. The work is massive in scope. Part 1 (pages 19–164) consists of the anatomy and physiology of the external ear, middle ear, and internal ear. Part 2 ("Diseases and Treatment") has seven sections: "Examination of patients"; "Auricle"; "External auditory canal"; "Membrana tympani"; "Middle ear"; "Diseases of the internal ear"; and "Deaf mutes and partially deaf children." A second edition was printed in 1884. Among his other books is *A text-book on diseases of the ear, nose and throat* (Philadelphia: J. B. Lippincott, 1901), written in collaboration with Ephriam Fletcher Ingals (1848–1919) and James Edward Newcomb (1857-1912). (See also OT19, OT52, and OT57.)

OT18. **FRANCKE HUNTINGTON BOSWORTH** (1843–1925). *Handbook upon diseases of the throat for the use of students.* New York: William Wood, 1879.

Bosworth is credited with having developed the science of laryngology and rhinology as a well-defined field of medical specialization. This volume is his first major book and remains an exceptionally scarce item. Bosworth received his undergraduate degree from Yale in 1862 and his M.D. from Bellevue Hospital Medical College six years later. He was a founder of the New York Laryngological Society in 1873, the first such association in the world devoted to the specialty. In 1871 he was appointed to the medical faculty at Bellevue Hospital Medical College. He became professor in 1881, and continued in that position after Bellevue merged with New York University in 1898 until retirement. His report on various forms of disease of the ethmoid cells is especially significant [G-M 3304]. His *Handbook* was based almost entirely on his own experience, as recorded in his carefully kept case records. Among Bosworth's other books are *Taking cold* (Detroit: G. S. Davis, 1891) and *The doctor in old New York* (New York: J. P. Putnam's Sons, 1898). (See also OT26, OT50, and OT61.)

OT19. **CHARLES HENRY BURNETT** (1842–1902). Hearing, and how to keep it. 152pp. Philadelphia: Lindsay & Blakiston, 1879.

Burnett was consulting aurist to the Pennsylvania Institution for the Deaf and Dumb, and aurist at the Presbyterian Hospital in Philadelphia. This book was the first volume in the Lindsay & Blakiston series of American Health Primers. Burnett's monograph consists of three parts: "Anatomy and physiology of the ear"; "The chief diseases and injuries of the ear, and the avoidance of their improper treatment"; and "General hygiene of the ear." The fourteen illustrations are all found in the first chapter on structure of the ear. This was the only one edition. (See also OT17, OT52, and OT57.)

The Lindsay & Blakiston American Health Primers series was edited by William Williams Keen (1837-1932) and consisted of twelve volumes. Other volumes are No. 2, *Long life and how to reach it* by Joseph G. Richardson (1836–86); No. 3, *The summer and its diseases* by James C. Wilson (1847-1934); No. 4, *Eyesight, and how to care for it* by George C.

Harlan (1835–1909) (OP29); No. 5, *The throat and the voice* by Jacob Da-Silva Solis Cohen (1838–1927) (OT20); No 6, *The winter and its dangers* by Hamilton Osgood (1839–?); No. 7, *The mouth and the teeth* by James William White (1850–1916); No. 8, *Our homes* by Henry Hartshorne (1823–97); No. 9, *The skin in health and disease* by L. Duncan Bulkley (1845–1923); No. 10, *Brain work and overwork* by H. C. Wood (1841-1920); No. 11, *Sea-air and sea-bathing* by John Hooker Packard (1832–1907); and No. 12, *School and industrial hygiene* by D. F. Lincoln (1841-1916). Seven volumes were published in 1879 and five in 1880. They were pocket-sized and bound with hard covers. They were available for fifty cents each; a subscription to the entire series cost $5.00. Their subjects mainly concerned personal health education and public health problems. Although written mostly for lay readers, they were quite instructive. Keen describes the series in an advertisement:

> They are not intended (save incidentally) to assist in curing disease, but to teach people how to take care of themselves, their children, pupils, employees, etc. They are written from an American standpoint, with especial reference to our climate and modes of life; and in these respects we differ materially from other nations . . . .

Burnett's monograph comprises three parts: "Anatomy and physiology of the ear"; "The chief diseases and injuries of the ear, and the avoidance of their improper treatment"; and "General hygiene of the ear." This was the only edition. (See also OT17, OT52, and OT57.)

OT20. **JACOB DASILVA SOLIS COHEN** (1838–1902). *The throat and the voice.* 159pp. Philadelphia: Lindsay & Blakiston, 1879.

In addition to being lecturer on diseases of the throat and chest at Jefferson Medical College, Solis Cohen also taught physiology and hygiene of the voice at the National School of Elocution and Oratory in Philadelphia. Material from these classes was incorporated into this volume:

> There is no pretension, in the following pages, to teach either the art of practising medicine or the art of cultivating the voice. The aim of the writer has been to direct the attention of the general reader to some scientific facts concerning *The Throat And The Voice*, and to present for consideration some opinions and advice based upon an intelligent appreciation of those facts.

The first part (pages 9–86) discusses the throat in fifteen chapters. The second part consists of nine chapters on the voice. There are eighteen illustrations scattered throughout the text. This book was No. 5 in Lindsay & Blakiston's series American Health Primers. (See also OT8, OT11, and OT15.)

OT21. **CARL SEILER** (1849–98). *Handbook of diagnosis and treatment of diseases of the throat and nasal cavities.* 156pp. Philadelphia: Henry C. Lea, 1879.

Seiler was lecturer on laryngoscopy at the University of Pennsylvania and chief of the throat dispensary at the University Hospital. His interest in laryngology began as an office student of Jacob DaSilva Solis

Cohen (1838–1927). In 1879 Seiler was elected a member of the American Laryngological Association and later served as its vice-president. This volume was

> . . . intended to serve as a guide to students of laryngoscopy in acquiring the skill requisite to the successful diagnosis and treatment of diseases of the larynx and naso-pharynx. All purely theoretical considerations have therefore been omitted, and only points of practical importance have been discussed as concisely as possible, so that the work may be used as a ready book of reference on the subjects of which it treats . . . .

There are thirty-five illustrations and fourteen chapters. Chapter 14 consists of extensive tables of symptoms of the diseases of the larynx and naso-pharynx, based on the records of over 1,000 cases which Seiler had treated in his practice. Seiler's mother was a noted authority on the voice and author of *The voice in speaking* (Philadelphia: J. B. Lippincott, 1875), and undoubtedly her influence must have encouraged Seiler to study the larynx and to write his senior thesis, "Physiology of the voice." Additional editions of the *Handbook* were published in 1883, 1889, and 1893. It was originally available in cloth for $1.00. Seiler's other medical book is the *Compendium of microscopical technology; a guide to physicians and students in the use of the microscope and in the preparation of histological and pathological specimens* (Philadelphia: D. G. Brinton, 1881).

OT22. C. E. SHOEMAKER (?–1891). *The ear: its diseases and injuries and their treatment.* 375pp. Reading: B. F. Owen, 1879.

Shoemaker was an aural surgeon who practiced in Reading, Pennsylvania. He received his M.D. from Pennsylvania Medical College in 1860 but eventually specialized in aural operations. The volume consists of ten parts, including "Anatomy"; "Physiology"; "General hygiene of the ear"; "Pathology"; "Examination of ear patients"; "Diseases of the external ear"; "Diseases of the middle ear"; "Diseases of the internal ear"; and "Unclassified ailments." The final chapter has an interesting presentation on artificial eardrums. Shoemaker writes in the preface:

> The great want of a better understanding of the organ of hearing, its ailments and their treatment, is the motive impelling me to place before the public this book. This want is not confined to the laity, but unfortunately is also shared by a large class of physicians, many of whom are reputable practitioners, but failing, for want of time or inclination, to give to this branch of medical science that study and attention to which its importance so justly entitles it, are unprepared to treat the diseases of these organs, or advise properly on this subject. Hence a conviction rests upon the public mind that little can be done in the way of treatment for the relief of deafness or the removal of the causes producing it. Hence too we may account for the fact that charlatans enjoy such a liberal patronage from this class of sufferers, who, while they are not at all successful in benefiting such afflicted, are, nevertheless, in consequence of their want of knowledge and skill, quite successful, by their tamperings, in further injuring the organs they attempt to treat, and thereby prejudicing the minds of the people against the treatment of ear ailments . . . .

This was the only edition and was the only book Shoemaker wrote.

OT23. **ALBERT HENRY BUCK** (1842–1922). *Diagnosis and treatment of ear diseases.* 411pp. New York: William Wood, 1880.

Buck was the son of Gurdon Buck (1807-77) (GS83). He graduated from the College of Physicians and Surgeons, Columbia, in 1867. After studying the physiology of the ear in Europe, he became aural surgeon at the New York Eye and Ear Infirmary and instructor in otology at his alma mater. This volume is Buck's most important work and was a popular textbook in medical schools. It was No. 76 of Wood's Library of 100 Standard Medical Authors, and seven more editions were published through 1898. There are no plates, but the work contains twenty-eight wood engravings. The eleven chapters include "Physiology of the organ of hearing"; "Examination of the patient"; "Diseases of the middle ear"; "Fractures of the temporal bone"; "Diseases of the mastoid process"; and "Different forms of aural disease in which the labyrinth is believed to be involved." Among Buck's other medical works are the two-volume *A treatise on hygiene and public health* (New York: William Wood, 1879); the nine-volume *A reference hand-book of the medical sciences, embracing the entire range of scientific and practical medicine and allied science by various writers* (New York: William Wood, 1886–93), *A vest-pocket medical dictionary; embracing those terms and abbreviations which are commonly found in the medical literature of the day, but excluding the names of drugs and of many special anatomical terms* (New York: William Wood, 1896); the eight-volume *American practice of surgery* (New York: William Wood, 1906–11) [G-M 5805], jointly edited with Joseph Decatur Bryant (1845–1916); *The growth of medicine from the earliest times to about 1800* (New Haven: Yale University Press, 1917); and *The dawn of modern medicine* (New Haven: Yale University Press, 1920). (See also OT51 and OT68.)

OT24. **BEVERLEY ROBINSON** (1844–1924). *A practical treatise on nasal catarrh.* 182pp. New York: William Wood, 1880.

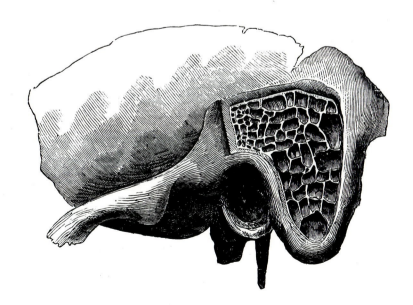

Fig. 72. (OT23) This engraving shows the temporal bone and mastoid process (number 24, page 298). Buck points out that the temporal bone shown here is unusual in the distribution of its pneumatic cells, since the cells extend farther than normal.

Robinson practiced in New York City after receiving an M.D. from the University of Paris in 1872. Soon after his graduation, he spent six months at the Throat Hospital in London and considered himself a specialist in laryngology for a short time. However, he eventually pursued general practice and became lecturer upon clinical medicine at Bellevue Hospital Medical College. His *Treatise* was dedicated to John Forsyth Meigs (1818–82), and he did not

> . . . attempt to make it learned in bibliographical research, and, indeed, to some instruments and methods of treatment adopted by others I have not even referred. I have wished especially to write a succinct, though complete account of personal experience and convinctions and thus, if possible, render it valuable as a practical guide to others.

There are nine chapters, including "Anatomy, physiology and pathology"; "Instruments for examination of the nasal cavities"; "Anterior and posterior rhinoscopy"; "Treatment of coryza"; "Hypertrophy of turbinated bones"; and "Follicular disease of the naso-pharyngeal space." A second edition was published in 1885. (See also OT46.)

OT25. **THOMAS FRAZIER RUMBOLD** (1830–1901). *Hygiene and treatment of catarrh; hygienic and sanitive measures for chronic catarrhal inflammation of the nose, throat, and ears.* Part 1. 174pp. St. Louis: G. O. Rumbold, 1880.

Rumbold was a member of the American Rhinological Association and practiced in St. Louis. His practice was limited to diseases of the nose and ears, and he contributed much to the periodical literature on these subjects. The text was written as a summation of his many years in practice, and he notes:

> I had been but a few years in the practice of this specialty, when I discovered that the successful management of this most common and tenacious complaint, depended on the faithful observance of the laws of health by my patients . . . . It is absurd to expect a patient can be successfully treated, while he continues to violate the laws of health. One might as consistently ask a physician to cure him of a burn, while he continues to expose himself to the fire, as to ask to be relieved of a catarrh, while he neglects to employ the means to prevent a renewal of its cause. For these reasons, I commenced in 1862, to give such rules to my patients as observation had taught me were useful in aiding them to take care of themselves during those seasons of the years in which they were most liable to take cold . . . . I do not claim that what is written here on hygienic and sanitive measures are new, but I do say that it has not been given sufficient detail and earnestness by any writer on this subject . . . .

The section of hygienic measures is divided into eleven chapters, including such titles as "Wrappings for the neck"; "Frequent changes of the under-clothing"; "The feet"; and "Disposition of the mind." The section on sanitive measures consists of six chapters, including "Removal of hardened secretions from the nasal passages"; "Application of oil to the surface of the body"; and "Tobacco—its mental and physical effects." This last chapter is an interesting diatribe against the use of tobacco and the ill effects it has on an individual's health. A second edition of this work was published in 1882 by the Medical Journal Publishing Company of St. Louis. (See also OT29, OT42, OT48, and OT66.)

OT26. **FRANCKE HUNTINGTON BOSWORTH** (1845–1925). *A manual of diseases of the throat and nose.* 427pp. New York: William Wood, 1881.

This book is a pioneering effort that helped establish the science of laryngology. It was written when Bosworth was lecturer on diseases of the throat at Bellevue Hospital Medical College and physician-in-charge of the clinic for diseases of the throat in the out-door department of Bellevue Hospital. Immediately after its publication, he was named full professor at Bellevue. When Bellevue merged with New York University Medical College in 1898, Bosworth became its initial professor of laryngology. The *Manual* was dedicated to James Rushmore Wood (1813–82), and Bosworth writes in the preface:

> I have embodied in the following pages the results of an experience, in dealing with throat affections, extending now over nearly ten years, and which has embraced the observation, treatment, and, in the large proportion of instances, the observed results of treatment, of something over eight thousand recorded cases . . . . In making these results public, I have endeavored to confine myself to my own personal experience, recording, with candor and fidelity, both the method and measure of my success in those affections in which success has followed treatment, and, at the same time, and with the same candor, acknowledging the difficulties and disappointments which have attended the management of those diseases in the treatment of which I have failed of full success.

Later in the preface Bosworth pays special tribute to Jacob DaSilva Solis Cohen (1838–1927) and his *Diseases of the throat* (OT11). In addition, he confesses:

> I am also under obligation to Dr. Morrell Mackenzie, for the woodcuts which I have appropriated, without permission, from his recent work on *The Throat and Nose*. My excuse for this is, that his work appeared in this country after my manuscript had been sent to the printer, and the cuts have been inserted while the book has been going through the press; my time was too limited to await a response, and it would not have been a very gracious act to seek his permission to use them after I had already appropriated them.

MacKenzie's work, *A manual of diseases of the throat and nose* (London: J. & A. Churchill, 1880–84) [G-M 3287] along with Solis Cohen's work and Bosworth's book, are considered the three works that launched laryngology on its own as a discipline. Bosworth goes on to summarize the book's major findings:

> Acute catarrhal inflammation may occur in the nose, pharynx, or larynx, resulting in acute coryza, pharyngitis, acute laryngitis, etc. Chronic catarrhal inflammation may occur in any portion of the air-passages, resulting in chronic coryza, chronic pharyngitis, chronic laryngitis, etc. Acute follicular inflammation may occur in the upper or lower pharynx, or in the tonsils, resulting in acute follicular tonsillitis, acute follicular pharyngitis, etc. Chronic follicular inflammation may occur in the pharynx or tonsils, resulting in chronic follicular pharyn-

gitis, enlarged tonsils, etc. Croupous inflammation may occur in the pharynx or larynx, resulting in croupous pharyngitis or membranous sore throat; or in croupous laryngitis, or true croup. Diphtheritic inflammation may occur in any portion of the upper air tract, as a local manifestation of the blood disease, diphtheria.

There are twenty-four chapters and 175 illustrations. This was the only edition published. (See also OT18, OT50, and OT61.)

OT27. **GERSHOM NELSON BRIGHAM** (1820–86). *Catarrhal diseases of the nasal and respiratory organs.* 112p. New York: A. L. Chatterton, 1881.

A homeopathic physician, Brigham initially practiced in Montpelier, Vermont. He graduated in 1845 from Vermont Medical College and also matriculated at the College of Physicians and Surgeons in New York. He was introduced to the principles of homeopathy soon after beginning practice. He later moved to Grand Rapids, where he practiced until his death. Brigham advocates a homeopathic approach to the subject in the book's preface:

> The frequency with which the mucous membranes of the nasal, aural, and respiratory tracts are affected with catarrhal inflammations, and the very general failure in successfully treating the same, together with the fact that our medical literature fails to furnish any treatise written from the homeopathic standpoint, are sufficient reasons, in the judgement of the author, for the appearance of this monograph.

The most interesting section of this work is a repertory of homeopathic medicine applicable to nasal and respiratory organs in part 4. A second edition was published in 1884. (See also OT32.)

OT28. **EPHRAIM FLETCHER INGALS** (1848–1918). *Lectures on the diagnosis and treatment of diseases of the chest, throat, and nasal cavities.* 437pp. New York: William Wood, 1881.

Ingals was an 1871 graduate of Rush Medical College. In 1874 he became lecturer on diseases of the chest and physical diagnosis and on laryngology in the postgraduate course at his alma mater. From 1883 to 1890, he served as professor of laryngology. At the time of the publication of his *Lectures*, he was also clinical professor of diseases of the throat and chest at Northwestern University Woman's Medical College. He is best remembered for devising the operation of partial excision of the septum for the correction of septum deflection [G-M 3289]. The *Lectures* grew out of a series of talks which he gave to medical students at various Chicago medical institutions. There are thirty-three chapters on the following major areas: physical diagnosis, and diagnosis and treatment of many types of diseases, such as diseases of the lungs, of the heart, of the aorta, of the throat and nasal passages, of the fauces, of the larynx, and of the nasal passages. There are 135 illustrations. Further editions were published in 1892, 1894, 1898, and 1900. Ingals's other book is *A textbook on diseases of the ear, nose and throat* (Philadelphia: J. B. Lippincott, 1901), written with Charles Henry Burnett (1842–1902) and James Edward Newcomb (1857-1912).

OT29. **THOMAS FRAZIER RUMBOLD** (1830–1901). *The hygiene and treatment of catarrh. Part 1. Hygienic and sanitive measures. Part 2. Therapeutic measures.* 473pp. St. Louis: G. O. Rumbold, 1881.

This book was a greatly expanded edition of Rumbold's previous work from 1880. It is included as a separate selection because of the addition of a 300-page section on therapeutic and operative measures. Forty illustrations are included in the thirteen chapters. Among the headings are "Instruments"; "The method of air-supply to the middle ear"; "Operative measures"; and three chapters reporting on numerous cases. He notes in the preface:

> If it is urged against me, that I have differed very materially from many who are recognized by the profession as being well informed on this subject, I have only to say that what has been given here, is the result of an honest search after facts, and that these facts are stated as I saw them, not fearing to question the correctness of long acknowledged theories, my only guide being my patients' reports—this has been my educator . . . .

There were no further editions of this work. (See also OT25, OT42, OT48, and OT66.)

OT30. **LAURENCE TURNBULL** (1821–1900). *Imperfect hearing and the hygiene of the ear; including nervous symptoms, tinnitus aurium, aural vertigo, diseases of the naso-pharyngeal membrane, middle ear, and mastoid region; with home instruction of the deaf.* 147p. Philadelphia: J. B. Lippincott, 3rd edition, 1881.

This is an interesting work that started out as little more than a pamphlet in its first two editions. These were published in 1874 and 1875 under the title *Tinnitus aurium, or noises in the ears.* When the third edition was published, Turnbull was aural surgeon at Jefferson Medical College and physician in the department of diseases of the eye and ear at Howard Hospital in Philadelphia. He notes in the preface:

> This little work having been out of print for some years, and a constant desire having been expressed for it, the author has felt it to be a pleasant task to publish a third edition. He has been favored with unusual knowledge by a visit to Europe, while there, acting as president to the subsection of Otology, of the British Medical Association . . . and later, August, 1879, as a member of the otological section at Amsterdam . . . . He has also on his return acted as chairman of the section of ophthalmology, otology, and laryngology at the meeting of the American Medical Association, which was held in New York City, June, 1880 . . . .

There were a few rudimentary illustrations. The chapters consist of "The limit of perception of musical tones by the human ear"; "Tinnitus aurium and observations on aural or auditory vertigo"; "The importance of treatment of the naso-pharyngeal space, tonsils, and uvula in acute and chronic catarrh of the middle ear"; "Artificial perforation of the membrana-tympani"; "The mastoid region and its diseases"; "The hygiene of the apparatus of hearing"; "On the method of educating the deaf-mute at home"; and "A comparison between the audiophone, dentaphone, etc., and the various forms of ear trumpets." There were no further editions. (See also GS93, GS124, and OT12.)

OT31. **CLINTON WAGNER** (1837–1914). *Habitual mouth-breathing; its causes, effects, and treatment.* 52pp. New York: G. P. Putnam's Sons, 1881.

This small treatise was a pioneering effort to understand and treat what was regarded as a serious medical condition. Wagner was professor of diseases of the throat at the University of Vermont, and this work was his first major monograph. It had initially been read as a paper before the New York County Medical Society on April 25, 1881. Wagner expanded it, included three plates, and had it published in book form. There is no table of contents, making the work somewhat difficult to read. It was well received, justifying publication of a second edition in 1884. (See also OT38.)

OT32. **GERSHOM NELSON BRIGHAM** (1820–86). *Phthisis pulmonalis; or, tubercular consumption.* 241pp. New York: Boericke & Tafel, 1882.

Although he was not an otorhinolaryngologist, Brigham considered his general homeopathic practice to be weighted toward the treatment of these conditions. While living in Grand Rapids, Michigan, Brigham wrote the *Phthisis* in reaction to the fact that

> from the homeopathic standpoint no very exhaustive treatise has yet appeared. Upon histological and pathological questions, much has been written of late, and yet the profession have come to no agreement . . . . We have endeavored to present in a succinct manner the salient points advanced by leading pathologists, not doubting that there may be much truth in what is advanced by each of them, but doubting if any presents the whole matter . . . .

The book has no table of contents or index. This was the only edition. (See also OT27.)

OT33. **GEORGE MOREWOOD LEFFERTS** (1846–1920). *A pharmacopoeia for the treatment of diseases of the larynx, pharynx, and nasal passages, with remarks on the selection of remedies and choice of instruments and on the methods of making local applications.* 101pp. New York: G. P. Putnam's Sons, 1882.

Lefferts was clinical professor of laryngoscopy and diseases of the throat at the College of Physicians and Surgeons in New York. He was a prolific contributor to medical journals. His other major medical monograph is the forty-nine page *Diagnosis and treatment of chronic nasal catarrh, three clinical lectures* (St. Louis: Lambert & Co, 1884). Lefferts writes in the preface to the *Pharmacopoeia*:

> The experience of a number of years in clinical teaching has convinced me that the time which is ordinarily devoted, during a limited course of lectures on a special subject, in dictating to the student in the first instance, and repeating in detail from time to time during the course, the necessarily large number and variety of formulae that are requisite for intelligent treatment, can be more profitably employed, and the subject itself better and more clearly understood

without laborious and too often imperfect note-taking, by collecting the commoner and more reliable ones in a systematic but simple form . . . . In pursuance of this conviction I have prepared this little volume for the use of my students . . . .

There are twelve chapters: "Pigmenta"; "Cleansing and disinfecting solutions"; "Medicated sprays"; "Medicinal solutions for local application"; "Powders for insufflation"; "Nasal bougies"; "Medicated cotton wools"; "Inhalations"; "Gargles"; "Lozenges-pastils"; "Caustics"; and "Miscellaneous." A second edition was published in 1884.

OT34. **WILLIAM H. WINSLOW** (?–?). *The human ear and its diseases; a practical treatise upon the examination, recognition, and treatment of affections of the ear and associate parts.* 526pp. New York: Boericke & Tafel, 1882.

Winslow was oculist and aurist at Pittsburgh Homeopathic Hospital. This massive work has ten chapters: "Anatomy of the ear"; "Physiology of the ear"; "Examination of the ear"; "Diseases of the external ear"; "Injuries and diseases of the membrana tympani"; "Diseases of the middle ear"; "Complications of chronic purulent inflammation of the tympanum"; "Diseases of the middle ear"; "Electricity in aural disease"; and "The internal ear." There are 138 illustrations in this, the only edition.

OT35. **JOSEPH MOSES WARD KITCHEN** (1846–1931). *Student's manual of diseases of the nose and throat; a digest, descriptive of the more commonly seen diseases of the upper air-tract, with the methods of their treatment.* 127pp. New York: G. P. Putnam's Sons, 1883.

Kitchen was an assistant surgeon at the Metropolitan Throat Hospital in New York when this volume was written. He writes in the preface:

> The medical student soon becomes sorrowfully aware that there is no royal road to medical knowledge. Yet there are some paths that are less difficult than others. In his undergraduate, as well as in his post-graduate days, the writer has often deplored the fact that so many authors find it proper to clothe, and perhaps even hide, a few ideas in a great flow of words. In this day, when so much study is required of even the average graduate, that very hard-worked individual has very little time to sift out the important points from the mass of words and discussion, even if he were able to differentiate the one from the other, and hence results much mental confusion; and it would seem that there should be room for many digested and easily absorbable books relating to all branches of medical science. This little work, written with the primary intention of confirming and condensing his own knowledge of Throat Diseases, the writer has thought, with some additions and change in its make-up, might be of service to the overworked student, and even be of value as a handy book for quick reference to the general practitioner. He has tried to incorporate in it nothing less than should be known of Throat and Nasal Disease by every graduate in medicine . . . .

Each of the forty chapters averages three to four pages in length. Among the contents are "Pharmacopoeia"; "Rhinitis atrophica"; "Epistaxis"; "Hay fever"; "Elongated uvula"; "Spasm of the glottis"; "Membranous

Fig. 73. (OT38) This rudimentary engraving (page 136)
depicts a forty-year-old woman
with a nasopharyngeal tumor.
The growth was attached to the
base of the skull and extended
downward below the soft palate. Its eventual effects included separation of the nasal
bones to such an extent that a
"frog-like face characteristic"
became evident.

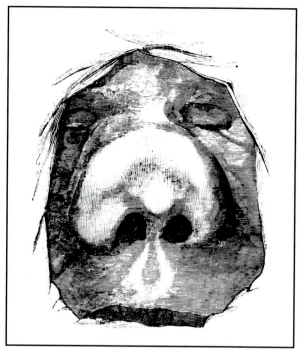

laryngitis"; and "Cancer of the larynx." This was the only edition.
Among Kitchen's other books are *Consumption; its nature, causes, prevention and cure* (New York: G. P. Putnam's Sons, 1885). (See also OT36.)

OT36. **JOSEPH MOSES WARD KITCHEN** (1846–1931). *Catarrh, sore-throat
and hoarseness; a description of the construction, action, and use of the
nasal passages and throat.* 80pp. New York: G. P. Putnam's Sons,
1884.

This small work comprises just eight chapters. Among them are
"The anatomical construction and healthy action of the nasal passages
and throat"; "Hygienic conditions necessary for the maintenance of
health in the parts"; "A brief mention of the more common diseases
producing catarrh, sore throat, and hoarseness"; "The productive causes
of nasal and throat disease"; and "The surgical and medical professional
treatment of diseases of the upper air-tract." The book was published in
only one edition. (See also OT35.)

OT37. **OREN DAY POMEROY** (1834–1902). *The diagnosis and treatment
of diseases of the ear.* 392pp. New York: Bermingham, 1883.

An 1860 graduate of the College of Physicians and Surgeons,
Pomeroy devoted his practice to diseases of the eye and ear. At the time
this volume was written he was surgeon at the Manhattan Eye and Ear
Hospital. He later became its full-time director. He was an important
figure in specialty surgery, and was a charter member of the American
Otological Society, becoming its president in 1872. This volume was
Pomeroy's most important work, but he excluded from it any mention
of anatomy and physiology. The nine chapters are "Instruments used in
the examination of the ear, with hints as to methods"; "Diseases of the
auricle"; "Diseases of the external auditory canal"; "Instruments for the

examination of the throat and nares, with suggestions as to the best method of making the examination"; "Diseases of the middle ear"; "Mastoid affections"; "Unclassified diseases"; "Diseases of the ear mostly or wholly confined to the labyrinth or acoustic nerve"; and "Instruments for aiding the hearing." There are 100 wood engravings. The book was originally available in cloth for $3.00. A second edition was pub-lished in 1886.

OT38. **CLINTON WAGNER** (1837–1914). *Diseases of the nose.* 252pp. New York: Bermingham, 1884.

Wagner graduated from the University of Maryland School of Medicine in 1858, and settled in New York in 1873. He was one of the founding members of the New York Laryngological Society, which stimulated the organization of the American Laryngological Association in 1878. These two societies were the earliest in the world devoted strict-ly to the specialty. At the time this volume was published, Wagner was professor of the diseases of the nose and throat in the New York Post-Graduate Medical School. This book was dedicated to William A. Hammond (1828–1900), who served as surgeon general in the United States Army. Wagner comments in the preface:

> In an experience extending over twenty-five years, nearly fourteen of which have been devoted exclusively to the study of the diseases of the nose and throat, I have enjoyed unusual opportunities in private, hospi-tal, and dispensary practice, for gathering and utilizing material upon which to base this work . . . . Modern rhinoscopy has made nasal sur-gery comparatively easy for the operator; unlike laryngoscopy, it has originated no operation requiring that high order of skill which only the trained eye and hand possess, for the removal, per vias naturales, of foriegn bodies lodged in the larynx. Any one competent to make ex-aminations properly by the present known methods, who has a fair knowledge of the anatomy of the parts, requires no special skill or train-ing for performing the operations on the nose daily undertaken by specialists.

There are seventeen chapters and an interesting appendix of cases on pages 200–33. An extensive bibliography appears on pages 234–44. There are fifty-four figures but no plates. This was the only edition. (See also OT31.)

OT39. **HENRY CLARKE HOUGHTON** (1837–1901). *Lectures on clinical otol-ogy.* 260pp. Boston: O. Clapp & Son, 1885.

Born in Roxbury, Massachusetts, Houghton received his M.D. from the University of the City of New York in 1867. He later became a homeopath and in 1885 was senior aural surgeon at New York Ophthal-mic Hospital and professor of clinical otology at the New York Homeopathic College. He also served as president of the American Homeopathic Ophthalmological and Otological Society. This work was dedicated to the allopathic physician Daniel Bennett St. John Roosa (1838–1908), with whom Houghton had studied, and Timothy Field Allen (1837-1902), professor of materia medica and therapeutics at New York Homeopathic Medical College, "in the hope of the abolition of all division-walls between educated physicians and surgeons." The preface states:

> My duties as professor of clinical otology . . . have given occasion for a request for the substance, in book-form, of the lectures given to the senior class. The manuscript has been rewritten from the notes of a stenographer; and no alterations have been made, except of errors in the structure of sentences, such as are liable to occur in extemporaneous speaking. The book is not written for the specialist, but for the student and the busy practitioner, who will find in it suggestions for the treatment of aural diseases, and indications for remedies that have proved effective in a large clinical practice . . . .

The book consists of twelve lectures, with an extensive homeopathic repertory on pages 193–252. The two chromolithographs are reproduced from the plates of Adam Politzer's (1835–1920) *Monograph on the membrana tympani* and Roosa's *Diseases of the ear* (OT14). There are also thirty-one illustrations of various aural instruments. This was Houghton's only major book; no further editions were issued.

OT40. **THOMAS NICHOL** (?–?). *Diseases of the nares, larynx and trachea in childhood.* 308pp. New York: A. L. Chatterton, 1885.

Nichols was a homeopathic physician who was trained in the United States, but who practiced in Montreal. The eleven essays in this volume are based on his thirty years of clinical experience. Some of the work was serialized earlier in the *American observer.* Among the topics are "Acute coryza"; "Purulent coryza"; "Spasm of the glottis"; "Acute catarrhal laryngitis"; "Pseudo-membranous croup"; "Diphtheritic croup"; "Scarlatinal croup"; and "Tracheitis."

OT41. **HOMER I. OSTROM** (1852–?). *Epithelioma of the mouth.* 120pp. New York: A. L. Chatterton, 1885.

Ostrom was a member of the American Institute of Homeopathy. He writes that this

> . . . monograph is the out growth of a series of investigations entered into in the course of professional study, for the purpose of elucidating to the author, some obscure points in the pathology, etiology, and treatment of epithelioma of the mouth. Originally designed for personal use only, the notes made, early assumed the character of a study of the subject, which, in accordance with urgent requests, is now presented to the profession.

There are two chapters: "Epithelium of the mouth" and "Epithelioma of the mouth." This was the only edition. Ostrom was quite prolific and also wrote *The diseases of the uterine cervix* (New York: Boericke & Tafel, 1904) and *Leucorrhoea and other varieties of gynaecological catarrh; a treatise on the catarrhal affections of the genital canal of women; their medical and surgical treatment* (New York: Boericke & Tafel, 1910). (See also GS86.)

OT42. **THOMAS FRAZIER RUMBOLD** (1830–1901). *Pruritic rhinitis (hay-fever, autumnal catarrh, etc.). Its medical and surgical treatment.* 167pp. St. Louis: Medical Journal Publishing, 1885.

Rumbold dedicated this monograph to the fellows of the American Rhinological Association. He notes in the preface:

> The subject of this little monograph is not new, yet but comparatively little has been written on it until the last two or three years. Within this short period, rapid progress has been made in the methods of treatment . . . . The first rational step toward the cure of this complaint, is its treatment as a sequence of chronic inflammation of the nasal passages . . . . The removal of a hyperaesthetic membrane can not arrest the inflammatory process that was the producing cause of the hyperaesthesia; this is self-evident, consequently the ultimate recovery of the patient will certainly depend upon hygienic and constitutional measures and the sprayproducers . . . . The manuscript of this little book has been on my table for several years. The reason for the delay in its publication, was owing to the fact that within a few years, a surgical operation was proposed for the immediate relief of the most prominent symptoms of this complaint, and I desired to test whether the claims of its efficacy were well founded . . . . While freely acknowledging that surgical interference will cut short the pruritic nasal symptoms, yet, as I freely say, I fear many patients will be operated upon, who ought to be cured without the formation of cicatricial tissue in the nasal passages, by being treated for the originating disease, the chronic catarrhal inflammation of the nasal cavities. That this latter course is successful, I know from experience.

The book has eleven chapters plus a lengthy appendix. An extensive review of surgical treatment is found in chapter 11. There are eight illustrations. This was the only edition. (See also OT25, OT29, OT48, and OT66.)

OT43. **CHARLES EUCHARISTE DE MÉDICIS SAJOUS** (1852–1929). *Lectures on the diseases of the nose and throat.* 439pp. Philadelphia: F. A. Davis, 1885.

Sajous was a lecturer on rhinology and laryngology in the Spring Course of Jefferson Medical College when this volume was published. A fellow of the American Laryngological Association, he had previously served as president of the Philadelphia Laryngological Society. This treatise had eight plates consisting of 100 chromolithographs from oil paintings by Sajous and ninety-three wood engravings. The book was dedicated to Samuel D. Gross (1805–84). As Sajous writes in the preface:

> To do justice to such an undertaking, coloring was obviously of prime importance, the difference between the normal and pathological states frequently being only appreciable in the change of color. With this object in view, the author has performed the part of artist, as well as anatomist, believing that, though deficient in the former capacity, he might be able to furnish more accurate representations than if the task were confided to a capable artist, unfamiliar with the special subject. Ninety-seven out of the hundred illustrations are original. . . . Most of the anatomical plates, notably those on the larynx, were copied from nature.

There are twenty-nine chapters ranging in subject from "Illumination"; "Rhinoscopy"; "Diseases of the anterior nasal cavities"; "Pharyngoscopy"; "Diseases of the pharynx"; "Laryngoscopy"; and "Diseases of the

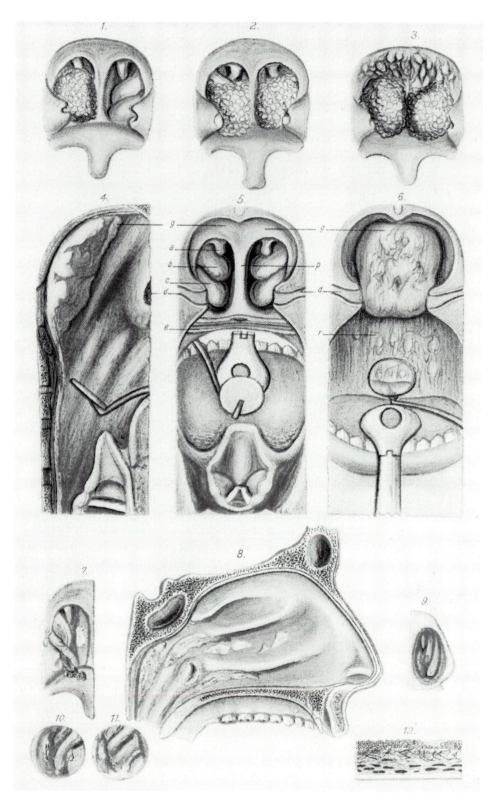

Fig. 74. (OT43) Sajous personally prepared these color plates from nature and used the services of W. H. Butler as lithographer. This plate, figure 3 on page 120, depicts various pathologic processes of the nasopharynx.

larynx to artificial openings into the larynx and trachea." A second edition was published in 1890. Among Sajous's other medical books are the six-volume *Annual and analytical cyclopaedia of practical medicine* (Philadelphia: F. A. Davis, 1898–1901) and the two-volume *The internal secretions and the principles of medicine* (Philadelphia: F. A. Davis, 1903–07). (See also OT44.)

OT44. **CHARLES EUCHARISTE DE MÉDICIS SAJOUS** (1852–1929). *Hay fever and its successful treatment by superficial organic alteration of the nasal mucous membrane.* 103pp. Philadelphia: F. A. Davis, 1885.

After having been promoted to instructor of rhinology and laryngology in the post-graduate and Spring courses of Jefferson Medical College, Sajous wrote this monograph as an expanded version of an essay read before the Philadelphia Laryngological Society on April 24, 1885. It is illustrated with thirteen wood engravings but has no table of contents or index. The bulk of the text is a review of a "comparatively large number of cases of so-called 'hay-fever' treated by the author within the last four years, having enabled him to note the value of certain practical points in connection with its successful treatment." (See also OT43.)

OT45. **CHARLES FREDERICK STERLING** (?–?). *The disease of the ear and their homoeopathic treatment, with a brief outline of the anatomy, physiology, and pathology.* 167pp. New York: A. L. Chatterton, 1885.

Sterling was a homeopath who was assistant surgeon at New York Ophthalmic Hospital and assistant to the chair of clinical otology at New York Homeopathic Medical College. The book contains fourteen chapters, with homeopathic remedies being noted in almost every section. Sterling writes in the preface:

> This little work is the outgrowth of a want felt by myself when first commencing the practice of medicine, for a small handy treatise on the examination and diagnosis of the more common diseases of the ear, and their homeopathic treatment. None such was at hand.... Dr. Winslow's book has since made its appearance, but while excellent, it is also elaborate and expensive, so that it seemed to me a little aid might perhaps be given to those who were similarly situated to myself, and possibly to another class; i.e., those physicians, who in practice before otology had reached its present development, wished for practical directions, and conscise statement, without theory....

There was only one edition.

OT46. **BEVERLEY ROBINSON** (1844–1924). *A manual on inhalers, inhalations, and inhalants, and guide to their discriminating use in the treatment of common catarrhal diseases of the respiratory tract.* 72pp. Detroit: G. S. Davis, 1886.

Robinson was clinical professor of medicine at Bellevue Hospital Medical College. His *Manual* was part of Series I of Davis's Physicians' Leisure Library. It was originally available in paper for twenty-five cents or cloth for fifty cents. The book consists of just five chapters: "Medicated sprays"; "Steam atomizers"; "Steam inhalers"; "Vapor inhalations"; and "Medicinal formulae." A second edition was printed in 1888. (See also OT24.)

OT47. **SAMUEL SEXTON** (1833–96). *The classification and treatment of over two thousand consecutive cases of ear diseases at Dr. Sexton's aural clinic, New York Eye and Ear Infirmary.* 95pp. Detroit: G. S. Davis, 1886.

Sexton was an 1856 graduate of the University of Louisville School of Medicine. An early member of the American Otological Society, he served as vice-president in 1886 and 1887. Sexton's practice was almost entirely devoted to the New York Eye and Ear Infirmary, where he was the dominant aural surgeon. This particular volume lacks a table of contents and index, making it difficult to read. It was published as part of Series I of Davis's Physicians' Leisure Library, and was available bound in paper for twenty-five cents or in cloth for fifty cents. A second edition was published in 1890. (See also OT49 and OT53.)

OT48. **THOMAS FRAZIER RUMBOLD** (1830–1901). *A practical treatise on the medical, surgical and hygienic treatment of catarrhal diseases of the nose, throat, and ears; including anatomy, physiology, pathology, etiology, and symptomatology.* 1,054pp. St. Louis: Medical Journal Publishing, 1887.

A massive work, the *Practical treatise* contains 148 illustrations and thirty-two lithographic plates, showing anatomical sections of the nasal and pharyngo-nasal cavities, and the cells and sinuses connected with them. The plates were taken from Emil Zuckerkandl's (1849–1910) *Anatomy of the nasal passages.* The *Practical treatise* contains five parts: "Anatomy, physiology, pathology, etiology and symptomatology"; "Instrumentation"; "The therapeutic and operative measures for catarrhal diseases of the nose, throat and ears"; "Hygienic and sanitary measures"; and "Detailed statements of cases and remarks on different methods of treatment." Rumbold writes in the preface:

> My attempt has been to discuss catarrhal disease of the nose, throat and ears as a unit. I contend that throat complaints can be more successfully treated in connection with the pharyngo-nasal and nasal inflammation, which always exists, than when treated alone; because the disease of the throat is a disease of the nasal passages extended to the throat; and that diseased ears can be more successfully treated by treating the rhinal inflammation which always exists since the ear disease is a rhinal inflammation extended to these organs . . . .

A second edition was published in 1888. (See also OT25, OT29, OT42, and OT66.)

OT49. **SAMUEL SEXTON** (1833–96). *The ear and its diseases; being practical contributions to the study of otology.* 461pp. New York: William Wood, 1888.

Sexton practiced in New York City, where he was aural surgeon at New York Eye and Ear Infirmary. He notes in the preface:

> The author has not attempted to present to the profession a treatise on the ear embracing the entire field of otology . . . . To the author's early

acquired vogue of noting in detail matters of practical interest in private and hospital practice is due the accumulation of the records of some ten thousand aural cases, or about one-third of all such that have passed through his hands during the past twenty years. It is at the earnest request of his professional friends, and many of the practitioners and students who have attended his aural clinics at the New York Eye and Ear Infirmary, and formerly at the New York Ear Dispensary, that he has been induced to select from this and from his published writings, the material of which this work is composed . . . . The following subjects introduced in the work are considered as worthy of special mention here, inasmuch as they present features not usually made so prominent in works on the war: Catarrh of the upper air tract; Oral irritation, specially dentition and diseased teeth, and Sea bathing—their causative influences on the ear. Wounds and injuries of the ear, occurring in warfare and civil life. Rupture of the drum-head from boxing the ears, and its medico-legal aspect. Concussion from the blast of great guns and explosives, etc. Anomalies of audition, noises in the ears and their connection with insane hallucinations and delusions. The effects of false hearing on singers, actors, lecturers, and musicians are also considered in this connection. Othaematoma occurring among lunatics, pugilists, and others has been presented very fully, and will, it is believed, be of special interest to alienists and examiners in lunacy. The operation of excision of the drum-head and ossicles for otorrhoea, and deafness due to chronic catarrh of the middle ear, including a full account of the literature of the subject. The results of this operation have been satisfactory, and it is hoped that its usefulness will be confirmed by experience. The effect of high atmospheric pressure on the ear in tunnels, caissons, and in diving, and the increase of submarine labor of late years makes it very important that the effect of such work on the ear be understood. The subject of pension claims of soldiers, sailors and marines on account of disability from deafness is discussed . . . .

The book is divided into four parts: "Remarks on the anatomy and physiology of the auricles, external auditory canal and contiguous parts, and the membrana tympani"; "Causes of ear disease"; "Wounds, injuries, and diseases of the ear and their treatment"; and "Miscellaneous articles." There are numerous illustrations but no plates. This was the only edition. (See also OT47 and OT53.)

OT49.1. **FRANK E. WAXHAM** (1852–1911). *Intubation of the larynx.* 110pp. Chicago: Charles Truax, 1888.

This book is unusual in that the publisher Charles Truax was actually a surgical instrument maker (GS189). Waxham was professor of otology, rhinology and laryngology at the College of Physicians and Surgeons in Chicago, where he was an early advocate of intubation in the treatment of diphtheria and croup in children. In the process of perfecting his intubation technique, Waxham began to use tubes made according to his instructions by Charles Truax and Company of Chicago. From this designer-manufacturer relationship emerged this monograph on intubation. It provides a lengthy history of efforts by physicians to devise intubation tubes and graphically portrays the process of intubation. Without these forty-five engravings, physicians could not easily grasp all the details necessary for the procedure to be successful. The book is dedicated to Joseph O'Dwyer (1841-98). Waxham states in the preface:

> Intubation has now become so thoroughly recognized as a practical and successful operation, that I believe it to be a duty the medical profession at large owe to the public, that at least one physician in every village, town and city throughout this great country, should possess the necessary instruments, pluck and skill to successfully perform this operation . . . .

There are six chapters: "History of intubation"; "Anatomy of the larynx"; "Directions for performing intubation"; "After treatment"; "Record of cases"; and "Comparative value of intubation and tracheotomy." There were no further editions.

OT50. **FRANCKE HUNTINGTON BOSWORTH** (1845–1925). *A treatise on diseases of the nose and throat.* 2 vols., 670pp. and 832pp. New York: William Wood, 1889–92. [G-M 3298]

This monumental work is one of the classics of American surgery. It was an immediate publishing success and added to the immense prestige that Bosworth already enjoyed. At the time he wrote the *Treatise*, he was professor of diseases of the throat at Bellevue Hospital Medical College. It is interesting to note that in the decade since publication of his last major work (OT26), Bosworth had changed his emphasis from diseases of the throat to diseases of the nose by reversing their order in the title. The first volume contains four color plates and 182 woodcuts. The preface states:

> The following work was originally undertaken with the intention of preparing a second edition of the volume on "Diseases of the Nose and Throat" [*sic;* even Bosworth forgot the title of his previous work] published by myself in 1881, but it soon became evident that the great advances made in the study of diseases of the upper air passages during the period which had elapsed since that work was issued, had rendered it necessary to rewrite practically the whole volume. I therefore determined to abandon the attempt to base the present work on my former one, and to write an entirely new treatise . . . . It has been my endeavor to present a full and complete treatise on the subjects covered by the title, and in carrying out this endeavor the work has grown on my hands in proportions beyond, perhaps, my original conception, and in place of a single volume which I originally contemplated, I have been compelled to divide the work into two volumes . . . . At the end of the volume there will be found a number of colored plates, illustrative of some of the operations described. These have in each instance been made from colored sketches of operations on the cadaver . . . .

Volume 1 contains forty-eight chapters divided in three major sections: "Diseases of the nasal passages"; "Diseases of the naso-pharynx"; and "External surgery of the nose."

Volume 2 was issued in 1892. It contained three color plates and 125 woodcuts. Bosworth explains the plan of this volume in the preface:

> In the preparation of this, the second and concluding volume of this work, I have followed the same general plan that was observed in the

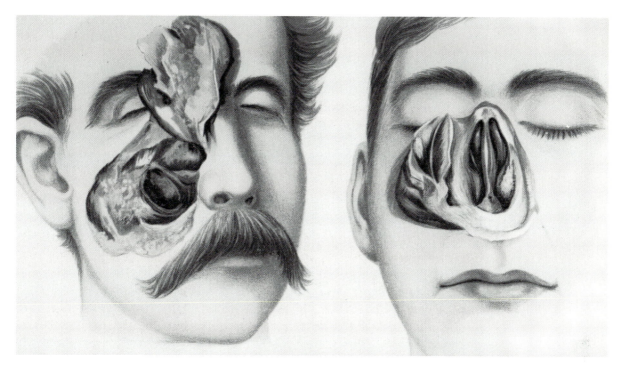

Fig. 75. (OT50) This chromolithograph plate from Bosworth's massive treatise, figure 4 on page 634 in volume 2, demonstrates Lagenbeck's operation for temporary resection of the upper portion of the superior maxilla and Brun's operation for the lateral osteo-plastic resection of the external nose.

arrangement of the first volume . . . . It is a source of regret that the appearance of this volume should have been so long delayed, the first volume having appeared two and a half years since. How unavoiable this delay has been will be fully appreciated when it is remembered that I have only been able to devote to its preparation the leisure intervals in my somewhat busy professional work. I can only bespeak for it the same friendly spirit in which the first volume was received.

Its three sections: "Diseases of the fauces"; "Diseases of the larynx"; and "External surgery of the throat"; contain fifty-one chapters. There were no further editions. (See also OT18, OT26, and OT61.)

OT51. **ALBERT HENRY BUCK** (1842–1922). *A manual of diseases of the ear.* 420pp. New York: William Wood, 1889.

As clinical professor of the diseases of the ear at the College of Physicians and Surgeons, Buck was an important individual in the history of American otorhinolaryngologic surgery. He served as president of the American Otological Society in 1879 and 1880. Buck writes in the preface:

Since the publication of my work in 1880, I have been led, by further experience, to modify the views therein expressed and the methods of treatment there advocated, in some important respects. The present time seemed therefore favorable for thoroughly revising the text and publishing it in a form adapted to the use as well of medical students as of practitioners of medicine. The manual now offered to the profession is the outcome of this effort. While a few chapters have been altered very little, others have been entirely rewritten, and considerable new matter has been added. The illustrations are also, in the majority

> of instances, different from those introduced in the earlier work . . . . In the present manual, as in the earlier treatise, I have made liberal use of my case-books for supplying brief descriptions of actual instances observed in practice . . . .

Among the fifteen chapters are "Fractures of the temporal bone"; "Diseases of the mastoid process"; "Syphilitic and tubercular disease of the deeper parts of the ear"; and "Different forms of aural disease in which the labyrinth is believed to be involved." The appendix (pages 389–412) provides an extensive anatomical and physiological sketch of the ear. Second and third editions were published in 1895 and 1898. (See also OT23 and OT68.)

OT52. **CHARLES HENRY BURNETT** (1842–1902). *Diseases and injuries of the ear: their prevention and cure.* 154pp. Philadelphia: J. B. Lippincott, 1889.

Part of Lippincott's Practical Lessons in Nursing Series, this small volume was written when Burnett was aural surgeon at Presbyterian Hospital in Philadelphia. He was also lecturer on otology at Woman's Medical College of Pennsylvania. Burnett had been president of the American Otological Society in 1884 and 1885. He writes in the preface:

> In the following pages the author has endeavored to present the important subject of "Diseases and Injuries of the Ear," in a form free from technical terms, so that it may be understood by any one . . . . The aim also has been to show the inexpert what to avoid in the treatment of ear-diseases, rather than what they may try to do for their relief. In this way it is believed the general reader can be best warned against error in treatment, and the hearing saved.

There were three parts: "Structure and function of the ear"; "Common diseases and injuries of the ear: their prevention and cure"; and "Aural hygiene of the deaf." This was the only edition and was available in cloth for $1.00. (See also OT17, OT19, and OT57.)

OT52.1. **CORNELIUS EVARTS BILLINGTON** (1844–1904) and **JOSEPH O'DWYER** (1841–98). *Diphtheria, its nature and treatment; and intubation in croup and other acute and chronic forms of stenosis of the larynx.* 326pp. New York: William Wood, 1889.

This work is actually two books in one, with Billington having persuaded O'Dwyer to write the portion on intubation. Billington explains in the preface:

> It affords me much pleasure that Dr. O'Dwyer has kindly consented to treat . . . that very important addition made by him to our therapeutical resources in dealing with the most distressing and fatal form of diphtheria,—intubation of the larynx.

O'Dwyer was an 1866 graduate of the College of Physicians and Surgeons in New York. From 1872 to 1897 he served as an attending physician at the New York Foundling Hospital. At a time when tracheotomy was the only, although ineffective, method of treating asphyxiation from diphtheria, O'Dwyer developed and pioneered laryngeal intubation [G-M 5057]. "O'Dwyer tubes" were widely used in cases of diphtheria before the availability of diphtheria antitoxin (1895) and later for other conditions, particularly laryngeal ulceration and stenosis. The portion of this work on diphtheria (pages 1-265) contains twenty-four black-and-white illustrations and one color plate with four figures. O'Dwyer's section (pages 265–309) has nine figures. An extensive index appears on pages 309–26. There was only one edition.

OT53. **SAMUEL SEXTON** (1833–96). *Deafness and discharge from the ear; the modern treatment for the radical cure of deafness, otorrhoea, noises in the head, vertigo, and distress in the ear.* 89pp. New York: J. H. Vail, 1891.

This small monograph, available for fifty cents, was written with the object of

> ... giving information concerning the modern treatment of ear diseases by radical measures to numerous inquirers, specially those whose letters I have not the necessary time at my disposal to answer, and indeed, could not answer satisfactorily within the limits of ordinary correspondence. This treatment of the ear is based upon modern surgical principles; but, like other advances in science, where ancient customs are displaced, it has met with strenuous opposition in some quarters and conservative indifference in others . . . .

The seven chapters are "History of former operations upon the ear, and the reason for their failure"; "The modern operation, what it is"; "Necessity of the operation, failure of the old methods for relieving deafness, noises in the head, vertigo, and discharge"; "The operation in catarrh of the middle ear"; "The operation in chronic discharge from the ear"; "Immediate and remote effects of the operation"; and "Summary and conclusions." There are a limited number of illustrations but no plates. (See also OT47 and OT49.)

OT54. **SAMUEL ELLSWORTH ALLEN** (?–?). *The mastoid operation, including its history, anatomy, and pathology.* 111pp. Cincinnati: R. Clarke, 1892.

Allen practiced in Cincinnati. This book is his only important contribution to surgical literature. He writes in the preface:

> In the little monograph here presented, the author does not lay any claim to originality. What knowledge he possesses was obtained at the fountain head, namely, at the clinic of Professor Schwartz, and the results of this instruction, supplemented by considerable thought and anatomical work of his own, are here made public. Of the defects of his literary style the author is only too well aware, but he trusts that the quality of the subject-matter will make up for the lameness in its presentation.

The four chapters are "Historical"; "Anatomical"; "Pathological"; and "The operation."

OT55. **FRANK E. MILLER** (1859–1932), **JAMES P. McEVOY** (?–?), and **JOHN E. WEEKS** (1853–1949). *Diseases of the eye, ear, throat, and nose.* 228pp. Philadelphia: Lea Brothers, 1892.

This work was part of Lea's Students' Quiz Series, which covered the essential subjects of a "thorough medical education arranged in form of question and answer." The volumes in the series were written by teachers and examiners in New York City and cost $1.00. Miller was an attending physician at St Joseph's Hospital and throat surgeon at the Vanderbilt Clinic. McEvoy was a throat surgeon at Bellevue Hospital, and Weeks practiced at the New York Eye and Ear Infirmary while also giving lectures on ophthalmology and otology at Bellevue Hospital Medical College. The contents include "The eye" (pages 17-126); "The ear" (pages 127-58); "The throat" (pages 159–94); and "The nose" (pages 195–228). There are two plates. This was the only edition. Among Weeks's other medical books is *A treatise on diseases of the eye* (New York: Lea & Febiger, 1910).

OT56. **ALBERT HENRY TUTTLE** (1861-?). *The surgical anatomy and surgery of the ear.* 96pp. Detroit: G. S. Davis, 1892.

Tuttle was a graduate of Harvard Medical School who practiced in Boston as a general surgeon. He writes in the preface:

> The following production is the outcome of special study to determine the topographical anatomy of the ear, with reference to the more modern surgical procedures. Some cases of ear disease having come under my treatment which I thought might be benefited by operative measures, I set to work on the skull, making sections and drawings to obtain, as nearly as possible, an accurate knowledge of the dangers and difficulties of the operations before me. As a result of this study, I soon had a collection of plates which were interesting, at least to me; and thinking they might perhaps be of some help to others, I have gathered them together in the following work, the scope of which I have extended somewhat, so as to make a short treatise on the surgery of the ear . . . .

There are twenty-five photographic plates reproduced from Tuttle's drawings from nature. The five chapters include "Anatomy of the ear"; "The external ear-diseases and treatment"; "Operations for the removal of the ossicles and membrana tympani"; "Diseases and operations on the mastoid, and necrosis of the temporal bone"; and "Meningitis, cerebral and cerebellar abscess, thrombosis of the cerebral sinuses, and phlebitis, with surgical treatment." This was the only edition.

OT57. **CHARLES HENRY BURNETT** (1842–1902). *System of diseases of the ear, nose, and throat.* 2 vols., 789pp. and 854pp. Philadelphia: J. B. Lippincott, 1893.

As the first multiauthor American textbook on otorhinolaryngology, this was an important work. It was also the first time that the specialty as it is practiced today was brought together in a single work. Burnett was emeritus professor of otology at the Philadelphia Polyclinic, clinical professor of otology at Woman's Medical College of Pennsylvania, and aural surgeon at Presbyterian Hospital. A graduate of Yale, he received an M.D. from the University of Pennsylvania in 1867. For many years he edited the department of progress of otology in the *American journal of the medical sciences.* Burnett writes in the *System's* preface:

> The close anatomical and pathological relations existing between the ear, the nose, and the throat often render it necessary that diseases of

these organs be treated by the same hand, whether it be that of the general practitioner or that of the specialist. And even in the practice of the aurist, the rhinologist, or the laryngologist, cases must present themselves where a knowledge of the morbid processes in all of these organs is absolutely necessary for the proper treatment of special maladies in any one of them. These weighty facts have rendered it very desirable that a systematic work should be prepared which should present at one view a consideration of the diagnosis and treatment of diseases of the ear, or the nose, and of the throat, thus freeing the practitioner from the necessity of referring to separate treatises upon any of these special departments of medical and surgical science . . . .

Volume 1 consists of part 1, "Diseases of the ear"; and part 2, "Diseases of the nose and naso-pharynx." Volume 2 continues with the concluding section of part 2, and part 3 , "Diseases of the pharynx and larynx." The book contains numerous plates and illustrations. Among the contributing authors are Edward B. Dench (1864–1936) on "Congenital malformations, cutaneous diseases, morbid growths, and injuries of the auricle"; Gorham Bacon (1855–?) on "Diseases and injuries of the membrana tympani and acute otitis media, including preventive hygiene"; Samuel Sexton (1833–96) on "Chronic catarrh of the middle ear"; Clinton Wagner (1837-1914) on "Local therapeutics in diseases of the nares, naso-pharynx, and larynx"; Francke Bosworth (1843–1925) on "Acute rhinitis"; Carl Seiler (1849–1905) on "Influenza and American grippe, or epidemic myxoidoedema"; E. Fletcher Ingals (1848–1918) on "Chronic pharyngitis"; Charles B. Nancrede (1847-1921) on "The surgical treatment of croup and diptheria"; Charles Huntoon Knight (1849–1913) on "Chronic diseases of the tonsils"; and Jacob DaSilva Solis Cohen (1838–1927) on "Tuberculosis and syphilis of the larynx." (See also OT17, OT19, and OT57.)

OT58. **HORACE FREMONT IVINS** (1856-99). *Diseases of the nose and throat.* 507pp. Philadelphia: F. A. Davis, 1893.

Ivins was a homeopath who lectured on laryngology and otology at Hahnemann Medical College, from which he had graduated in 1879. In addition, he was the laryngological editor of *The homeopathic.* The preface states:

> Although the following pages are especially intended for practical aids to the advanced medical student and general practitioner, it is hoped that they will also prove of value to the specialist in affections of the nose and throat . . . . In preparing the therapeutic indications it has been my endeavor to present a few remedies which are characteristic and reliable; it is, however, not always easy to separate the true from the spurious . . . . With few exceptions (cuts of instruments excluded), the illustrations are from my original photographs, drawings, or oil-sketches . . . .

The book contains thirty-eight chapters and has 129 illustrations and eighteen color plates. There was only one edition.

OT59. **EDWARD BRADFORD DENCH** (1864–1936). *Diseases of the ear.* 645pp. New York: D. Appleton, 1894.

Dench practiced otology in New York City, where he was professor of diseases of the ear at Bellevue Hospital Medical College. He served as president of the American Otological Society in 1911 and 1912. The *Diseases* contains eight color plates and 152 illustrations. Dench writes in the preface:

> In the preparation of the present work it has been my aim to adapt it to the needs both of the general practitioner and the special surgeon. For this reason minute pathology has not been considered extensively. In detailing the various manipulative procedures, I have preferred to err on the side of prolixity, for the benefit of those not familiar with the subject . . . . In advocating operative procedures upon the middle ear and in devoting much space to the subject of middle-ear operations, I am aware that I shall not have the support of many distinguished colleagues . . . . The absence of extensive bibliographical citations may seem a defect, but in a work intended as a clinical guide, a complete bibliography would be impossible, and unless complete it would be useless. No attempt has been made, therefore, to collate the entire literature of any subject, and the citations have been limited to those necessary to give individual investigators the proper credit for their researches.

There is an extensive table of contents which outlines each of the forty-eight chapters. The chapters are divided into five sections: "Anatomy and physiology of the ear"; "Diseases of the conducting apparatus";

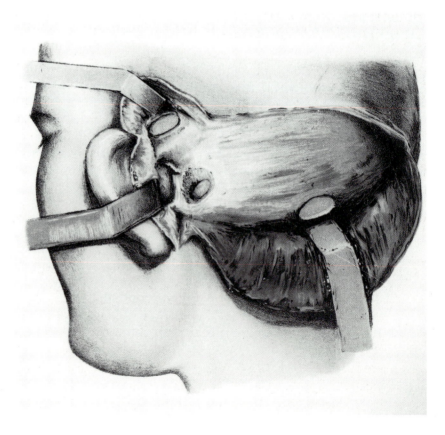

Fig. 76. (OT59) W. A. Holden prepared Dench's color plates from actual clinical cases. This plate, figure 8 on page 527, demonstrates exploration of the tympanic roof, lateral sinus, and cerebellum.

"Surgery of the conducting apparatus"; "Diseases of the perceptive mechanism"; and "Complicating aural affections." It was originally available in cloth for $5.00 or sheepskin for $6.00. Further editions were published in 1898, 1903 and 1909.

OT60. **E. BALDWIN GLEASON** (1854–1934). *Essentials of the diseases of the ear.* 147pp. Philadelphia: W. B. Saunders, 1894.

This book was No. 24 in Saunders' Question Compends Series. Gleason was clinical professor of otology at the Medico-Chirurgical College in Philadelphia. This book was

> ... written mainly for physicians who may desire to take a post-graduate course in otology, in order to enable them, with as little preliminary reading as possible, to acquire the rudimentary facts of otology which are essential to appreciate properly what is seen and heard in the actual work of an ear dispensary. For this purpose a quiz-compend is undoubtedly of greater value than is a large textbook, no matter how great is the excellence of the latter . . . .

The book comprises the following sections: "Anatomy of the ear"; "Tests for hearing"; "Diagnosis and treatment"; "Examination of patients"; "Diagnostic table of diseases of ear"; "Diseases of the external ear"; "Diseases of membrana tympani"; "Diseases of the middle ear"; "Operations upon the middle ear"; and "Formulae." It was available in cloth for $1.00. Further editions were published in 1897, 1902 and 1906. Gleason also wrote *A manual of diseases of the nose, throat, and ear* (Philadelphia: W. B. Saunders, 1907). (See also OP47.)

OT61. **FRANCKE HUNTINGTON BOSWORTH** (1845–1925). *A text-book of diseases of the nose and throat.* 814pp. New York: William Wood, 1896.

The immediate success of his *Diseases of the nose and throat* (OT50) prompted Bosworth to bring out this shorter textbook. It enjoyed great popularity and was for many years the vade mecum of American students and practioners of general medicine as well as those who specialized in the field. At the time of its publication, Bosworth was professor of diseases of the throat at Bellevue Hospital Medical College. He writes in the preface:

> My recent work on the nose and throat in two volumes having been considered somewhat too voluminous for the use of students, it has been thought best to prepare the following volume, designed especially for the use of the general practitioner and student. The work is mainly a condensation of my former two volumes into one, in which the effort has been to retain all that is of practical use so far as possible. This has been accomplished by eliminating those parts of the work which were of value only for reference, and I trust that it has been done to the satisfaction of the reader. Some new material has been added and some few changes made, but in essentials the single volume is the same as the larger edition.

There are ninety-nine chapters divided into six sections: "Diseases of the nasal passages"; "Diseases of the naso-pharynx"; "External surgery of the nose"; "Diseases of the fauces"; and "Diseases of the larynx." The book contains 186 engravings and seven full-page color plates. (See also OT18 and OT26.)

OT62. **JOSEPH HOWARD BUFFUM** (1849–?). *Manual of the essentials of diseases of the eye and ear.* 315pp. Chicago: Gross & Delbridge, 1896.

Buffum was professor of ophthalmology and otology at Chicago Homeopathic Medical College. He describes his purpose in writing the book in the preface:

> This manual, written at the request of the author's classes, presents the essential diagnostic and therapeutic points of the various diseases of the eye and ear in such concise form as to enable the student and general practitioner to readily obtain the more important details of the treatment of such diseases . . . . It is intended that the outlines here given will be supplemented by ophthalmological and otological lectures, clinical and didactic, as well as by reference to the larger text-books pertaining to the subjects.

There are numerous black-and-white illustrations and a few chromolithographs. Written in a concise fashion, it was quite well received. A second edition appeared in 1901. (See also OP36 and OP59.)

OT63. **LEVI COOPER LANE** (1830–1902). *The surgery of the head and neck.* 1,180pp. San Francisco: Privately printed, 1896.

This massive compendium is the first American textbook on head and neck surgery and the first American surgical textbook published in California. It was published when Lane was professor of surgery at Cooper Medical College in San Francisco. He is credited with having performed the first vaginal hysterectomy in this country. Lane wrote a most unusual and erudite preface:

> It has been the custom of authors in separating from their books to say a parting word to them; this, by some, has been a dedication to a father, brother or friend, and in one case to the author of nature. Horace warns his of coming abuse and final neglect; Martial hints to his scroll that it may serve the base use of wrapping fish, or the worse one of becoming a flaming festoon to illuminate and torture the criminal; but Ovid, more ambitious and hopeful, announced in advance the salutations of immortality with which the coming years would greet his *Metamorphoses*; but the medical writer of today, warned by the fortune of his contemporaries, may prudently contract the horizon of his expectation, and reckon on but a brief life for his book. He who thinks otherwise, reckons ill with futurity. Thus warned, with limited hope, should a few years of existence be granted to the following pages, the writer's expectations will be fully realized.

There are thirty-five chapters and 111 illustrations. The first edition is rather scarce, and a second edition was published in 1898.

OT64. **SETH SCOTT BISHOP** (1852–1923). *Diseases of the ear, nose, and throat and their accessory cavities.* 496pp. Philadelphia: F. A. Davis, 1897.

Bishop was an 1876 graduate of Northwestern University Medical School. He practiced in Chicago where he eventually became professor at Chicago Post-Graduate Medical School and Hospital and surgeon at

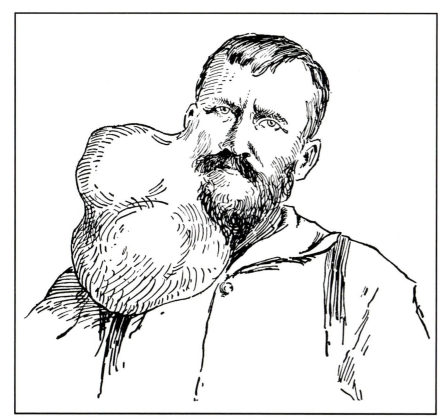

Fig. 77. (OT63) A sarcomatous tumor of the cervical glands which Lane successfully removed is shown in this engraving (number 94, page 875).

Illinois Charitable Eye and Ear Infirmary. He was one of the early editors of the journal *Laryngoscope* and was a vice-president of the United States Hay Fever Association. This volume was dedicated to Nicholas Senn (1844–1908) and

> . . . was designed, first, to help students in preparing for their degree; second, for those progressive practitioners who wish to acquire the proficiency necessary to properly treat those patients who are unable to visit specialists; and, third, for those who are gradually exchanging their general practice for special work in these branches. The subjects are simplified and condensed so as to constitute this book a key, or introduction, to the exhaustive treatises already in the field. The place of the latter is not expected to be filled by this unpretentious book, for it was not intended primarily for specialists . . . . Several subjects are treated in greater detail than characterizes the work as a whole, for the following reasons: No book, equivalent to this, is now available containing the latest developments concerning diphtheria, the blood-serum therapy, the medical and surgical management of mastoid diseases, the most successful treatment of hay fever, the improved con-pressed-air instruments, vaporizing apparatus, inhalents, etc . . . . Like works on general medicine and surgery, little space is devoted to the anatomy of the various organs . . . .

The first part deals with diseases of the ear and comprises seventeen chapters, the second part describes diseases of the nose and consists of nine chapters, the third part has eight chapters on diseases of the pharynx, and the final eight chapters deal with diseases of the larynx. There are 100 colored lithographs and 168 additional illustrations.

Included is a statistical table of 15,000 cases from Bishop's own clinical record books. The first printing was exhausted in a few months, and further editions were published in 1898, 1904 and 1908. Bishop also wrote *The ear and its diseases* (Philadelphia: F. A. Davis, 1906).

OT64.1. **GEORGE H. QUAY** (?–?). *A monograph of diseases of the nose and throat.* 214pp. Philadelphia: Boericke & Tafel, 1897.

Quay was a homeopathic physician who served as professor of rhinology and laryngology at Cleveland Medical College. He notes in the preface of this rather elusive volume:

> The book is the outcome of an experience in the general practice of medicine which was not small, supplemented by several years of exclusively nose, throat and ear work. During the last five years I have been in almost daily contact with students, in the capacity of teacher, and have especially felt the need of a condensed work on the subject. Few general practitioners have either the time or the inclination to wade through a volume on rhinology and laryngology which deals with exhaustive details, though a working knowledge of the diseases of the nose and throat is absolutely essential to the successful physician. I have, therefore, kept constantly in mind these two classes of readers . . . .

There are twenty chapters, including "Epistaxis"; "Syphilitic rhinitis"; "Tumors of the nose"; "Retro-pharyngeal abscess"; "Laryngeal tuberculosis"; and "Tumors of the larynx." The seventeen illustrations are all rather rudimentary engravings; most of them show surgical instruments. This was the only edition.

OT65. **GORHAM BACON** (1855–?). *A manual of otology.* 398pp. New York: Lea Brothers, 1898.

Bacon was one of America's most prominent otologists. He served as president of the American Otological Society from 1891 to 1894 and was professor of otology at Cornell University Medical College. In preparing this *Manual*, Bacon

> . . . tried to meet the demands of the student, by giving him a short and compact treatise of the subject, and at the same time affording him a book of easy reference, since he may not always find the time necessary for consulting the many excellent and more exhaustive treatises upon otology which have been published not only in this country but also in England and on the Continent . . . .

There were fourteen chapters, including "Otitis media purulenta acuta"; "Otitis media catarrhalis chronica"; "Brain abscess"; "Diseases of the sound-perceiving apparatus"; and "Deaf-mutism." A total of 110 illustrations and one color plate are included. The book was well received and went through further editions in 1900, 1902, 1906 and 1909.

OT66. **THOMAS FRAZIER RUMBOLD** (1830–1901). *The hygiene of the voice.* 144pp. St. Louis: Witt, 1898.

This is a little known and hard-to-find volume. Rumbold notes in the preface:

> Having had a long and large experience in the medical care of singers and speakers, I have made their health, the stability and purity of their voices, and the diseases that affect their upper respiratory and vocal or-

gans an earnest study. The result of this experience and study, . . . is here given for their benefit. No medical treatment is recommended, except a few simple remedies for temporary relief, and those only of such character as would not, under any circumstances, be harmful, however taken . . . . My long experience teaches me that none but medical men should attempt the treatment of voice-users. It is not an exercise of common sense to think that non-medical voice-users, or their teachers, can employ medical prescriptions, however circumstantially given, nearly as successfully as can a physician. Not only this, but no one but a specialist, one who has limited his practice to the diseases of the nose, throat and ears, should treat these diseases . . . .

The contents include "Nasal passages"; "Pharyngo-nasal cavity"; "Pharynx"; "Soft palate"; "Uvula and the azygos prominence"; "Tonsils"; "Epiglottis"; "Larynx and vocal cords"; "Causes of vocal disability"; "Care of the voice"; "Ears"; "Tongue"; "Lips"; "Teeth and gums"; "Lungs"; "Diaphragm"; "Corsets"; "The respirator"; "Protection and relief of the throat"; "Temperature of the stage"; "Diet"; and "The effect of tobacco on the mucuous membranes." The book has twenty-seven illustrations. This was Rumbold's last medical work, and only one edition was published. (See also OT25, OT29, OT42, and OT48.)

OT67. **WILLIAM SCHEPPEGRELL** (1860–?). *Electricity in the diagnosis and treatment of diseases of the nose, throat and ear.* 403pp. New York: G. P. Putnam's Sons, 1898.

An 1889 graduate of the Medical College of the State of South Carolina, Scheppegrell almost immediately took up the study of eye, ear, nose, and throat surgery. He eventually settled in New Orleans, where he became surgeon and head of the electrical department at the Eye, Ear, Nose and Throat Hospital. He also served as coeditor of the *Annals of otology, rhinology and laryngology. Electricity* is a massive compendium of thirty-seven chapters dealing with all facets of electricity in its relation to diseases of the nose, throat and ear. It is especially notable for chapters 36 and 37, which deal with the use of X rays in otolaryngology. This book was written within three years of Roentgen's discovery of X rays and is the first time that such information was noted in an American textbook of ear, nose and throat surgery. There are 161 illustrations. This was the only edition.

OT68. **ALBERT HENRY BUCK** (1842–1922). *First principles of otology.* 212pp. New York: William Wood, 1899.

The *Principles* was written while Buck was clinical professor of the diseases of the ear at the College of Physicians and Surgeons and in the Medical Department of Columbia University, and consulting aural surgeon to the New York Eye and Ear Infirmary. He notes in the preface:

> The complaint has frequently been made—and rightly, as I believe—that the larger treatises on otology contain a great deal of material which, however useful it may be to men who propose to treat diseases of the ear, is practically of little value to medical students, of whom a knowledge of only the first principles of this branch of surgery is required for graduation. For such readers, therefore, a much smaller

work—one that treats only of the fundamental facts and theories relating to the anatomy, physiology, pathology, and therapeutics of the ear—should amply suffice. The present little book is the outcome of an attempt to supply such a manual for the exclusive use of undergraduate medical students.

The volume, which contains thirteen chapters, is quite thorough in its presentation of the subject. A second edition was published in 1903. (See also OT23 and OT51.)

OT69. **CORNELIUS GODFREY COAKLEY** (1862–1934). *A manual of diseases of the nose and throat.* 536pp. Philadelphia: Lea Brothers, 1899.

Coakley received his M.D. from New York University Medical School in 1887. He served as president of the American Laryngological Association in 1918 and president of the New York Laryngological Society in 1933. Coakley's *Manual* was written when he was clinical professor of laryngology at his alma mater. This book became a standard text in many medical colleges, and further editions were published in 1901, 1905 and 1908. The eleven chapters include "Antisepsis in operations upon the upper respiratory tract"; "Nasal obstruction"; and a special chapter devoted to "Therapeutics" (pages 491-512); this chapter contains a classification of drugs according to their local actions and a number of useful prescriptions, together with indications for their employment. There are ninety-two engravings and two color plates.

OT70. **GEORGE EDMUND DE SCHWEINITZ** (1858–1938) and **BURTON ALEXANDER RANDALL** (1858–1932): An *American text-book of diseases of the eye, ear, nose and throat.* 1,251pp. Philadelphia: W. B. Saunders, 1899.

De Schweinitz was professor of ophthalmology at Jefferson Medical College and Randall was clinical professor of diseases of the ear at the University of Pennsylvania and professor of diseases of the ear at the Philadelphia Polyclinic. The book contains 766 engravings, 59 of them in color. It was available in either cloth for $7.00, or in sheepskin or half morocco for $8.00, and was part of Saunders' American Text-Book Series. Other titles in the series include *Diseases of children* by Louis Starr (1849–1925); *Legal medicine and toxicology* by Frederick Peterson (1859–1938); *Obstetrics*, edited by Richard C. Norris (1863–?); *Pathology* by Ludvig Hektoen (1863–1951); *Physiology* by William H. Howell (1860–1945); and *Theory and practice of medicine* by William Pepper (1843–98). De Schweinitz and Randall write in the preface that

> . . . it is unnecessary to discuss the "collaboration-method" thus employed, which has too often demonstrated its value to need either defence or explanation in this place, except to point out its greatest use, and the one to which no doubt it is indebted for its success—namely, that by its means, in the words of Dr. W. H. Howell, "the student gains the point of view of a number of teachers, reaping, in a measure, the same benefit as would be obtained by following courses of instruction under different teachers." This work is essentially a text-book on the

one hand, and, on the other, a volume of reference to which the practitioner may turn and find a series of articles written by men who are authorities on the subjects portrayed by them . . . . A word should be said with reference to the effort to comprise within one volume studies of the Eye, Ear, Nose, and Throat—an effort which may challenge criticism in this day of highly differentiated specialties. Yet it has seemed to the editors that each of these branches could receive text-book treatment within the space here assigned, while their important correlations could be better brought out by such juxtaposition. Specialism has often been carried much too far in the exclusion of attention to the adjacent fields . . . . Indeed, no practitioner, general or special, should be unfamiliar with all the types of disease and the most precise methods of their study, for it must often happen that he cannot avail himself of help from others. He should know a little of everything and all about some one thing . . . . It seems proper to note that there has been complete division of the editorial labor and responsibility, that of the ophthalmic portion being assumed by Dr. de Schweinitz, and that of the Otological and Laryngological sections by Dr. Randall.

Part 1 discusses the eye, and among the authors in this section are George Arthur Piersol (1856–1924), Edward Jackson (1856–1942), Swan Moses Burnett (1847-1906), Alvin Allace Hubbell (1846–1911), and Casey Albert Wood (1856–1942). Part 2 discusses the ear in thirteen chapters, including contributions by Christian Rasmus Holmes (1851-1920), Clarence John Blake (1843–1919), Edward Bradford Dench (1864–1936), Albert Henry Buck (1842–1922), and Hermann Knapp (1832–1911). The nose and throat are discussed in part 3 in twenty chapters by authors such as Harrison Allen (1841-97), Charles Euchariste de Médicis Sajous (1852–1929), and Jonathan Wright (1860–1928). There was only one edition. (See also OP52 and OP67.)

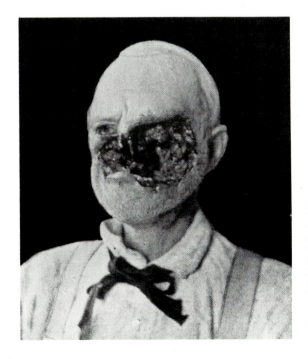

Fig. 78. (OT70) In this remarkable engraving from a photograph (number 174, page 251) de Schweinitz and Randall show the potential destructiveness of a rodent (basal cell carcinoma) ulcer. This patient, who was under the care of Dudley P. Allen of Cleveland, initially had the lesion in the left lower eyelid.

OT71. **DAVID BRADEN KYLE** (1863–1916): *A textbook of diseases of the nose and throat.* 536pp. Philadelphia: W. B. Saunders, 1899.

Kyle was educated at Muskingum College and at Jefferson Medical College, from which he graduated in 1891. In 1896 he was elected clinical professor of laryngology and rhinology at Jefferson. In 1900 he was president of the American Laryngological, Rhinological and Otological Society, and in 1911 he held the same office in the American Laryngological Association. Kyle's textbook was dedicated to William Williams Keen (1837-1932), professor of surgery at Jefferson. It contains 175 illustrations, 23 of them in color. Subsequent editions were published in 1900, 1904, 1907 and 1911. It was part of Saunders' New Aid Series and was available in cloth for $4.00 or in morocco for $5.00. Kyle writes in the preface:

> It has been my aim to present to the reader the subject of Diseases of the Nose and Throat in as concise a manner as is compatible with clearness. While the arrangement differs somewhat from many of the other text-books on this subject, it has been my aim to classify the diseases according to the pathological alterations caused by them . . . . The lithographs and original illustrations are made from specimens prepared by the authors in his own laboratory, and the drawings are from cases under his immediate observation . . . .

The book contains twenty-three chapters, including "Diseases of the anterior nasal cavities"; "Neuroses"; "Intubation of the larynx"; "Tracheotomy"; and "Operations on the larynx."

OT72. **FRANCIS NAULTEUS** (?–?): *Medical compendium on all acute and chronic, all female and children, eye, ear, nose and throat diseases.* 321pp. Hastings: E. Watkins, 1899.

Naulteus was born in Germany, where he received his medical education and training as a pupil and assistant at Albrecht von Graefe's (1828–70) eye clinic in Berlin. He eventually settled in Hastings, Nebraska. This work is unique in that the table of contents appears in both German and English. Naulteus writes in the preface:

> Long years of practice and experience brought me to the conclusion, that the long, many-sided text books and descriptions in the manuals with the long words, are well enough for future reference, but too long for the beginner and student to secure a quick, correct diagnosis. A much better foundation can be laid with brevity . . . . This book . . . is a welcome friend of the people in time of danger before the physician can be at hand . . . .

Although the title suggests otherwise, the book covers much more than just eye, ear, nose and throat diseases. In fact, only a small portion deals with otorhinolaryngology. Instead, almost every other organ system of the body is described relative to various disease states.

IV. ORTHOPEDIC SURGERY

OR1. **JOHN COLLINS WARREN** (1778–1856). *A letter to the honorable Isaac Parker, Chief Justice of the Supreme Court of the State of Massachusetts, containing remarks on the dislocation of the hip joint.* 142pp. Cambridge: Hilliard & Metcalf, 1824.

Published when Warren was professor of anatomy and surgery at Harvard University, this work presents testimony by Warren concerning a medical malpractice case. *The life of John Collins Warren* gives an interesting account of the genesis of this work (volume 1, pages 221–22):

> One of the most remarkable publications by Dr. Warren, upon surgical subjects, was his letter to Judge Parker, printed in 1824. It contains a very clear and minute description of the different forms of dislocation of the hip-joint, intended to explain, in terms intelligible to non-medical men, the injuries of this joint, which are often the most complicated and difficult to recognize of any that occur in the human body. With a great deal of research and close reasoning, he proves the possibility of a species of dislocation whose existence had been denied by Sir Astley Cooper, though recognized by some of the most distinguished

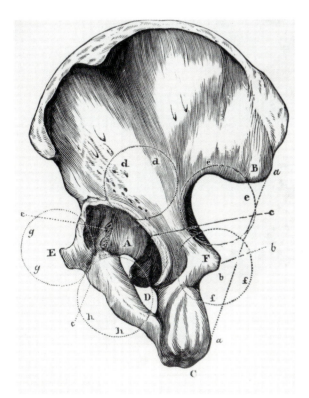

Fig. 79. (OR1) This was typical of all the illustrations in Warren's work. Simple in form, it provides a lateral view of the pelvic girdle with letters to explain various types of dislocations.

Continental surgeons. The occasional occurrence of this form of dislocation has since been proved by a specimen in St. Bartholomew's Hospital, and by cases published in the American edition of Sir Astley Cooper's work on dislocations.

This book is quite scarce. Five plates are included along with extensive accounts of the trial. (See also GS15, GS26, and GS27.1.)

OR2. **SAMUEL DAVID GROSS** (1805–84). *The anatomy, physiology, and diseases of the bones and joints.* 389pp. Philadelphia: John Grigg, 1830.

The *Anatomy* was Gross's first surgical textbook and was written when he was only twenty-five years old. He had graduated from Jefferson Medical College only two years before and was in private practice in Philadelphia and Easton, Pennsylvania. Gross describes the composition of the book in his autobiography (volume 1, pages 42–43):

> I commenced the composition of an original work, which was issued by Mr. Grigg in the autumn of 1830 under the title of *The Anatomy, Physiology, and Diseases of the Bones and Joints*. This work formed an octavo volume of nearly four hundred pages, and was written in the space of little more than three months. The title was unfortunate; it should have been *A Practical Treatise on Fractures and Dislocations, with an Account of the Diseases of the Bones and Joints*, which the profession, especially the younger members of it, would have better understood. The work was well received, and two thousand copies were exhausted in less than four years. Notwithstanding this, no other edition was ever issued; first, because I had no time to bestow upon it the requisite attention, and, secondly, because I had not the experience which was necessary to make the work what it should be. I need hardly add that, young as I was when the book was issued, I had to depend for the facts mainly upon the labors of others, though in the composition of it I used my own language. I have often thought that this work, if entirely rewritten and brought to a level with the existing state of the science, might be rendered useful to the younger members of the profession, to whom the subjects of which it treats are a stumbling-block, and who are so often prosecuted for malpractice in consequence of the mismanagement of cases of fractures and dislocations. For this book I never received a cent of remuneration!

The six chapters deal with the "General anatomy of the bones"; "Fractures or injuries of the bones"; "Diseases of the bones"; "General anatomy of the joints"; "Injuries of the joints"; and "Diseases of the joints." There are no illustrations or plates. (See also GS16, GS19, GS34, GS46, GS49, and GU5.)

OR3. **THOMAS DENT MÜTTER** (1811–59). *A lecture on loxarthrus or clubfoot.* 104pp. Philadelphia: Hooker & Claxton, 1839.

Mütter was not fond of writing, and this somewhat loosely written treatise is one of his few literary efforts. At its publication he was lecturer on surgery at and a fellow of the College of Physicians of Philadelphia. The work is difficult to read because it has neither table of contents nor index. It contains a number of wood engravings. Pages 79–103 give detailed reports of twenty-eight cases of loxarthrus. (See also GS20).

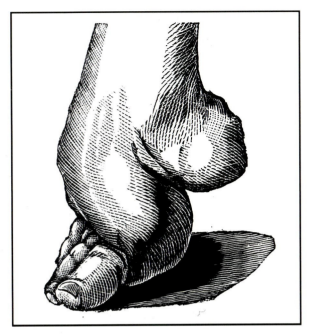

Fig. 80. (OR3) Mütter describes three varieties of clubfoot; this one was called "pes equinis." The engraving (page 24) shows a second-degree variation of this form in which the whole foot is bent upon itself.

OR4. **HENRY JACOB BIGELOW** (1818–90). *Manual of orthopedic surgery, being a dissertation which obtained the Boylston Prize for 1844, on the following question: "In what cases, and to what extent is the division of muscle, tendons, or other parts proper for the relief of deformity or lameness?"* 211pp. Boston: William D. Ticknor, 1845.

Bigelow graduated from Harvard Medical School in 1841 and spent most of his professional life on the Harvard medical faculty, being named professor of surgery there four years after publication of the *Manual*. However, he was in private practice when he wrote the *Manual*. Although Bigelow was one of America's major innovators in orthopedic surgery [G-M 4461], he made other contributions in urologic surgery [G-M 4292] and anesthesia [G-M 5651 and 5730]. This volume was the first comprehensive treatment of the subject in America and includes a superb summary of French orthopedic surgery of the day. Bigelow wrote in the preface that "The works I have consulted in writing the following dissertation, are chiefly those of Guerin, Bonnet, Velpeau, Phillips, Duval and Little . . . . " Interestingly, the first sixty-eight pages are devoted to operations for strabismus and stammering. There are six rather unimpressive plates, four of which picture surgical devices to treat clubfoot, torticollis, false anchylosis of knee-joint, and lateral curvature of the spine. A major source of information about Bigelow and his collective writings can be found in three volumes prepared anonymously by his son William (1849–1926): *I. The mechanism of dislocation and fracture of the hip, II. Litholapaxy; or, rapid lithotrity with evacuation* (Boston: Little & Brown, 1900), *Orthopedic surgery and other medical papers* (Boston: Little & Brown, 1900), and *Surgical anaesthesia; addresses and other papers* (Boston: Little & Brown, 1900). In addition, his son edited *A memoir of Henry Jacob Bigelow* (Boston: Little & Brown, 1900). (See also OR22.)

OR5. **GEORGE OGELVIE JARVIS** (1795–1875). *Lectures on fractures and dislocations, explaining new modes of treatment, founded on anatomy, physiology, and the laws of mechanics, together with concise instructions in the use of the "surgical adjuster."* 80pp. Derby: H. & G. Kellogg, 1846.

Jarvis practiced in Portland, Connecticut, where he paid particular attention to fractures and dislocations. He received his medical license in 1817 and was awarded an honorary M.D. from Yale University in the year this monograph was published. His major claim to fame was the development of his "surgical adjuster":

> By means of this instrument the surgeon has at his command an extending and counter-extending force, equal to that of twelve men, all or any part of which he can apply to any limb at pleasure, and yet the limb remain perfectly moveable and free for manipulation.

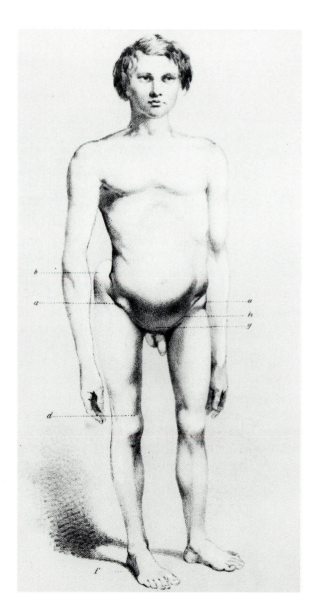

Fig. 81. (OR6) Carnochan's monograph contains finely detailed illustrations. This plate, figure 1, shows an anterolateral view in a case of double congenital dislocation of the head of the femur upon the dorsum of the ilium. The lithographer was Sarony & Major.

This volume is basically an advertisement for the "adjuster." It consists of five lectures on fractures and dislocations that Jarvis gave at the Royal Westminster Ophthalmic Hospital in London in November 1845. They were originally published in the March, April and May 1846 *Lancet* and later brought together in book form. The book does not have a table of contents or index but does present a number of illustrations, including twelve plates. The volume went through five editions by 1848.

OR6. **JOHN MURRAY CARNOCHAN** (1817–87). *A treatise on the etiology, pathology and treatment of congenital dislocations of the head of the femur.* 235pp. New York: S. S. & W. Wood, 1850.

Carnochan is listed on the title page of this work as lecturer on operative surgery with surgical and pathological anatomy. A year after this book was published he was named professor of surgery at New York Medical College. In this volume, Carnochan first introduced the most current European ideas on dislocation of the femur to American surgeons. He wrote in the preface that

> . . . it should embrace a general parallel between the state of British and French surgery, and the actual condition of the science in our own country . . . the subject of the present monograph being a novel one, and, indeed, quite new upon the American continent . . . it being the first attempt to introduce to the surgeons of this country a systematic account of this important affection of the human organism.

There are eight chapters, including "General observations"; "Anatomical remarks"; "Etiology"; "Symptomatology"; "Diagnosis"; "Prognosis"; "Pathology"; and "Treatment." The book is illustrated with nine plates which show skeletal abnormalties and four additional lithographs depicting various apparatuses for the treatment of dislocation. (See also GS40.)

OR7. **FRANK HASTINGS HAMILTON** (1813–89). *A practical treatise on fractures and dislocations.* 757pp. Philadelphia: Blanchard & Lea, 1860. [G-M 4420]

Hamilton's *Treatise* is the first American text to deal with fractures in depth. As professor of surgery at the University of Buffalo, Hamilton had previously published a well-received report on deformities after fractures [G-M 1742]. Shortly before publication of the *Treatises*, he was appointed to the chair of surgery at Long Island College Hospital. Hamilton writes in the preface:

> Very little space has been devoted to what is now only historical, except so far as was necessary to correct certain time-consecrated errors or to confirm and illustrate the practice of the present day; but, by a pretty full report of characteristic examples selected from more than one thousand cases already published by myself, by copious references to the examples recorded by others, and by a careful exclusion of whatever has not been confirmed by experience or established by dissection, I have endeavored to make this treatise useful both to the student and practical man, and a reliable exponent of the present state of our art upon those subjects of which it treats.

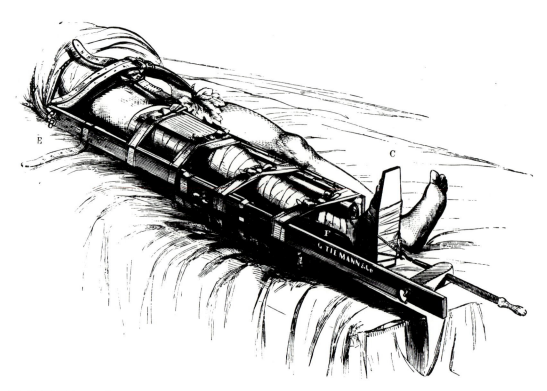

Fig. 82. (OR7) This wood engraving, figure 160 on page 424, demonstrates a splint for the lower extremity for which Hamilton had supplied a foot-piece.

The first part contains thirty-five chapters on numerous topics related to fractures. There are 210 woodcuts in this section. The second part has twenty-six chapters on dislocations and seventy-nine woodcuts. The book was initially available only in cloth for $4.25. Further editions were published in 1863, 1866, 1871, 1875, 1880, and 1884. (See also GS50, GS70, GS75, OR37 and OP8.)

OR8. **RICHARD MANNING HODGES** (1827–96). *The excision of joints.* 204pp. Cambridge: Welch & Bigelow, 1861.

This monograph was the recipient of the 1861 Boylston Prize. Hodges explains his reason for writing the book in his preface:

> Excisions of joints have been comparatively little practised in the United States. The personal experience of any one American surgeon in regard to them is therefore of a very limited character; and American medical periodicals, or systematic writings, furnish but little material calculated to throw light upon the questions connected with this class of operations. British, and, to a larger extent, European medical literature offer, however, a fertile field for their study . . . .

The work is divided into sections on the upper and lower extremities; a bibliography at its end provides an extensive list of all the principal works and articles on excisions of joints. There are no illustrations or plates, although several tables of operative cases are included. Hodges's writings on joints, spiroidal fractures and other surgical conditions became the authoritative texts. In 1862 the United States Sanitary Commission published a 23-page report, written by Hodges, as part of its

Medical and Surgical Monographs on excision of joints for traumatic cause. (See also GS43.)

OR9. **CHARLES FAYETTE TAYLOR** (1827–99). *Theory and practice of the movement-cure; or, the treatment of lateral curvature of the spine, paralysis, indigestion, constipation, consumption, angular curvatures and other deformities, diseases incident to women, derangements of the nervous system and other chronic affections by the Swedish system of localized movements.* 295pp. Philadelphia: Lindsay & Blakiston, 1861.

Taylor received his M.D. from the University of Vermont in 1856. He studied in London after graduation, where he was introduced to the concept of kinesipathy or the "Swedish movement" system of Per Henrik Ling (1776–1839) that became of great importance to orthopedic surgery. Ling developed the ancient Greek art of calisthenics to a science based on sound anatomic and physiological principles. He was among those who thought in terms of motions rather than muscles, and believed that the education of the locomotor system was the best way to prevent the occurrence of iodiopathic deformities such as scoliosis, round shoulders, hollow back, and weak feet. Taylor returned to New York City and became the first American to introduce this new system to the medical profession. His book was dedicated to Baron William de Wetterstedt, minister resident from Sweden and Norway to the United States

> . . . as a token of personal regard and as an expression of gratitude to the country he represents, which has produced, not least among her sons of unpretentious greatness, with a Celsius; a Linnaeus; a Berzelius; and a Retzius; Peter Henry Ling, poet and philosopher, to teach us not only to despise effeminacy and to emulate the physical nobleness of the old Norse heroes, but to banish disease by the beautiful system he originated.

Taylor writes in the preface:

> Having made a somewhat hazardous attempt to introduce a new and distinct practice and that a specialty, it is gratifying to know that the "Movement Cure" treatment has met with a cordial approbation of every physician whose attention has been directed to its merits. It is to supply an apparent demand that this work which at best can be considered as but an incomplete elucidation of the subject, has been prepared. In this circumscribed but new field of medical inquiry, there is a rich harvest to reward patient investigation. Such investigation I intend to continue and at a future day with ampler material, I hope to give to the profession a work of more lasting value than this unpretending book.

The volume contains fifteen chapters, plus an appendix on the life of Ling. Among the subjects are the "Nutritive process"; "Muscular contraction"; "Physiology of general exercise"; "Lateral curvature of the spine"; "Paralysis of motion"; "The circulation of the blood"; "Constipation of the bowels"; "Chronic diarrhea"; "Dyspepsia"; "Pulmonary consumption"; "Angular curvature of the spine"; "Deformities of the limbs";

"Chronic injuries to the foot and ankle"; "Diseases incident to women"; and "Derangements of the nervous system." There are seventy-one line drawings. Some of these depict several pieces of apparatus that Taylor had designed for exercising. A second edition was published in 1864. Among Taylor's other books are *Official formulae of American hospitals* (Philadelphia: Medical World, 1885) and *Manual of treatment* (Philadelphia: Medical World, 1887). (See also OR12 and OR30.)

OR10. **CHARLES HARLEY CLEAVELAND** (1820–63). *Causes and cure of diseases of the feet; with practical suggestions as to their clothing.* 111pp. Cincinnati: Bradley & Webb, 1862.

Cleaveland was an early eclectic physician who graduated from Dartmouth Medical College in 1843. He organized the College of Eclectic Medicine in Cincinnati and held the chair of materia medica and therapeutics until the college was merged into the Eclectic Medical Institute in 1859. This paperbound volume is the earliest work in America to deal strictly with problems of the feet. Cleaveland writes in the preface:

> The large armies of the nation which have been in the field during the past year, have suffered so much from various diseases of the feet, that not only the attention of surgeons has been specially directed to that part of the system, but the people have realized the very great importance which attaches to those derangements, and are ready to be instructed in their causes and cure. To supply, in part, the information

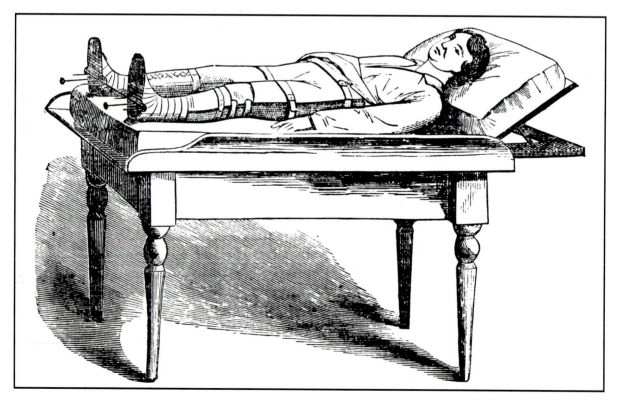

Fig. 83. (OR11) Bauer described the application of a lower body splint to treat deformities arising from hip-joint diseases in this wood engraving, figure 42 on page 56.

which was not readily attainable, even by physicians, a portion of the following work was published in the *Journal of Rational Medicine*. Those articles having attracted considerable attention, I have thought the interests of the profession and of the people would be subserved by republishing them, with additions, in the present form, particularly as no work covering the same ground had been published in America.

The book has an alphabetized seven-page table of contents detailing numerous ailments and treatments of the feet. It is illustrated with a number of engravings. Cleaveland's other books are *Galvanism; its application as a remedial agent* (New York: S. W. Benedict, 1853) and *Pronouncing medical lexicon, containing the correct pronunciation and definition of most of the terms used by speakers and writers on medicine and the collateral sciences* (Philadelphia: Lindsay & Blakiston, 1865).

OR11. **LOUIS BAUER** (1814–98). *Lectures on orthopedic surgery.* 108pp. Philadelphia: Lindsay & Blakiston, 1864. [G-M 4334]

Bauer was born in Prussia. He settled in the United States in 1853, where the following year he wrote a small pamphlet of thirty-nine pages entitled *Outlines of the principles and practice adopted in the Orthopaedic Institution of Brooklyn*. This institute, which Bauer had founded, was the first orthopedic hospital in the New York City area. Eventually he helped establish the German Dispensary, which later became the Long Island College Hospital and Medical School. A professor of anatomy and clinical surgery at his own school, Bauer also gave a series of lectures on orthopedic subjects at the Brooklyn Surgical and Medical Institute. In 1862 these were published in the *Philadelphia medical and surgical reporter*, and two years later were put in book form. Considered the first American textbook on orthopedic surgery, it consists of five major sections: "Deformities of the feet"; "The knee-joint"; "The hip-joint"; "The spine"; and "The neck." The book is dedicated to Joseph Pancoast (1805–82). There are eighty-two wood-engraved illustrations. An enlarged edition (336 pages) was brought out in 1868. Two years later the book was translated into German and soon into Italian and Swedish. (See also OR21.)

OR12. **CHARLES FAYETTE TAYLOR** (1827–99). *Infantile paralysis, and its attendant deformities.* 119pp. Philadelphia: J. B. Lippincott, 1864.

Taylor was a founder of the New York Orthopedic Dispensary and Hospital and a charter member of the American Orthopedic Association. This book was a continuation of his promotion of the Swedish movement cure and how it could help treat deformities caused by infantile paralysis. Taylor's experience with therapeutic exercises directed his attention to the neglected state of sufferers from chronic joint and spinal troubles and other deformities. He improved their treatment by the pioneering application of local rest and protection by proper splinting and the abundant use of fresh air. He devised a series of corrective and protective devices, and proposed a system of exercising machines for the weak and paralyzed. (See also OR9 and OR30.)

OR13. **JOSIAH C. NOTT** (?–?). *Contributions to bone and nerve injury.* 85pp. Philadelphia: J. B. Lippincott, 1866.

Nott was professor of surgery at the Mobile Medical College. This scarce volume contains no table of contents, index, or illustrations, making it difficult to read. There was only one edition. Nott writes in the preface:

> This little volume is intended simply as a contribution to a department of surgery which has been strangely neglected, and in which there is a remarkable want of medical literature, viz., the sequelae of gunshot and other injuries of bones. We have works in profusion of field surgery, primary and secondary operations, organization of hospitals, camp diseases, etc., but little on the class of cases to which I ask attention. Although the war has been over for some months, there are still thousands of soldiers scattered throughout the United States who are suffering from injuries of bones, and for years to come many of them will be seeking surgical assistance. I have been called on to treat a great many such cases and not a few of them dating their injuries back two, three, and even four years, to the first battle of Manassas. The principles I have endeavored to inculcate are equally applicable in civil as in military surgery, and if I can aid in directing other minds to this important field, my object will be fully attained.

OR14. **DAVID PRINCE** (1816–89). *Orthopedics; a systematic treatise upon the prevention and correction of deformities.* 240pp. Philadelphia: Lindsay & Blakiston, 1866.

Prince received his medical education at the Medical College of Ohio and received his degree in 1838. In 1852 he settled in Jacksonville, Illinois, where he spent the remainder of his life in the practice of general medicine and surgery. Prince writes in the preface:

> This treatise has been prepared with special reference to the wants of physicians engaged in general practice. Outside of the large cities, the majority of patients needing attention on account of deformities, or diseases or accidents that lead to them, must find relief at the hands of the profession in their near vicinity, or not find it at all . . . . This renders it important that there should be a general prevalence, in the profession, of a knowledge of prevention and treatment; to bring the means of relief within the pecuniary resources of the majority of sufferers . . . an attempt has been made to connect the medical treatment with the mechanical . . . .

The book was divided into two parts, the first deals with classification of orthopedic diseases, and the latter with "particular diseases and deformities not yet noticed, or only incidentally referred to." Approximately half of the ninety-two illustrations are original to Prince. (See also OR26.)

OR15. **JOHN ASHHURST** (1839–1900). *Injuries of the spine; with an analysis of nearly four hundred cases.* 127pp. Philadelphia: J. B. Lippincott, 1867.

Ashhurst's monograph was written while he was surgeon at the Episcopal Hospital in Philadelphia. Having previously served in the Army of the Potomac, he was well acquainted with the personal devastation of traumatic injuries to the spine suffered by soldiers in the Civil War. Ashhurst's *Injuries* treated the subject in the then novel statistical manner and described the morbid anatomy in detail. There is an extensive list of 368 cases of spinal injury and their primary treatment on pages 72–121. A unique discussion on pages 122–27 records the treatment of twenty-six individuals on whom resection of the spine was performed for traumatic causes. (See also GS72 and GS100.)

OR16. **HENRY GASSETT DAVIS** (1807–96). *Conservative surgery, as exhibited in remedying some of the mechanical causes that operate injuriously both in health and disease.* 314pp. New York: D. Appleton, 1867.

Having received an M.D. from Yale Medical School in 1839, Davis practiced medicine first in Millbury, Massachusetts, and later in New York City. His most important work was *Conservative surgery*, which was based on his nearly thirty years of practice. A passage from the book's introduction provides insight into Davis's philosphy concerning mechanical causes in health and diseases:

> We, as a profession, have never studied, as we ought, man as a machine, neither have we investigated the influence that mechanical causes exert in health and disease upon its structure. The absence in some, and the neglect to cultivate them in others, of those faculties which are so important and necessary to constitute an expert in this field of investigation, is a great hindrance to the ready comprehension and acceptance of any truths discovered by such researches . . . . If there is no necessity for specialists in any other department, there certainly is in that of conservative or mechanical surgery, as distinguished from operative surgery. There are so few in any sphere, much less among professional men, who possess large mechanical ingenuity, that all programs in this direction must necessarily be limited to those endowed by nature with this capacity.

The chapters contain extensive discussions of "The nature and treatment of clubfoot"; "Bowleg"; "Wry neck"; "Congenital dislocation of the hip"; "Lateral curvature of the spine"; "Chronic disease of the joints"; and "Deformities resulting from poliomyelitis," outlining Davis's beliefs on the treatment of these conditions. There are hundreds of illustrations depicting mechanical devices which he designed for his patients. The book was initially available in cloth for $3.00. Only one edition was published.

OR17. **BENJAMIN LEE** (1833–1913). *Contributions to the pathology, diagnosis, and treatment of angular curvature of the spine.* 129pp. Philadelphia: J. B. Lippincott, 1867.

Lee received his M.D. from New York Medical College in 1856. In 1863 he became associated with Charles Fayette Taylor (1827–99) in the treatment of deformities and spinal diseases by mechanical means. In 1865 Lee moved to Philadelphia, where his practice was limited to orthopedics and the development of mechanical therapeutics. Active in many medical organizations, Lee was president of both the American Public Health Association and the American Orthopedic Association.

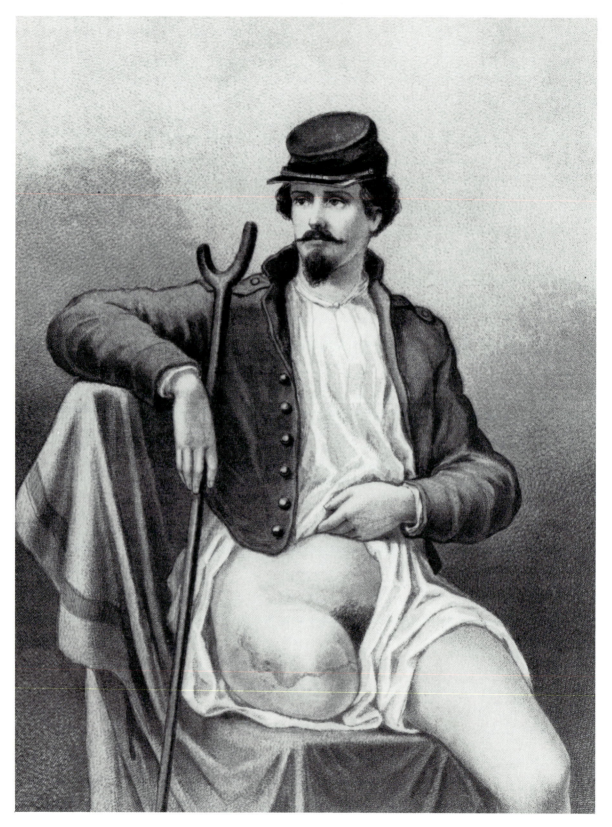

Fig. 84. (OR18) This magnificent chromolithograph by F. Moras after a drawing by Faber, demonstrates a successful secondary amputation at the hip joint by Dr. George C. Blackman.

His most important book is *Contributions*, which consists of four major sections: "Initial gastralgia"; "False views"; "Correct principles"; and "Types of cases." Lee notes in the introduction that the first three sections had been published previously in medical periodicals. The section on correct principles was awarded a prize by a committee of New York physicians. There was only one edition. (See also OR27.)

OR18. **GEORGE ALEXANDER OTIS** (1830–81). *A report on amputations at the hip-joint in military surgery. Circular No. 7, 1867.* 87pp. Washington: Government Printing Office, 1867.

Otis was an assistant surgeon and brevet lieutenant colonel in the U.S. Army who worked in the Office of the Surgeon General. By assisting John H. Brinton (1832–1907), curator of the Army Medical Museum, Otis participated in gathering material for a surgical history of the Civil War. Otis writes about this *Report*:

> Compared with the immense aggregate of major amputations, the number of amputations at the hip-joint during the war was not large; but considered with reference to the previously recorded examples of this amputation as performed for gunshot injury, they constitute a great accession to the statistics of the operation. It would be difficult, indeed, to find in the annals of military surgery a hundred and twenty authentic instances of amputation at the hip-joint for injuries inflicted by weapons, or to produce half that number in which even meager histories of the cases have been preserved .... The list of operations includes not only those that were performed in the army of the United States, but those done in the Rebel army.

This monograph is divided into four sections: "A historical summary"; "An account of individual cases"; "A citation of the opinions of surgeons"; and "A discussion of results." There are thirty figures, but the strength of this work is in the spectacular plates, five of which are chromolithographs. More important, some of the plates are engravings taken from actual photographs. These are among the earliest examples of such a process in American surgical texts. Otis ends by summarizing:

> 1. We have learned that the primary operation for traumatic causes is not uniformly fatal .... 2. Much evidence has been brought to controvert the prevailing doctrine that disarticulation at the hip is an exception to the general rule requiring all amputations deemed indispensable to be performed immediately .... 3. We have proved that secondary amputations at the hip for necrosis of the whole of the femur or for chronic osteomyelitis following gunshot injury, may be performed with as successful results as hip-joint amputations for other pathological causes. 4. It has been shown that when, after amputations in the continuity of the thigh, the stump has become diseased, reamputations at the hip may be done with comparative safety.

(See also GS62, GS63, GS74, and OR23.)

OR19. **NATHAN RYNO SMITH** (1797–1877). *Treatment of fractures of the lower extremity by the use of the anterior suspensory apparatus.* 70pp. Baltimore: Kelly & Piet, 1867. [G-M 4423]

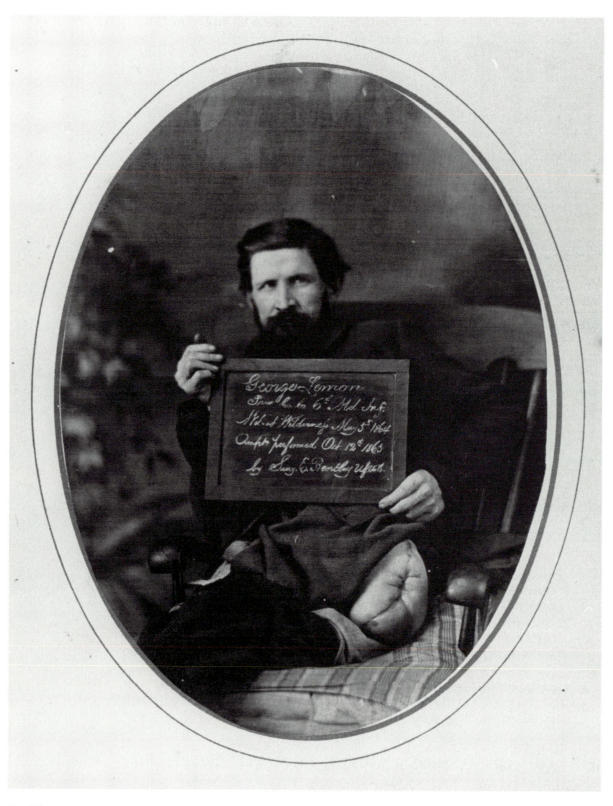

Fig. 85.

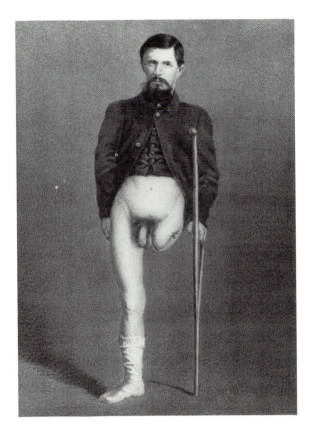

Figs. 85–86. (OR18) This original lithograph by Julius Bien after the drawing by E.M. Wells illustrating a successful secondary amputation at the hip joint is found in all copies of Otis's monograph. The original mounted cameo photograph bound in a copy of the book depicts the same patient (Fig. 85). On the blackboard held by the patient we learn that he was George Lemon, a private in the 6th Maryland Infantry. His left femur was fractured by a musket ball at the battle of the Wilderness, May 5, 1864. Surgeon Edwin Bentley, U.S. Volunteers, amputated October 12, 1865, nearly a year and a half after the injury.

Smith was professor of clinical surgery and surgery of the skeleton at the University of Maryland when this monograph was published. He is well known as the founder of the University of Vermont Medical School and aided in the establishment of Jefferson Medical College. His reputation in the history of orthopedic surgery was established by his invention of the anterior splint for use in the treatment of fractures of the femur [G-M 4422]. He took over thirty years to perfect it, and in his *Treatment* claims that the splint can be used for all fractures of the thigh and leg. This volume was kept purposely short, as Smith wrote in the preface:

> The author of the following monograph does not undertake a complete treatise of Fractures of even the lower extremity. His object is to describe, and illustrate, the usefulness of the Anterior Suspensory apparatus in the treatment of all fractures of that portion of the skeleton. For a knowledge of the causation and diagnosis of those injuries, he refers to the systems of Surgery in the hands of all pupils and practitioners.

The book has no table of contents or index, and the few engravings are quite rudimentary. The volume was available in cloth for $3.00. (See also GS8.)

OR20. **PHILIP SKINNER WALES** (1837–1906). *Mechanical therapeutics, a practical treatise on surgical apparatus, appliances, and elementary operations; embracing bandaging, minor surgery, orthopraxy, and the treatment of fractures and dislocations.* 685pp. Philadelphia: Henry C. Lea, 1867.

Wales entered the Navy as an assistant surgeon in 1856 and was promoted to surgeon in 1861. During the Civil War he served at the Naval Hospital in Norfolk. From 1879 to 1884 he was surgeon-general of the Navy. The book presented few original ideas and, as Wales writes in the preface:

> In offering to the profession the present volume on mechanical thera-peutics, the author would state that his design is to place in the hands of students and practitioners of medicine a systematized and condensed description of surgical dressings, apparatus, and elementary operations, drawn from the writings and teaching of the ablest surgeons in Amer-ica and Europe. In its preparation care has been taken to adapt it also to the necessities of those wishing to enter the public service, inasmuch as the rigid and thorough examinations of our Military and Naval Medi-cal Boards require more minute and extended information upon these subjects than can be obtained from the ordinary text-books.

The work is exhaustive in scope with thirty-one chapters and 642 il-lustrations. On pages 666–67 is a short description of local anesthesia, which according to the text can be obtained in three ways: "compres-sion, local narcotization, and refrigeration." The book was available in extra cloth for $5.75 or in leather for $6.75. This book is the only one Wales wrote.

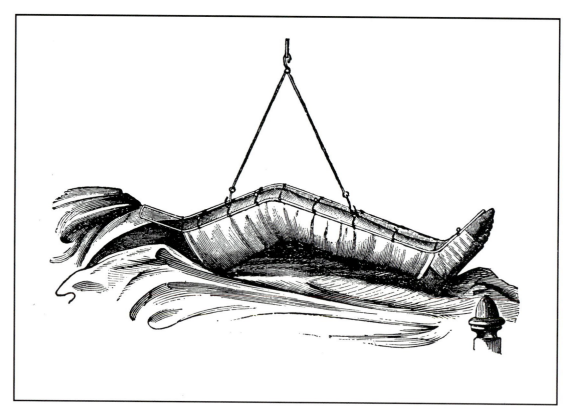

Fig. 87. (OR19) This simple wood engraving, figure 3 on page 45, is typical of the illustrations in Smith's monograph. It demonstrates the anterior splint which was devised for the treatment of fractures of the lower extremity.

OR21. LOUIS BAUER (1814–98). *Lectures on causes, pathology, and treatment of joint diseases.* 96pp. New York: William Wood, 1868.

Bauer was the first pupil of Georg Stromeyer (1804–76) to come to America. He practiced in Brooklyn from 1853 to 1869, when he moved to St. Louis and started the College of Physicians and Surgeons, where he was professor of surgery. This volume consists of a series of lectures delivered at McGill University Medical College in 1867. Bauer expressed strong and definite opinions concerning the etiology and treatment of numerous joint conditions. His first axiom of treatment for all joint diseases was "rest—absolute and unconditional." He then made certain there was proper positioning of the affected articulation. There was only one edition. (See also OR11.)

OR22. HENRY JACOB BIGELOW (1818–90). *The mechanism of dislocation and fracture of the hip with the reduction of the dislocation by the flexion method.* 150pp. Philadelphia: Henry C. Lea, 1869. [G-M 4424]

Bigelow was professor of surgery and clinical surgery at Harvard Medical School. In this classic treatise, he describes in detail the structure and function of the accessory Y (iliofemoral) ligament of the acetabulum, which clarified the pathology of dislocation of the hip. Among the topics covered are "Dislocation of the hip"; "Anatomy of the hip";

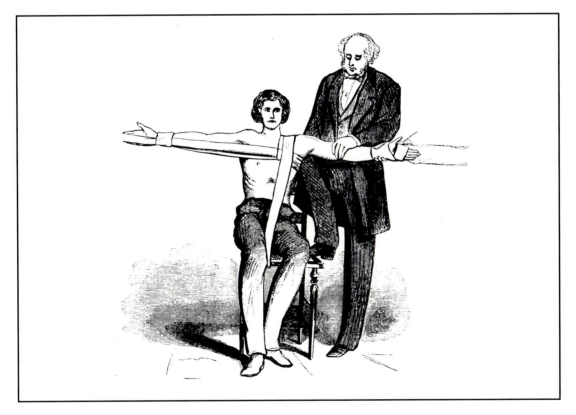

Fig. 88. (OR20) Wales shows Nathan Ryno Smith's method of treating dislocation of the humerus. In the illustration (number 464, page 527) a counter-extending band is being used to secure the wrist of the sound arm before fixing the scapula.

Fig. 89. (OR22) Bigelow was the first to describe in detail the mechanism of the ilio-femoral (the Y or Bigelow's) ligament, and to show its importance in the reduction of dislocation by the flexion method. This wood engraving depicts the ligament showing its inner and outer fasciculi (figure 1 on page 18).

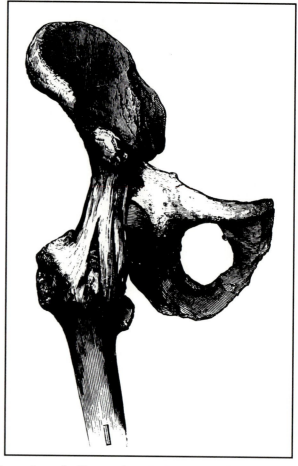

"Dislocations"; "Regular dislocations"; "Irregular dislocations"; "Special conditions of dislocations"; "Angular extension"; "Fracture of the neck of the femur"; and "Fracture of the pelvis." The work has fifty-two illustrations but no plates. (See also OR4.)

OR23. **GEORGE ALEXANDER OTIS** (1830–81). *A report on excisions of the head of the femur for gunshot injury. Circular No. 2, January 2, 1869.* 141pp. Washington: Government Printing Office, 1869.

This report is a companion piece to Otis's monograph on amputations at the hip-joint in military surgery. He collected the material both during and after the Civil War and had planned to incorporate it into an extensive work on military surgery. Otis notes:

> I describe the operations in three categories: primary, intermediate, and secondary excisions . . . . If a study of the histories of over twenty thousand major amputations, and of more than four thousand excisions of the larger joints, performed during the late war, may permit me to speak authoritatively on this point, I would say that no doctrine in military surgery is supported by more ample evidence than that which teaches that in operations for traumatic cases, there is a wide difference in the results of those performed immediately after the reception of the injury, those performed during the existence of inflammatory action, and those done after the symptomatic fever and inflammatory symptoms have abated . . . .

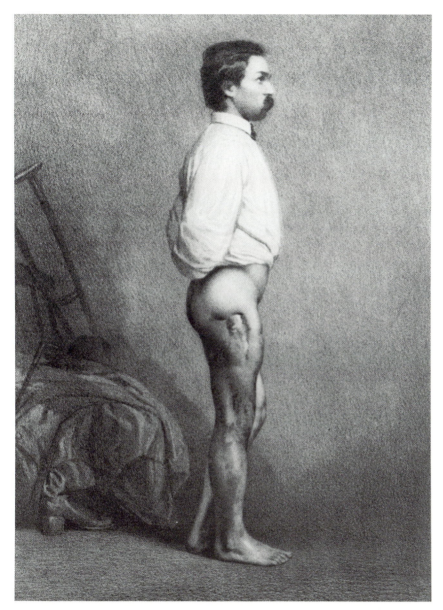

Fig. 90. (OR23) Otis described the case of Lieutenant Dwight Beebe, who suffered a gunshot wound to his hip. This plate, figure 1 on page 32, taken from a photograph by Ward and lithographed by J. Bien, shows the result of a successful primary excision of the head of the femur.

Over 270 cases are discussed in depth, and Appendix A provides tables which summarize the various excisions. Appendix B is particularly useful because of its extensive bibliography of excisions at the hip. There are three black-and-white plates and seventy-one other illustrations. The plates have particular historical significance since they are among the earliest examples of engravings taken directly from photographs (by E. J. Ward and William Bell) in a surgical text. The report was paperbound and published in only one edition. (See also GS62, GS63, GS74, and OR18.)

OR24. LEWIS ALBERT SAYRE (1820–1900). *A practical manual of the treatment of club foot.* 91pp. New York: D. Appleton, 1869.

A graduate of the College of Physicians and Surgeons of New York in 1842, Sayre was one of the chief organizers of Bellevue Hospital

Medical College. As professor of orthopedic surgery at Bellevue, he occupied the first chair of orthopedic surgery in America. Sayre is remembered for performing one of the earliest resections of the hip for ankylosis [G-M 4331], and the first to utilize plaster-of-paris as a support for the spinal column in scoliosis and Pott's disease [G-M 4344]. The *Manual* was Sayre's first book. It is written in a clear and succinct fashion, for he believed that clubfoot was a result of a muscle paralysis and strongly advocated that "treatment commence the instant the child is born." He explained that "the more frequent the manipulations, the more benefit there is to be derived from treatment." The book had numerous illustrations, including Sayre's clubfoot shoe and its modified version. He wrote in the preface:

> ... experience in the treatment of club-foot has proved that ... in all cases of congenital club-foot the treatment should commence at birth, as at that time there is generally no difficulty that can not be overcome by the ordinary family physician; and that, by following the simple rules laid down in this volume, the great majority of cases can be relieved, and many cured, without any operation or surgical interference. If this early treatment has been neglected, and the deformity has been permitted to increase by use of the foot in its abnormal position, surgical aid may be requisite to overcome the difficulty; and I have here endeavored to clearly lay down the rules that should govern the treatment of this class of cases.

When initially published it was available in cloth only for $1.00. Further editions were published in 1874, 1875, 1882, and 1894. The book was also translated into French and German. (See also OR33 and OR34.)

OR25. **ANDREW JACKSON HOWE** (1825–92). *A practical and systematic treatise on fractures and dislocations.* 424pp. Cincinnati: C. F. Wilstach, 1870.

Howe was the most prominent surgeon in the resurgent eclectic movement following the Civil War. This was his first textbook and was written when he was professor of anatomy at the Eclectic Medical Institute of Cincinnati. The first part consists of twenty-eight chapters and 105 illustrations dealing mainly with fractures of different bones. The second part has sixteen chapters and twenty-three engravings on dislocations of various joints. Howe writes in the preface:

> The improvements and modifications which have recently taken place in the management of fractures and dislocations, and the fact that the ordinary textbooks to be found in every physician's library contain too little on the nature and treatment of these lesions, and the special treatises too much, have induced me to venture upon the task of preparing a work specially adapted to the wants of the great mass of medical men .... In preparing this work, I have taken the liberty of drawing from every available source of information, and have not always given credit for material employed. This omission did not arise from a reckless disposition to appropriate the ideas of others; but in an early attempt to give each author his due, I found that A had drawn from B, and B from C, and so on, and therefore I abandoned an undertaking which at best must have been imperfect, laborious, and unsatisfactory ....

A second edition was published in 1873. (See also GS84, GY37 and OP21.)

OR26. **DAVID PRINCE** (1816–89). *Plastics and orthopedics.* 240pp. Philadelphia: Lindsay & Blakiston, 1871.

This is Prince's major work and was one of the earliest textbooks in America to treat plastic surgery as a separate specialty. It is actually a compendium of three reports that he had made to the Illinois State Medical Society, in 1864, 1867, and 1871. These consisted of a reprint of his textbook *Orthopedics; a systematic treatise upon the prevention and correction of deformities* (OR14) and *Plastics: a new classification and a brief exposition of plastic surgery.* The latter was reprinted from the *Transactions of the Illinois State Medical Society* for 1867. In addition, there is an untitled report on plastic and orthopedic surgery from 1871 that discusses three areas of plastic surgery: "Principles"; "Expedients"; and "Specialties," including "Rhinoplasty"; "Canthoplasty"; "Genyoplasty"; "Cheiloplasty"; and "Intestinal and urinary plastics." The orthopedic topics include "Cicatricial contraction"; "Spinal curvature"; "Joint inflammation"; "Talipes"; and "Artificial hands." There are thirty-eight illustrations in this section of the book. The preface to the previously published *Plastics* declares that

> a successful classification of any branch of knowledge, is such an arrangement of its component parts, as not only to make the whole easy of comprehension, but to secure for each minute division, a name showing its relations to the other divisions, and enabling it to be easily designated in descriptions. The present essay, is an attempt to reduce the subject of Plastic Surgery to such a classification, as to give it an intelligible language.

Plastics contains fifty illustrations. Chapter headings include "Classification"; "Cicatrix"; "Rhinoplasty"; "Otoplasty"; "Blepharoplasty"; "Operations involving the mouth"; "Extroverson of the bladder"; and "Autoplasty of the penis." (See also OR14.)

OR27. **BENJAMIN LEE** (1833–1913). *The correct principles of treatment for angular curvature of the spine.* 77pp. Philadelphia: J. B. Lippincott, 1872.

This monograph is a follow-up to Lee's previous work on angular curvature of the spine. He writes in the preface:

> The little volume entitled "Contributions to the Diagnosis, Pathology, and Treatment of Angular Curvature of the Spine," which I had the honor to lay before the profession a few years since, has been for some time out of print. In the mean time our knowledge of this affection and our means of treating it have not made such advances as to render the doctrines then advanced obsolete on the one hand, nor, on the other, has the great body of practicing physicians become so familiar with them as to make their repetition unnecessary. It has occurred to me, however, that the information which appears to be called for by the frequent inquiries addressed me by members of the profession, in regard to the subject, might be placed within still smaller compass, omitting much that was merely argumentative or indirectly personal.

Fig. 91. (OR30) It was Taylor's belief that almost all diseases of the hip joint could be cured by mechanical treatment. This wood engraving, figure 5 on page 30, depicts such a lower extremity splint.

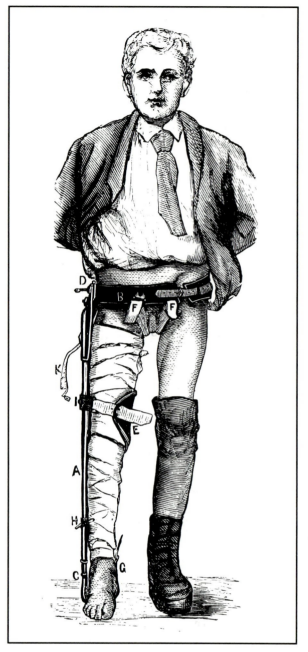

I have, therefore, determined to reproduce only that one of the former collection of papers which was devoted to the consideration of the principles on which the disease can be most successfully combated and the means for their practical application, supplementing it with a more complete and minute explanation of one of the modes of treatment there alluded to . . . . I confess, not unwillingly, that I find myself able to improve in not the slightest degree on the principles unfolded in the first essay, and to but a very trifling extent on the details of their material embodiment . . . .

The most interesting aspect of the book is a table in an appendix that indicates what diseases angular curvature is most frequently confused with in its initial stage. This was the only edition. (See also OR17.)

OR28. **THOMAS MASTERS MARKOE** (1819–1901). *A treatise on diseases of the bones.* 416pp. New York: D. Appleton, 1872.

Markoe was professor of surgery at the College of Physicians and Surgeons in New York after having graduated from that school in 1841. In addition, he was surgeon at New York Hospital from 1852 to 1892. This volume is the only textbook he wrote. It discusses structural changes of bones as affected by various diseases and their clinical history and treatment as well as various tumors. No injuries of bone were included, nor were joint diseases except where the condition of the bone was a prime factor in the problem of the disease. The preface states:

> The book which I now offer to my professional brethren contains the substances of the lectures which I have delivered during the past twelve years at the college . . . . I have followed the leadings of my own studies and observations, dwelling more on those branches where I had seen and studied most, and perhaps too much neglecting others where my own experience was more barren, and therefore to me less interesting. I have endeavored, however, to make up the deficiencies of my own knowledge by the free use of the materials scattered so richly through our periodical literature, which scattered leaves it is the right and the duty of the systematic writer to collect and to embody in any account he may offer of the state of a science at any given period.

There are three parts: "Diseases of bone"; "Tumors of bone"; and "Malignant disease of bone." The book was available in cloth for $4.50. This was the only edition published.

OR29. **WALTER ELA** (1848–?). *Fractures of the elbow joint. Boylston Prize essay.* 57pp. Cambridge: Welch & Bigelow, 1873.

Ela was a surgeon who practiced in Massachusetts. This short essay was awarded the second prize of the Boylston Medical Society for 1873. Most of the statistics and case reports were obtained from the fracture books of the outpatient department of the Massachusetts General Hospital. A few woodcuts are included. There is no table of contents or index.

OR30. **CHARLES FAYETTE TAYLOR** (1827–99). *On the mechanical treatment of disease of the hip-joint.* 62pp. New York: William Wood, 1873.

Taylor was a surgeon at the New York Orthopedic Dispensary and Hospital. He wrote in his preface:

> This little monograph is to be just what its name implies—an exposition of the Mechanical Treatment of Disease of the Hip-Joint—and nothing more. Even the minor details of treatment have been purposely left out, in the hope that the general principles involved might impress the mind more deeply and with a clearer force than if buried in a multitude of explanations. There has been no need to discuss pathology in all its bearings. If, in the opinion of any one, there be cases in which the mechanical treatment, on account of pathological conditions, is not applicable, let such be left out of consideration. But that it does apply with immense advantage to vast numbers, of which a large majority, when taken in time and properly treated, are as curable as cases of simple inflammations in any other location, is the conviction which I desire to impress on the reader's mind.

There is no table of contents nor index, and the fifteen illustrations are crude at best. A German translation was published the same year. In 1881 Taylor wrote a monograph of seventy-seven pages entitled *Sensation and pain* (New York: G. P. Putnam's Sons). Indirectly related to orthopedic surgery, it deserves mention as his last major work. (See also OR9 and OR12.)

OR31. **ROBERT WILLIAM TAYLOR** (1842–1908). *Syphilitic lesions of the osseous system in infants and young children.* 179pp. New York: William Wood, 1875.

Taylor was an 1868 graduate of the College of Physicians and Surgeons of New York. This was his first major published work, which he wrote while a surgeon at the New York Dispensary. It consists of thirty chapters which provide a comprehensive look at the subject. Later in his career he was appointed clinical professor of genitourinary surgery at his alma mater. Taylor writes in the preface:

> When my attention was primarily drawn to lesions of a syphilitic nature occurring in the osseous system of infants, so little was known upon the subject that I was soon compelled to turn my inquiries from the few works in which, indeed, it was but casually mentioned, to the disease itself, as presented in the sick, to a number exceeding a dozen, the details of which I have been careful to give at length. In a word, the volume of nature was before me, and in that I studied . . . . In fact, the field I entered upon was almost untrod . . . .

This was the only edition. Among Taylor's most prominent other books is *A clinical atlas of venereal and skin diseases* (Philadelphia: Lea Brothers, 1889). (See also GU33 and GU37.)

OR32. **HOWARD CULBERTSON** (1828–90). *Excision of the larger joints of the extremities.* 672pp. Philadelphia: Collins, 1876.

After graduating from Jefferson Medical College in 1850, Culbertson began practicing in his native city of Zanesville, Ohio. In 1862, he entered the army as an assistant surgeon. After serving for seven years he returned to his private practice in Zanesville. He devoted most of his time to ophthalmology and was professor of ophthalmology at Columbus Medical College. His *Excision* is the most important work he wrote. It won a prize from the American Medical Association and was published as an individual supplement to the *Transactions* of the organization. It was considered the most exhaustive treatise on the subject of its time, and was highlighted by numerous "tabular statements" which indicated when and who had performed joint excisions in the past. It is a gold mine of bibliographic information. The volume contains fifteen plates. Culbertson's other book is *Essay on the use of anaesthetics in obstetrics* (Cincinnati: S. G. Cobb, 1862).

OR33. **LEWIS ALBERT SAYRE** (1820–1900). *Lectures on orthopedic surgery and diseases of the joint.* 476pp. New York: D. Appleton, 1876.

Sayre served as president of the American Medical Association in 1880. He was one of the major forces behind the eventual establishment of the *Journal of the American Medical Association*. Sayre was professor of orthopedic surgery, fractures and dislocations, and clinical surgery at Bellevue Hospital Medical College. His *Lectures* was his foremost written work and was based on his clinical experiences. He stated in the preface:

> As many of my views were so directly at variance with the standard authorities, I hesitated to write until a larger experience should either confirm my observations or prove them to be erroneous. In the latter case, of course, I should have no occasion for publishing. A more extended experience has confirmed my original views; but constant professional occupation has prevented me from complying with the request of my friends . . . . I therefore employed . . . a stenographic reporter, to follow me during the course of last winter's lectures, . . . and the present work is the result.

The twenty-nine lectures deal with such varied topics as "Deformities"; "Talipes"; "Diseases of the joints and spine"; and "Anchylosis". There are 274 engravings, but no plates are included. It was available in either cloth for $5.00 or sheepskin for $6.00. Further editions were printed in 1883, and the second edition was reprinted in 1892. It is known to have also been translated into German, Spanish and French. (See also OR24 and OR34.)

OR34. **LEWIS ALBERT SAYRE** (1820–1900). *Spinal disease and spinal curvature, their treatment by suspension and the use of the plaster of Paris bandage.* 121pp. Philadelphia: J. B. Lippincott, 1877.

This book was written and first published in London while Sayre was visiting England in 1877. He was a delegate from the American Medical Association to the British Medical Congress, held in Manchester, England. His fame in the treatment of spinal disease had preceded him [G-M 4344], and he was asked to lecture and give demonstrations of his methods of treating tuberculosis of the spine and scoliosis. This work was dedicated to the medical profession of Great Britain:

> To the British physicians and surgeons who have received me with such great personal and professional cordiality, who have thoroughly scrutinized the merits of this plan of treating diseases and deformities of the spine, and given me abundant opportunity of publicly testing its practical value.

Sayre describes in detail the head suspension apparatus and the jury-mast used for high dorsal and cervical spine lesions. The patient was literally suspended by an overhead traction apparatus attached to a specially constructed chin and occiput halter. Only his toes touched the ground, and this was permitted just enough to keep discomfort from becoming too serious. While under this severe traction, a snugly fitted plaster-of-paris jacket was applied. Lateral traction bands were later added to the suspended body according to the nature of the deformity, and the plaster applied around them. These bands were removed before the finishing layer was applied. This method of treatment persisted well into the first quarter of the twentieth century. This book is a landmark in American medical photography since it was the first known surgical textbook to contain actual mounted photographs. The photographs consist of twenty-one albumen prints on eight plates, most of which are presented in series of photographs of the same subjects. They are remarkable for their artistic qualities. There are also engraved illustrations from photographs. The photography was performed both in New York and London. The photographer at Bellevue Hospital and at the New York Academy of Medicine sessions was O.G. Mason, who later became one of the most noted medical photographers of his time. In London, many of the photographs were taken by J. R. Mayall, a transplanted Philadelphian. The London edition which preceded the American edition was published by Smith & Elder. Both are as much sought after by photography collectors as by collectors of early American surgery. There were no other editions. (See also OR24 and OR33.)

OR35. **EDWARD CARROLL FRANKLIN** (1822–85). *The homoeopathic treatment of spinal curvatures according to the new principle.* 80pp. St. Louis: H. C. G. Luyties, 1878.

Franklin wrote this monograph while he was professor of surgery at the Homeopathic Medical College of Missouri, and it was initially read at the Western Academy of Homeopathy in Indianapolis in 1877:

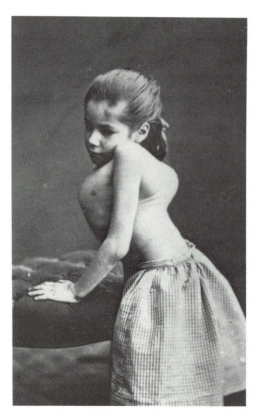 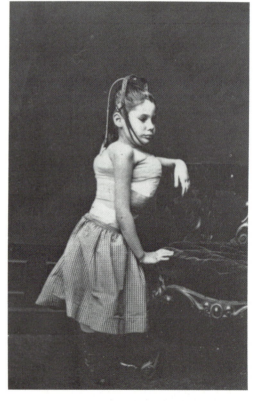

Figs. 92–94. (OR34) These albumen prints (pages 82, 86, and 117) are the earliest tipped-in photographs used in an American surgical textbook, and are exceptional for their artistic value as photographs. The child was the ten-year-old daughter of an English physician; she had had Pott's disease of the cervical and upper dorsal vertebrae since the age of nineteen months. When first examined by Sayre (July 1877 in Guy's Hospital, London), she could neither sit nor stand except by bearing her weight upon her hands. After placement of a plaster-of-paris bandage, she was able to ambulate alone. The final photograph shows Sayre with a young woman in his self-suspension device for treatment of her lateral curvature of the spine.

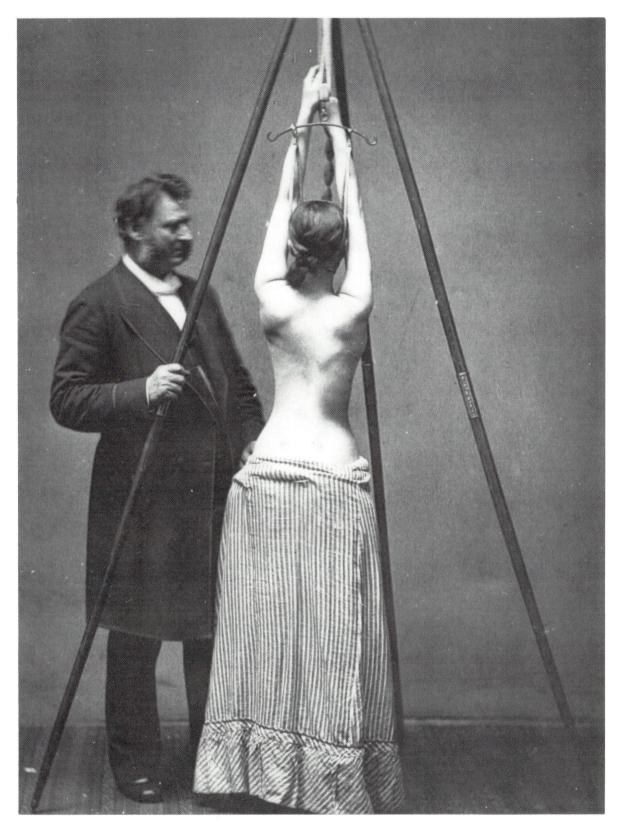

Fig. 94.

Since then, it has been considerably enlarged and illustrated for the use of practitioners and students of medicine . . . . The intention of the author has been, therefore, to present the more prominent and salient features of the disease, and the curative means demanded for their rectification rather than a learned and elaborate treatise covering this subject . . . .

The index lists twenty-two topics, including "Artificial sacrum"; "Artificial spine"; "Lateral curvatures"; "Antero-posterior curvature"; "Mechanical appliances"; and "Occipito-mental apparatus." There are a few crude illustrations. This was the only edition. (See also GS65, GS107, GS108, and GU16.)

OR36. **NEWTON MELMAN SHAFFER** (1846–1928). *Pott's disease, its pathology and mechanical treatment, with remarks on rotary lateral curvature.* 82pp. New York: G. P. Putnam's Sons, 1879.

Shaffer received his M.D. from New York University Medical College in 1867. He succeeded Charles Fayette Taylor (1827–99) as surgeon-in-chief at New York Orthopaedic Dispensary and Hospital in 1876. In 1900, he became the first professor of orthopedic surgery at Cornell University Medical College. This small monograph was Shaffer's initial contribution to American orthopedic surgery. In it, he criticized the conservative writings of James Knight (1810–87), which he felt amounted practically to a surgical nihilism. Shaffer believed that more recoveries occur from a plan of non-interference with a tubercular abscess than from surgical opening of the abscess. He was an opponent of recumbency in the treatment of Pott's disease, and believed in protection of the diseased part, with the maintenance of functional activity of the other parts of the body. He opposed Lewis Sayre's (1820–1900) plaster-of-paris jacket and claimed in this monograph that it was not adapted to the treatment of Pott's disease. The work has only two chapters dealing with pathology and treatment. The volume had originally been intended for publication in *The hospital gazette*, but grew in length until Shaffer decided to publish it in its present form. Figures 6–11 are interesting line drawings of spinal deformities. (See also OR39 and OR58.)

OR37. **FRANK HASTINGS HAMILTON** (1813–86). *Fracture of the patella: a study of one hundred and twenty-seven cases.* 106pp. New York: L. Bermingham, 1880.

Hamilton was visiting surgeon at Bellevue Hospital and consulting surgeon at the Hospital for the Ruptured and Crippled at the time this monograph was published. It contains neither a table of contents nor an index, which makes it difficult to read. Of the cases discussed, fifty-four had been under Hamilton's direct care, while the remainder had been admitted to Bellevue Hospital. (See also GS50, GS70, GS75, OR7, and OP8.)

OR38. **JOSEPH CHRISMAN HUTCHISON** (1827–87). *Contributions to orthopedic surgery; including observations on the treatment of chronic inflammation of the hip, knee, and ankle joints, by a new and simple method of extension, the physiological method; and lectures on club-*

foot. 121pp. New York: G. P. Putnam's Sons, 1880.

An 1848 graduate of the University of Pennsylvania Medical School, Hutchison moved to Brooklyn in 1853, where he eventually became attending surgeon at Brooklyn Hospital and surgeon-in-chief at the Orthopedic Dispensary. From 1860 to 1867 he served as professor of operative and clinical surgery at Long Island College Hospital. The book is dedicated to Edward R. Squibb (1819–1900). The section on treatment of chronic inflammation of the hip, knee, and ankle joints was initially published in the January 1879 *American journal of the medical sciences* and the April 1879 *Proceedings of the Kings County, New York, Medical Society.* Because these papers were so well received, Hutchison revised them for publication in book form. The lectures on clubfoot were based on his personal experience in both hospital and private practice. They were originally delivered before the medical class of the New York College of Physicians and Surgeons and eventually published in the *Medical record of New York, 1878–79.* They too were revised and expanded for this volume. The section on clubfoot comprises five chapters (pages 45–121), while that on joints contains only one (pages 8–44). There are thirty-one illustrations but no plates. Hutchison's other book is *A treatise on physiology and hygiene for educational institutions and general readers* (New York: Clark & Maynard, 1870).

OR39. **NEWTON MELMAN SHAFFER** (1846–1928). *The hysterical element in orthopaedic surgery.* 66pp. New York: G. P. Putnam's Sons, 1880.

Shaffer was surgeon-in-charge of the New York Orthopaedic Dispensary and Hospital and orthopedic surgeon at St. Luke's Hospital. This essay was originally read before the New York Neurological Society on December 1, 1879. It was later serialized in three consecutive numbers of the *Archives of medicine.* Several footnotes and remarks were added to prepare the manuscript for this book,. Among its topics are "Nervous mimicry of knee-joint disease"; "Hip-joint disease"; "Pott's disease"; "Lateral curvature of the spine"; and "Hysterical clubfoot." Twelve different cases were presented which were of functional rather than of organic origin. Shaffer then presented their differential diagnosis. There is only one illustration (page 58), which depicts a hysterical clubfoot, and no plates. Unfortunately, the book does not contain an index, which makes it difficult to peruse. (See also OR36 and OR58.)

OR40. **LEWIS ATTERBURY STIMSON** (1844–1917). *A treatise on fractures.* 539pp. Philadelphia: Henry C. Lea's Son, 1883.

This was Stimson's first major orthopedic work. At the time of its publication he was professor of surgical pathology in the medical faculty of the University of the City of New York and attending surgeon at Bellevue and Presbyterian hospitals. Only one edition was published. The book is divided into twenty-eight chapters, with the first eleven covering general topics and the final seventeen discussing specific types of fractures. Massive in scope, it was considered the foremost textbook on fractures in America at that time. The book contains 360 illustrations on wood. (See also GS91, OR45, and OR61.)

OR41. **VIRGIL PENDLETON GIBNEY** (1847–1927). *The hip and its diseases.* 412pp. New York: Bermingham, 1884.

Gibney received his M.D. from Bellevue Hospital Medical College in 1871. After graduation he obtained a position at the Hospital for the Ruptured and Crippled under James Knight (1810–87). Gibney lived in the hospital for thirteen years and eventually found himself having frequent clinical disagreements with Knight. Gibney published this work without Knight's knowledge. Knight immediately asked for his resignation. Gibney went into private practice but after Knight's death Gibney was asked to return to the hospital as surgeon-in-chief.

In 1894 Gibney was appointed as the first professor of orthopedic surgery at Columbia's College of Physicians and Surgeons. As professor of orthopedic surgery at New York Polyclinic and assistant surgeon at the Hospital for the Ruptured and Crippled, Gibney's most significant work was this book. He writes in the preface:

> For nearly thirteen years I have resided in the Hospital for the Ruptured and Crippled, all of my time being devoted to daily service in both the in-door and the out-door departments. This hospital is well known for the large number of orthopedic cases that come under observation and treatment. For instance, during my term of service the annual reports show that up to the present time 2048 cases of "hip-disease" alone have been treated, and a very large proportion of this number have been under my own observation. The hospital is further known as an extremely conservative institution. Dr. Jas. Knight, its founder and surgeon-in-chief, has been led by his extensive experience to adopt a plan of treatment which coincides, in many respects, with the definition I have elsewhere given of the term "expectant." It will therefore be readily seen that the writer of this book has enjoyed unusual facilities for the study of the clinical history of bone and joint diseases. A large number of our cases in the wards are of this nature, and many remain in hospital for two or three years . . . . My observations have not been confined especially to cases under the non-mechanical treatment. My relations with those gentlemen who are fully committed to mechanical therapeutics have been close enough to permit from time to time personal examinations of their own cases . . . . I feel that I can thus present a pretty accurate picture of the clinical features of bony lesions of the hip, both under the expectant and the mechanical forms of treatment.

The volume has eighteen chapters and is quite comprehensive in scope. The largest number of cases concerned bone and joint tuberculosis, and Gibney wrote that in the early days of the Hospital, over one-half of the inpatients suffered from some form of this infectious process. The book contains sixty-four illustrations. There was only one edition.

OR42. **JAMES KNIGHT** (1810–87). *Orthopaedia or a practical treatise on the aberrations of the human form.* 364pp. New York: G. P. Putnam's Sons, 1874.

Knight graduated from Washington Medical College in Baltimore in 1832. He soon began to devote himself to the study of orthopedic surgery, having come under the influence of Valentine Mott (1785–1865). Knight is remembered for having founded the Hospital for the

Ruptured and Crippled in New York, presently known as the Hospital for Special Surgery, which was America's first permanent orthopedic institution. One-third of the fourteen chapters discuss nonorthopedic subjects such as "Electricity as a therapeutic agent"; "Hernia"; "Procidentia uteri"; "Ectropion vesicae"; "Relaxed abdomen"; "Hemorrhoids"; "Varicose veins"; and "Tonics and their effect upon the body." In orthopedic cases, Knight advocates using the so-called conservative, or expectant, plan of treatment for joint lesions. There is a rather extensive description of lateral curvature of the spine, with numerous illustrations of cases involving the Knight spinal brace. Considerable material discusses the treatment of bowleg and knock-knee. Knight mentions the need for cutting contracted and superficial tendons and muscles, rather than manipulating them or taking a chance of tearing them apart. This work contains a great deal of information, but it covers only what Knight thought and practiced. There is little mention of many of the other, more common forms of treatment then in use. There are five chromolithograph plates and 135 engravings. Knight's *Orthopaedia* went through a second edition in 1884. Knight also wrote *The improvement of the health of enfeebled children and adults by natural means, including a history of food and a consideration of its substantial qualities* (New York: Sackett and Mackay, 1868).

OR43. **CHARLES TALBOT POORE** (1846–1911). *Osteotomy and osteoclasis for deformities of the lower extremities.* 187pp. New York: D. Appleton, 1884.

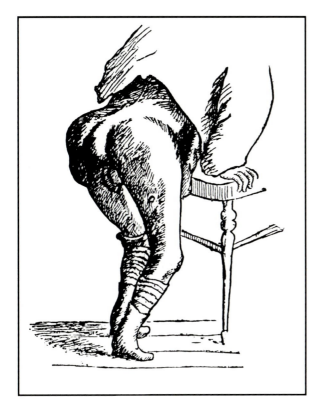

Fig. 95. (OR41) The illustrations in Gibney's work were comparatively crude. This engraving, figure 33 on page 335, shows bilateral articular ostitis.

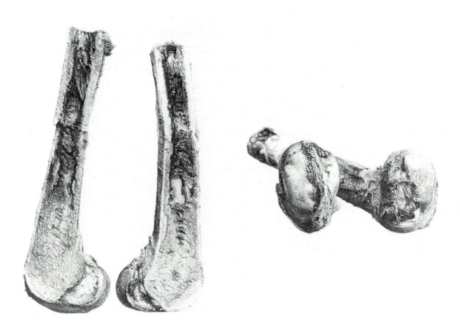

Fig. 96. (OR44) This lithograph from Watson's textbook shows a case of osteo-myelitis (figure 2 on page 680).

Poore was surgeon at St. Mary's Free Hospital for Children in New York. The book is dedicated to his uncle Charles N. Talbot, a lawyer from New York. The preface states:

> The author of this volume has had considerable experience both in the mechanical and in the operative treatment of the deformities considered in this book. That there is a want of a concise treatise on osteotomy—one in which the methods of operating and the management of the wound and limb after section are considered—there can be no doubt . . . . Very free use has been made of Dr. Macewen's excellent work on Osteotomy, as well as of Campenon's thesis *Du redressement des membres par l'ostéotomies* . . . .

There are ten chapters, including "Osteotomy for deformities at the hip joint"; "Osteotomy for genu valgum"; "Osteotomy for anchylosis of the knee joint"; and "Osteotomy for tibial curves." This monograph was originally available in cloth for $2.50 and contained fifty woodcuts and five plates. There was only one edition.

OR44. **BERIAH ANDRE WATSON** (1836–92). *A treatise on amputations of the extremities and their complications.* 762pp. Philadelphia: P. Blakiston & Sons, 1882.

Watson received his M.D. from New York University in 1861. Following the Civil War, he settled in Jersey City, where he was instrumental in the formation of the Jersey City hospitals. In 1873, he was named surgeon at St. Francis Hospital and later at Christ Hospital. This volume was dedicated to Joseph Lister (1827–1912): "The father of antiseptic surgery, whose labors mark a new era in the treatment of wounds, . . . this work is humbly inscribed by one of his disciples. " It is significant that this work predates Arpad Gerster's (1848–1923) *The rules of aseptic and antiseptic surgery*, commonly acknowledged as the first American surgical textbook based on Listerian principles, and Henry Marcy's (1837–1924) *The anatomy and surgical treatment of hernia.* (GS133 and GS155.) Marcy was considered Lister's first American pupil, and his *Anatomy* was also dedicated to Lister. Watson writes in the preface:

> The Author's desire to familiarize himself with all the questions pertaining, directly or indirectly, to the subject of this work, had its origin in our late War of the Rebellion, in which he was actively engaged as a medical officer . . . . These studies have been pursued under favorable circumstances, inasmuch as the Author has had access to a large surgical library in which the works of the great masters of the art and science of surgery have been constantly open to him, as well the hospital wards of a large city in which terminate a greater number of railroads than in any other in the United States . . . . It may not be amiss here to call the reader's attention to the fact, that the scope of this work is much broader than might be at first inferred from the title, inasmuch as the complications of amputation wounds are essentially the same as those which pertain to any solution of continuity involving the various tissues of the body . . . .

Among the eleven chapters are "History of amputations"; "Selection and application of artificial limbs"; and "Complications of wounds." Chapter 7 is important because in it Watson provides one of the earliest descriptions of Lister's antiseptic treatment to be found in an American surgical text. There are 255 illustrations and two plates. This volume was originally available in cloth for $5.50 or paperbound for $1.00. (See also NS3.)

OR45. **LEWIS ATTERBURY STIMSON** (1844–1917). *A treatise on dislocations.* 539pp. Philadelphia: Lea Brothers, 1888.

When this volume was published, Stimson was professor of clinical surgery at the University of the City of New York and surgeon at New York, Presbyterian, and Bellevue Hospitals. He wrote in the preface:

> The interval of nearly five years that has elapsed between the publication of the volume on Fractures and the completion of this one on Dislocations is longer than was anticipated, and the delay is in the main due to the great amount of material that had to be collected and examined in the preparation of the work . . . . An effect of this increase in the amount of material appears in the accounts given of the rarer forms of injury, of some of which I have been able to give systematic descriptions, instead of simply quoting the one or two cases which have heretofore embodied all that was known upon the subject. So far as possible, I have always gone to original reports, and have subjected them to careful scrutiny; this has resulted in the rejection of some cases, and in the transfer of others to different groups. A number of errors— some of them of long standing and wide circulation—have thus been corrected, some of which arose through reliance upon incomplete or faulty abstracts or reports, and other through faulty diagnoses which have been corrected by the aid of post-mortem examination or by critical review of the history in the light of later researches and accumulated evidence . . . .

Part 1 consists of eight chapters on traumatic dislocations. Part 2 contains two chapters on non-traumatic dislocations. Part 3, on special dislocations, contains twenty-two chapters. A total of 163 illustrations are included. There was only one edition. (See also GS91, OR40, and OR61.)

OR46. EDWARD HICKLING BRADFORD (1848–1926) and **ROBERT WILLIAMSON LOVETT** (1859–1924). *A treatise on orthopedic surgery.* 783pp. New York: William Wood, 1890. [G-M 4353]

Bradford graduated from Harvard Medical School in 1872. In 1880 he was appointed clinical instructor in orthopedic surgery at Harvard, and in 1903 he became the first John Ball and Buckminster Brown Professor of Orthopedic Surgery. Lovett graduated from Harvard in 1885. He soon met Bradford, and, after advancing through the academic ranks, was named Bradford's successor in 1915. The *Treatise* was the most notable contribution of both men. Further editions were published in 1899, 1905, 1910, and 1915. It was considered the standard textbook of its day in most medical schools and had no competition until Royal Whitman (1857–1946) published his *Treatise on orthopaedic surgery* (Philadelphia: Lea Brothers, 1901). Massive in scope, Bradford and Lovett's *Treatise* is illustrated with 789 wood engravings. They wrote in the preface:

> The writers of previous works on Orthopedic Surgery have confined themselves to a consideration of the treatment of existing deformities, such as club-foot, lateral curvature, and bow legs. The only conspicuous exception to this is found in the excellent book of Dr. Sayre. But the term Orthopedic Surgery, if it is properly defined, should include the prevention as well as the cure of deformity. For this reason the diseases of the joints have been considered by us at considerable length, inasmuch as they are among the most common sources of deformity and disability. We have endeavored throughout to include such subjects as are likely to come to the attention of those who interest themselves in the practice of this branch of surgery, without perhaps adhering too closely to the definition of the term orthopedic surgery. In this way, besides the consideration of joint disease and Pott's disease, we have added a brief description of some disabling and deforming nervous affections, which we have only attempted to discuss in their practical surgical aspect. The deformities resulting from fractures, dislocations, and burns are so fully treated in works on general surgery that they have not been considered here.

Within the twenty-five chapters are extensive descriptions of the Bradford frame. Among Lovett's other medical books is *Lateral curvature of the spine and round shoulders* (Philadelphia: P. Blakiston's Son, 1907). (See also OR47.)

OR47. ROBERT WILLIAMSON LOVETT (1859–1924). *The etiology, pathology, and treatment of diseases of the hip joint.* 220pp. Boston: G. H. Ellis, 1891.

Lovett was outpatient surgeon at Boston City Hospital and assistant surgeon to outpatients at the Children's Hospital. He wrote the winning forty-second Fiske Prize Fund Dissertation, which this volume presents. He later became professor of orthopedic surgery at Harvard Medical School and coauthor with Robert Jones (1858–1933) of the monumental *Orthopaedic surgery* (London: H. Frowde, 1923) [G-M 4391]. The *Etiology* consists of thirteen chapters, including "Acute arthritis"; "Acute synovitis"; "Chronic serous synovitis"; "Tuberculous ostitis"; "Gummatous ostitis"; "Arthritis deformans"; "Charcot's disease"; "Malignant and other tumors"; "Loose bodies"; "Congenital dislocations"; and "Hysterical affections." A total of fifty-six photographic figures are presented. There was only one edition. (See also OR46.)

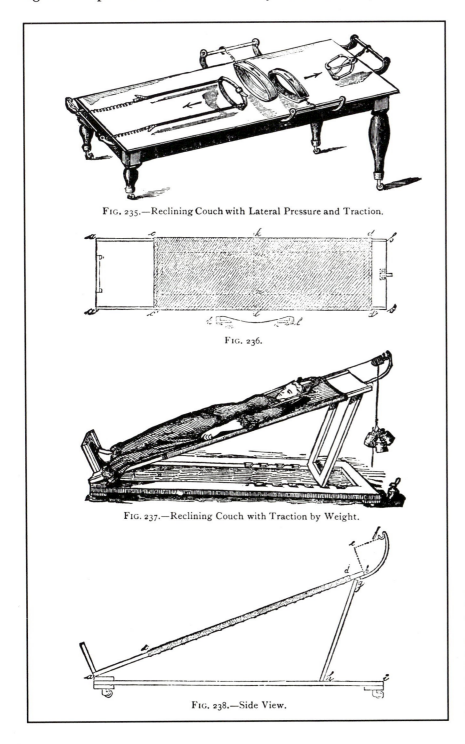

Fig. 235.—Reclining Couch with Lateral Pressure and Traction.

Fig. 236.

Fig. 237.—Reclining Couch with Traction by Weight.

Fig. 238.—Side View.

Fig. 97. (OR46) In his textbook Bradford described the frame now synonymous with his name. Unfortunately, the authors did not provide any illustrations of it. These engravings, figures 235–38 on page 181, demonstrate various forms of a reclining couch used to provide lateral pressure and a traction force in spinal deformities.

Fig. 98–99. (OR47) In one of
the earliest examples of actual
operative photographs, Lovett
demonstrates the incision exposing the trochanter and neck
of the femur, and the head of
the femur thrown out of the
socket prior to its resection
(numbers 45 and 46, page 139).

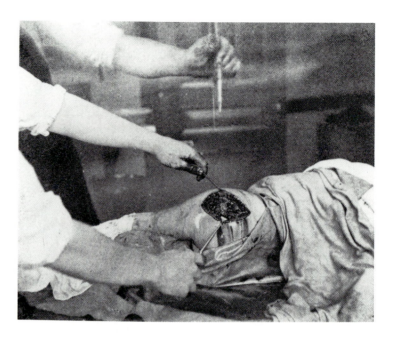

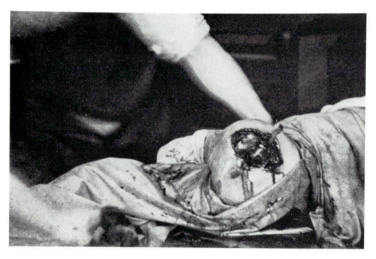

OR48. **CHARLES FREDERICK STILLMAN** (1853–92). *A practical resumé of
modern methods employed in the treatment of chronic articular ostitis
of the hip.* 118pp. Detroit: G. S. Davis, 1891.

An 1876 graduate of the College of Physicians and Surgeons of New
York, Stillman later became professor of orthopedic surgery at the
Chicago Polyclinic. This volume was part of Davis's Physicians' Leisure
Library. Stillman wrote in the preface:

> This work has been compiled with the object of acquainting prac-
> titioners and medical students with the most recent views held by or-
> thopaedic writers upon the management of hip disease. It also aims to
> familiarize them with the methods they advocate and employ in prac-
> tice, and to secure accuracy and reliability the author has made as few

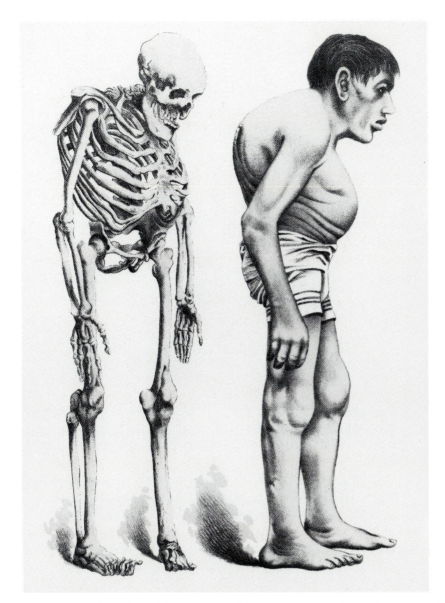

Fig. 100. (OR49) Senn illustrates osteitis deformans in this lithographic plate (number 6, figure 31, page 177). Burk & McFetridge of Philadelphia were the lithographers.

changes as possible in the publications and private letters which have been utilized in its preparation . . . .

Among the surgeons whose treatment is discussed are Hugh Owen Thomas (1834–81), DeForest Willard (1846–1910), Louis Bauer (1814–98), Lewis Sayre (1820–1900), Newton Shaffer (1846–1928), and Robert Lovett (1859–1924). The book contains sixty engravings. It was available either paperbound for twenty-five cents or in cloth for fifty cents. Stillman's other book is *The life insurance examiner, a practical treatise upon medical examinations for life insurance* (New York: Spectator, 1888).

OR49. NICHOLAS SENN (1844–1908). *Tuberculosis of bones and joints.* 504pp. Philadelphia: F. A. Davis, 1892.

Senn was professor of the practice of surgery and clinical surgery at Rush Medical College when this treatise was completed. He was president-elect of the American Surgical Association and dedicated this work to "the fellows of the American Surgical Association, who have contributed so much toward the advancement of surgery in the United States." He goes on to explain in the preface that

> ... the tubercular nature of most of the chronic affections of bones and joints is not as freely accepted and as fully realized as it should be by the mass of the profession, and consequently a correct diagnosis is often not made before the disease has become incurable .... The object of the author in writing this book has been to collect from recent literature the modern ideas on tubercular disease of bones and joints and present them to the reader in a condensed form, mingled, in appropriate places, with the results of his own experience.

There are thirty-seven chapters and 107 illustrations, including seven plates. Plates 1, 4, and 7 are important because they are copied from the work of Koch and demonstrate tubercle bacilli less than seven years after the enunciation of his famous postulates. (See also GS138, GS139, GS140, GS144, GS162, GS168, and GU36.)

OR50. **JOHN RIDLON** (1852–1936) and **ROBERT JONES** (1858–1933). *Chronic joint disease; some preliminary papers.* 179pp. Chicago: C. J. Burroughs, 1894.

Ridlon's association with Jones dates back to 1887, when Ridlon visited Liverpool and made the acquaintance of Hugh Owen Thomas (1834–91) [G-M 4340 and 4348], Jones's uncle. Ridlon was an 1878 graduate of the College of Physicians and Surgeons of New York. In 1889 he was made instructor in orthopedic surgery at Northwestern University in Chicago. A year later he was named professor and served at Northwestern for sixteen years. Ridlon was a charter member of the American Orthopedic Association. Jones was one of the most prominent English orthopedic surgeons of his time. He is probably best remembered for the first published report of the clinical use of X rays [G-M 2684]. The Ridlon-Jones relationship has been described in depth by Hiram Winnett Orr (1877–1956) in *On the contributions of Hugh Owen Thomas of Liverpool, Sir Robert Jones of Liverpool and London, John Ridlon, M.D., of New York and Chicago, to modern orthopedic surgery* (Springfield: C. C. Thomas, 1949) [G-M 4483]. As a result of their acquaintance and mutual esteem, Ridlon and Jones cooperated between 1892 and 1893 on a number of articles, both in America and England, dealing with orthopedic conditions of hips, spine, knees, shoulders, elbows, and wrists. The most important were those on spondylitis in the December 10, 1892, *Journal of the American Medical Association,* and that on hip disease in the February 18 and March 4, 1893, editions of the *Journal.* A number of these jointly written reports were reprinted and serve as the basis for this book. (See also OR59.)

OR51. **JAMES KELLY YOUNG** (1862–1923). *A practical treatise on orthopedic surgery.* 446pp. Philadelphia: Lea Brothers, 1894.

Young was an 1883 graduate of the University of Pennsylvania Medical School. He was instrumental, along with De Forest Willard (1846–1910), in establishing the orthopedic department of the

University of Pennsylvania, and eventually held the chair of orthopedics at the university's Graduate School of Medicine. The book was dedicated to David Hayes Agnew (1818–92), John Ashhurst (1839–1900), William G. Porter (1846–1906), DeForest Willard (1846–1910), and Algernon S. Roberts (1855–96), who Young described as his surgical teachers. Most of the *Treatise* was based on Young's personal clinical experience. He also devoted a large portion of the volume to orthopedic pathology. There are twenty-eight chapters covering a wide range of orthopedic topics. This was the only edition and was available in cloth for $4.00 or leather for $5.00. Among Young's most important other books is *A manual and atlas of orthopedic surgery, including the history, etiology, pathology, diagnosis, prognosis, prophylaxis, and treatment of deformities* (Philadelphia: P. Blakiston's Son, 1905). (See also GS141.)

OR52. **OSCAR H. ALLIS** (1836–1921). *An inquiry into the difficulties encountered in the reduction of dislocations of the hip. The Samuel D. Gross Prize Essay.* 171pp. Philadelphia: W. Dornan, 1896.

Allis graduated from Jefferson Medical College in 1866 and was one of the original staff surgeons at the Presbyterian Hospital in Philadelphia. Allis wrote this monograph in 1895, and won the $1,000 Samuel D. Gross Prize from the Philadelphia Academy of Surgery. He wrote in the preface that

> . . . clinical difficulties have suggested and directed experimental work. To no class of affections has clinical experience contributed so little. To anesthesia, to knowledge gained from dissection, to the study of fatal cases of traumatic dislocations, and to experimental work in the dissection-room do we owe all the progress we have made in this department of surgery. The clinic has really been the amphitheatre for the display of skill for the relief of the living which was gained upon the cadaver in the dissecting-room. Some have fancied that they have found in experimental work, the solution of all conceivable difficulties, and have spoken with confidence upon the subject. For my part, I have been too often and too sadly disappointed in dogmatic assertions to venture upon the same course myself. I have everywhere striven to be clear and candid. My oft-repeated failures have left me no room for boasting. They have not, however, been an unmixed evil; for, while they have been a constant menace to over-confidence, they have also been a constant spur to exertion.

There is no table of contents, and the index is minimal at best. The book contains 159 wood engravings.

OR53. **JOHN BINGHAM ROBERTS** (1852–1924). *A clinical, pathological, and experimental study of fracture of the lower end of the radius, with displacement of the carpal fragment toward the flexor or anterior surface of the wrist.* 76pp. Philadelphia: P. Blakiston & Son, 1897.

Roberts was professor of anatomy and surgery at the Philadelphia Polyclinic and professor of surgery at the Woman's Medical College of

Pennsylvania when he published this work. This rather small monograph consists of six chapters: "Cases and specimens"; "Experimental observations"; "Causes and mechanism"; "Symptoms"; "Diagnosis"; and "Treatment." There are thirty-three illustrations. (See also GS99, GS102, GS143, OR60, and NS1.)

OR54. **EDWARD JAMES FARNUM** (1860–?). *Deformities; a textbook on orthopedic surgery.* 544pp. Chicago: Medical Press, 1898.

Farnum was an eclectic surgeon who was professor of orthopedic surgery and clinical surgery at Bennett Medical College in Chicago and attending surgeon at Cook County Hospital. He also served as president of the National Eclectic Medical Association. Farnum writes in the preface:

> During the writer's experience as a teacher he has felt the great necessity of a comprehensive work on deformities. To produce a book with subjects systematically arranged, and with a clear and concise delineation; brief, yet sufficiently elaborate to cover the ground, has been the aim of the author in preparing this work . . . . Theoretical matter, and much technical matter, has been purposely omitted, and practical facts elucidated which are in accordance with the writer's experience in practice . . . .

There are nine sections: "Orthopedic surgery"; "Congenital deformities"; "Deformities of the spine"; "General joint diseases"; "Special joint diseases"; "Rickets, paralysis"; "Talipes"; "Affections of the toes and fingers"; and "Hernia." The work is massively illustrated and includes 209 figures. This was the only edition.

OR55. **JAMES EDWARD MOORE** (1852–1918). *Orthopedic surgery.* 354pp. Philadelphia: W. B. Saunders, 1898.

Moore was professor of orthopedia and of clinical surgery at the College of Medicine of the University of Minnesota. He was quite active in the American Surgical Association and served as its vice-president in 1906. Moore explains in the preface that

> this book is written as a text-book for students and as a ready-reference book for general practitioners. A studied effort has been made to reduce its size by eliminating all that is not of practical value. Special stress is laid upon early diagnosis, and, instead of giving in detail every method of treatment that has even been employed, only such methods are given as in the writer's experience have yielded the best results. The simplest kinds of apparatus, such as can most readily be applied by the general practitioner, are recommended. The book is written by a general surgeon who has taught orthopedic surgery for the past decade, and who believes that the orthopedic surgeon should know when and how to operate . . . .

The twenty-four chapters cover numerous topics, but no X rays are used. The 177 illustrations include multiple clinical photographs. The book was published in cloth as an octavo volume for $2.50. There was only one edition.

OR56. **STUART LEROY MCCURDY** (1859–1931). *Manual of orthopedic surgery.* 339pp. Pittsburgh: Nicholson Press, 1898.

McCurdy was professor of anatomy and oral surgery at Pittsburgh Dental College and orthopedic surgeon at Presbyterian Hospital. He had formerly served as professor of orthopedic surgery at Ohio Medical University. This work has no table of contents or index. McCurdy states in the preface:

> It is not the object of the author to treat exhaustively the subject of orthopedic surgery. This book is intended for the busy practitioner as an aid in diagnosis and treatment, and for the student who finds little time to pursue the larger works. It is thought an advantage to group cuts illustrating similar conditions in order that comparison may be more easily made. The sole aim has been to consider as much in one sentence as possible, to eliminate speculation, and to present what the author believes the most modern and accepted views of pathology and treatment.

The work has 145 illustrations. This was the only edition. Among McCurdy's other books are *Oral surgery; a textbook on general medicine and surgery as applied to dentistry* (Pittsburgh: Calumet, 1901); *Anatomy in abstract* (Pittsburgh: Medical Abstract, 1905); *Surgical and medical emergencies in abstract* (Pittsburgh: Medical Abstract, 1906); and *Arthrosteopedic surgery* (Pittsburgh: Medical Abstract, 1909).

OR57. **ALGERNON SYDNEY ROBERTS** (1855–96). *Contributions to orthopedic surgery; with a brief biographical sketch by James K. Young.* 298pp. Philadelphia: W. J. Dornan, 1898.

Roberts was an 1877 graduate of the University of Pennsylvania Medical School. He took graduate training under Newton Shaffer (1846–1928) in New York City. Having returned to Philadelphia to begin practice, Roberts was named surgeon at Philadelphia Hospital and instructor in orthopedic surgery at his alma mater. Among his pupils in Philadelphia was James Young (1862–1923). Roberts died prematurely, and it is through the efforts of Young that his orthopedic writings were collected in this volume. According to the preface, "The present collection is undertaken for private distribution only, for the sole purpose of increasing the interest in the subjects of which it treats . . . . " Some of the topics discussed are "Clubfoot"; "Pott's disease"; "Spinal arthropathies"; "Chronic articular osteitis of the knee joint"; and "Deformity of the forearm and hands." Pages 5–21 contain a biography of Roberts written by Young. There are seventy-eight illustrations.

OR58. **NEWTON MELMAN SHAFFER** (1846–1928). *Brief essays on orthopedic surgery, including a consideration of its relation to general surgery, its future demands, and its operative as well as its mechanical aspects, with remarks on specialism.* 81pp. New York: D. Appleton, 1898.

Surgeon-in-chief at the New York Orthopedic Dispensary and Hospital, Shaffer was a charter member and one of the early presidents of the first orthopedic organization in America, the New York Orthopedic

Society. He was also one of the principal organizers and a charter member of the American Orthopedic Association and its second president in 1887. Shaffer writes in the preface:

> At the request of a few friends, who have been kind enough to take considerable interest in my work, these essays, which have appeared at various periods during the past fourteen years, are now presented in their present form, and they are submitted to the medical profession and the public with the hope that orthopaedic surgery may be benefited by their publication.

This volume consists of seven nonclinical essays, which Shaffer had written for medical journals between 1884 and 1897. The contents consist of the definition, scope, status, operative side, present needs of, and future demands on orthopedic surgery. In addition, one chapter explores the relationship between orthopedic and general surgery. The last essay is entitled "Is orthopaedic surgery to become an obsolete specialty? Remarks on specialism." (See also OR36 and OR39.)

OR59. **JOHN RIDLON** (1852–1936) and **ROBERT JONES** (1858–1933). *Lectures on orthopedic surgery.* 358pp. Philadelphia: E. Stern, 1899.

This volume consists mainly of lectures by Ridlon delivered while he was professor of orthopedic surgery at Northwestern University, as added to or commented upon by Jones. This particular book was originally intended to be published as a multivolume set. One volume of approximately 250 pages was published by the Philadelphia Medical Press. However, there was a change in management of the company, and a decision was made not to complete the project. As a consequence volume 2 was never printed. Instead, the entire work was reprinted in expanded form and sold as this textbook. Ridlon writes in the preface:

> The authors of this volume have undertaken to preserve the things of most value in the writings on orthopedic surgery by the late Hugh Owen Thomas, modified by their own personal experience and convictions; they have endeavored to make a volume for the use of the student and the general practitioner and have omitted much that would be of interest and inserted much that may not be of interest to the orthopedic specialist . . . .

There are eighteen chapters covering such topics as "Spondylitis"; "Hip disease"; "Great toe disease"; "Rachitic deformities"; and "Clubfoot." This was the only edition. (See also OR50.)

OR60. **JOHN BINGHAM ROBERTS** (1852–1924): *Notes on the modern treatment of fractures.* 162pp. New York: D. Appleton, 1899.

Roberts, professor of surgery in the Philadelphia Polyclinic, was among the most widely published of nineteenth-century American surgeons. He writes in the preface:

> No injuries require more careful and judicious treatment than fractures: and in no branch of surgical therapeutics is the exercise of common sense followed by more satisfactory results than in the treatment of these lesions. A blind reliance upon therapeutic dogmas and the adoption of routine measures, without due consideration of the mechanical and pathological problems presented, have led to many disasters in this

department of surgery . . . . the author has always believed that independent thinking leads to the abandonment of false theories, and aids in the search for truth.

There are nineteen chapters and thirty-nine illustrations. Figures 11–13 depict X rays of experimental fractures on cadavers. (See also GS99, GS102, GS143, OR53, and NS1.)

OR61. **LEWIS ATTERBURY STIMSON** (1844–1917): *A practical treatise on fractures and dislocations.* 822pp. New York: Lea Brothers, 1899.

Stimson was professor of surgery at Cornell University Medical College when this *Treatise* was published. He explains in the preface why he wrote the book:

Although this work is, in one sense, a second edition of the volumes published in 1883 and 1888, it has been so largely rewritten that it is

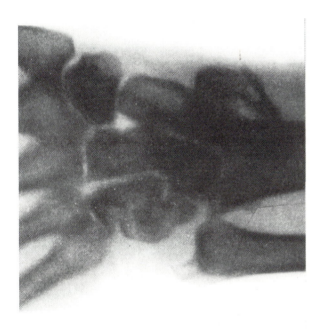

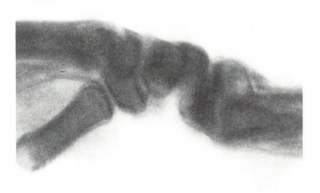

Fig. 101. (OR61) Some of the earliest examples of X rays in orthopedic texts are found in Stimson's work. This plate, figure 7 on page 272, demonstrates two views of a Colles's fracture in a 26-year-old male.

practically new. The wider experience gained through eleven years of service in charge of the House of Relief (Hudson Street Hospital) where traumatic cases are very numerous . . . gave the opportunity and seemed to justify a recasting of the work in a more personal form, with a corresponding reduction in the number of quotations of histories and of opinions based on single cases. This has enabled me not only to introduce such additions as have been made to our knowledge of the subject in the interval, but also to adapt the work more specifically to the needs of the practitioner, especially in respect to diagnosis and treatment, while those of the student of special subjects have been heeded in the bibliographical references, which have been largely added to. The portion treating of fractures has been almost wholly rewritten, the most marked change in classification and arrangement being that made in the chapter on fractures of the skull . . . . In the portion treating of dislocations the most notable changes . . . are those dealing with operative reduction of both old and recent injuries.

Stimson goes on to discuss X rays:

Shortly after the discovery of the x-rays an apparatus for their utilization was set up in the hospital, and some of the results are shown in the skiagrams introduced as plates. In studying these photographs it must be remembered that they are the reproductions of shadows, not, like ordinary photographs, of the appearance of illuminated surfaces, and that the apparent modelling of the bones is inexact because it is due to differences in thickness and opacity to the rays. While the x-rays have been of interest and value in showing details of certain fractures, especially at the wrist, elbow, and ankle, yet it cannot fairly be said that they have yielded much information of practical value which could not have been obtained by palpation. Probably their usefulness will be increased by improvements in methods and apparatus, but at present the information which they give needs to be sifted with great care from among many misleading appearances.

The volume contains fifty-eight chapters and 326 illustrations. Twenty monotint plates of X rays are included. The book was initially available in cloth for $5.00 or leather for $6.00. The first edition was also published in a two-volume set. Further editions were printed in 1899, 1900, 1905, 1907, and 1910. (See also GS91, OR40, and OR45.)

V. GYNECOLOGY

GY1. **WILLIAM POTTS DEWEES** (1768–1841). *A treatise on the diseases of females.* 557pp. Philadelphia: H. C. Carey & I. Lea, 1826.

Primarily known as an obstetrician, Dewees contributed to the evolution of obstetrics from midwifery to its establishment as an academic discipline. It has been stated that in Dewees's day no pregnant woman in Philadelphia considered herself safe in other hands. Like most publications of its time, the *Treatise*, although considered the first gynecologic textbook in America, was concerned almost completely with medical gynecology. Operative surgery for gynecologic disease was still in its infancy. Ephraim McDowell's (1771–1830) introduction of ovariotomy had only occurred in 1809 and was not reported in medical journals until 1817 [G-M 6023].

Dewees was an 1806 graduate of the University of Pennsylvania, where he received his M.D. Dewees wrote this volume while he was adjunct professor of midwifery at his alma mater. In 1834 he was promoted to full professor. The *Treatise* is dedicated to Nathaniel Chapman (1780–1853) and contains twenty-one chapters, including "Of tumours and excrescences of the external parts" (chapter 3); "Of the displacement of the uterus" (chapter 10); and "Of prolapsus uteri, when not impregnated" (chapter 13). Chapter 20 discusses milk abscess of the breast along with some rudimentary surgical treatments, including puncturing and seton.

The book was quite well received, with eleven editions being printed; the last appeared in 1860, almost two decades after the author's death. There are twelve copperplate engravings (four of which are foldouts) at the end of the text. An additional unnumbered plate is bound in front of the index. A detailed description of this plate, which depicts a small wire crochet used to remove a hemorrhaging placenta, appears on page 316.

Among Dewees's other writings are his inaugural dissertation for the M.D. degree, published in book form as *An essay on the means of lessening pain, and facilitating certain cases of difficult parturition* (Philadelphia: Thomas Dobson, 1819); *Essays on various subjects connected with midwifery* (Philadelphia: Carey & Lea, 1823); *A compendious system of midwifery* (Philadelphia: Carey & Lea, 1824); the first American textbook on pediatrics, *Treatise on the physical and medical treatment of children* (Philadelphia: H. C. Carey & I. Lea, 1825) [G-M 6331]; and *A practice of physic, comprising most of the diseases not treated in "Diseases of females" and "Diseases of children"* (Philadelphia: Carey & Lea, 1830).

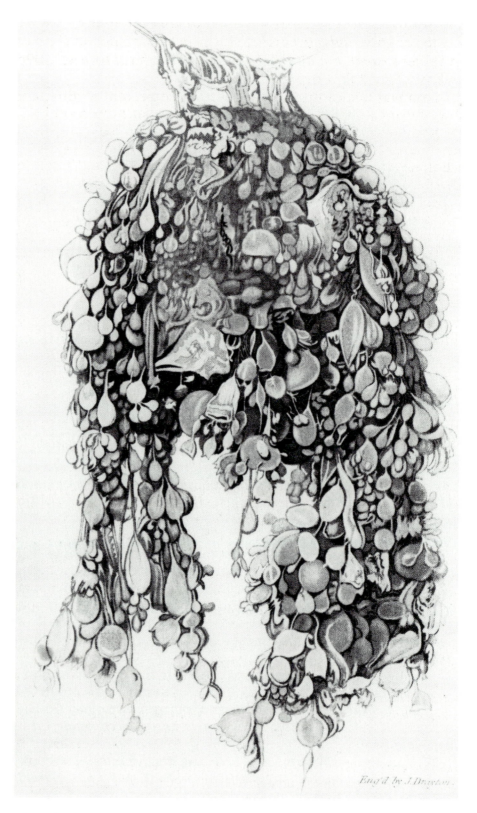

Fig. 102. (GY1) In this uncolored plate Dewees shows a portion of hydatids of the uterus. He states that the quantity passed by the patient "would have filled a gallon measure." The figure was engraved by J. Drayton.

GY2. **EDWARD H. DIXON** (1808–80). *Woman, and her diseases, from the cradle to the grave: adapted exclusively to her instruction in the physiology of her system and all the diseases of her critical periods.* 309pp. New York: Privately Printed, 1847.

Dixon was one of the more interesting and eccentric nineteenth-century American physicians. He studied under Valentine Mott (1785–1865) and later became known as an able genitourinary surgeon. He never held an academic post, and eventually left scientific medicine to concentrate on writing satiric magazine articles and books. His writings made him into a medical pariah of sorts, and he was shunned by the members of his own profession.

Dixon's *Woman* is a massive compendium of twenty-two chapters outlining numerous diseases related to females. Gynecology is discussed in chapters 14 and 15 ("Prolapse and displacements of the uterus and bladder"), chapter 16 ("Rectal prolapse"), and chapter 17 ("Inflammation and cancer of the uterus"). Chapter 19 is of some interest because of its discussion of breast cancer. The work contains no plates because, as Dixon notes in the introduction, "Although they would serve a useful purpose in illustrating derangements of natural position in some important organs, their effect might be injurious to the youthful mind; and we would fondly hope our book will never communicate evil, should it fail in imparting wholesome instruction." The work proved quite popular and went through ten editions, the last in 1860. Among Dixon's other books are *Scenes in the practice of a New York surgeon* (New York: DeWitt & Davenport, 1855) and *Back-bone; photographed from "The scalpel"* (New York: R. M. DeWitt, 1866). (See also GU2.)

GY3. **CHARLES DELUCENA MEIGS** (1792–1869). *Females and their diseases; a series of letters to his class.* 670pp. Philadelphia: Lea & Blanchard, 1848.

As professor of midwifery and the diseases of women and children at Jefferson Medical College, Meigs was one of Philadelphia's best-known physicians. Highly regarded as a teacher, he did much to elevate standards of care and the practice of obstetrics. Meigs is best remembered for drawing attention to embolism as a cause of sudden death in labor [G-M 6177].

Females and their diseases consists of forty-four lectures delivered to classes at Jefferson. Among the gynecological topics are "Wounds and lacerations of the labia" (pages 64–68); "Uterine displacements" (pages 127–63); "Ovariotomy" (pages 299–323); and "The breast" (pages 643–61). There are no plates. Further editions were published in 1851, 1854, and 1859. Among his other medical books are *The Philadelphia practice of midwifery* (Philadelphia: James Kay & Brother, 1828), *Obstetrics: the science and the art* (Philadelphia: Lea & Blanchard, 1849), *Observations on certain of the diseases of young children* (Philadelphia: Lea & Blanchard, 1850), and *On the nature, signs, and treatment of childbed fevers* (Philadelphia: Blanchard & Lea, 1854). (See also GY5.)

GY4. **GEORGE HINCKLEY LYMAN** (1819–91). *Non-malignant diseases of the uterus; an essay which obtained the Boylston Prize for 1854.* 76pp. Boston: Ticknor & Fields, 1854.

Lyman was an 1843 graduate of the University of Pennsylvania. He died in London, after having practiced obstetrics and gynecology in Boston. He was one of the earliest members of the American Gynecological Society. This monograph lacks a table of contents and an index and is therefore difficult to read. Lyman notes in the preface that:

> The following dissertation is published for more convenient distribution among professional friends, who have taken sufficient interest in the matter to desire its perusal. It professes to be nothing more than a concise sketch of those non-malignant diseases of the uterus which are most frequently met with, and of their surgical treatment, as described and advocated by many distinguished modern writers . . . .

(See also GY7.)

GY5. **CHARLES DELUCENA MEIGS** (1792–1869). *A treatise on acute and chronic diseases of the neck of the uterus.* 116pp. Philadelphia: Blanchard & Lea, 1854.

Meigs received his M.D. from the University of Pennsylvania in 1817, and within ten years was one of the editors of the *North American medical and surgical journal.* Always active in medical politics, he was appointed by the American Medical Association to present a report on the subject of acute and chronic diseases of the cervix and uterus. This report, which had been partially published in the *Transactions of the American Medical Association,* constitutes the bulk of his *Treatise.* Dedicated to Robert Huston (1795–1864), professor of therapeutics and materia medica at Jefferson, this separate work was published in the hope that it would receive a wider circulation among "our professional brethren." There is no table of contents, although an exhaustive index is found on pages 109–16. The text contains only five figures, but the most prominent portion of the work is the twenty-two superb chromolithograph plates. Unfortunately, there are no separate captions. Instead, descriptions of the plates are incorporated into the text. Meigs's son was the pioneer Philadelphia pediatrician, John Forsyth Meigs (1818–82), and his grandson was Arthur Vincent Meigs (1850–1912), whose greatest contribution was accurate chemical analysis and comparison of human and cow's milk to make the latter more suitable for infant consumption. (See also GY3.)

GY6. **GUNNING S. BEDFORD** (1806–70). *Clinical lectures on the diseases of women and children.* 602pp. New York: Samuel S. & W. Wood, 1855.

Bedford founded the first obstetrical clinic in America in the medical department of the University of New York. He was also a founder of the New York Academy of Medicine. Bedford received his M.D. from Rutgers Medical College in 1829, and soon departed for two years of study in Europe. He was named professor of obstetrics, the diseases of women and children, and clinical midwifery at the University of New

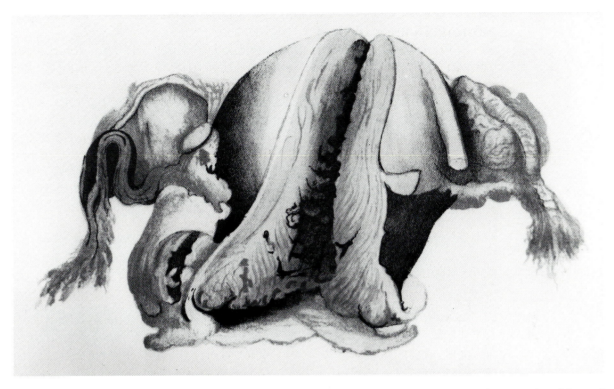

Fig. 103. (GY5) This plate drawn from a specimen in Meigs's personal collection, demonstrates hypertrophy of the neck of the uterus with consequent blockage of the cervical canal. W. Dreser executed the plate and T. Sinclair of Philadelphia was the lithographer.

York. Bedford's works were always among the most popular of the day. His *Lectures* is a compendium of clinical material which he presented to classes at the University of New York. Most of the information came from the more than 8,000 obstetric and gynecologic cases that Bedford treated from 1850 to 1855. The first twenty-four chapters are devoted to diseases of women. The volume went through at least ten editions by 1870. Bedford's other medical book is *The principles and practice of obstetrics* (New York: S. S. & W. Wood, 1861).

GY7. **GEORGE HINCKLEY LYMAN** (1819–91). *The history and statistics of ovariotomy and the circumstances under which the operation may be regarded as safe and expedient.* 146pp. Boston: John Wilson & Son, 1856.

Lyman received a prize from the Massachusetts Medical Society for writing this monograph. It provides an exhaustive review of all aspects relating to the surgical removal of the diseased ovary. Unfortunately, the work has neither a table of contents nor an index. However, Lyman's extensive footnotes prove quite valuable, since they provide important information in this first American book detailing ovariotomy. There was only one edition. (See also GY4.)

GY8. **JOHN MILTON SCUDDER** (1829posed to.–94). *A practical treatise on the diseases of women; and a paper on the diseases of the breasts.* 525pp. Cincinnati: Moore, Wilstach & Keys, 1857.

One of the most prominent of eclectic physicians, Scudder graduated from the Eclectic Medical Institute in Cincinnati in 1856. He almost immediately began to teach and was named professor of general, special, and pathological anatomy at the institute. The *Treatise* is massive in scope and was the first of many books that Scudder wrote; it eventually went through fifteen editions, the last in 1891. Among his other contributions are *The American eclectic materia medica and therapeutics* (Cincinnati: Moore, Wilstach & Keys, 1858), jointly written with Lorenzo E. Jones; *The eclectic practice of medicine* (Cincinnati: Moore, Wilstach & Keys, 1864); *Domestic medicine: or, home book of health* (Cincinnati: J. R. Hawley, 1865); *On the use of medicated inhalations, in the treatment of diseases of the respiratory organs* (Cincinnati: Moore, Wilstach & Baldwin, 1866); *The eclectic practice in diseases of children* (Cincinnati: American Publishing, 1869), *Specific medication and specific medicine* (Cincinnati: Wilstach & Baldwin, 1870); *On the reproductive organs, and the venereal diseases* (Cincinnati: Wilstach & Baldwin, 1874); and *Specific diagnosis: a study of diseases with specific reference to the administration of remedies* (Cincinnati: Wilstach & Baldwin, 1874). Scudder writes in the preface:

> On examination of the numerous allopathic works on this subject, I found that the pathology of uterine disease had been carefully and successfully studied, and that, in this respect, this branch of medical science was at least equal, if not in advance of the general practice of medicine: and yet, with this accurate knowledge of the nature and character of the diseased actions, their treatment was far less successful than our own, so far as medicinal agents were used for the cure, but where operative interference was required, nothing more could be desired than was given in these works . . . .

The book contains a chapter (No. 15) on "Diseases of the breast" by Robert S. Newton, professor of surgery at the institute. The other fourteen chapters include "Anatomy of the female organs of generation"; "Pathology and diagnosis"; "Diseases of the external organs of generation"; "Diseases of the urethra, vagina, and uterus"; "Laceration or rupture of the perineum"; "Pelvic cellulitis"; and "Venereal diseases." There are a few colored plates and numerous wood engravings.

GY9. **HUGH LENOX HODGE** (1796–1873). *On diseases peculiar to women, including displacements of the uterus.* 469pp. Philadelphia: Blanchard & Lea, 1860.

Hodge was professor of obstetrics and diseases of women and children at the University of Pennsylvania. He received his M.D. from that institution in 1818 and soon began to practice surgery in Philadelphia. Considered an outstanding teacher, he is best remembered for *The principles and practice of obstetrics* (Philadelphia: Blanchard & Lea, 1864) [G-M 6185], considered to be one of the most important textbooks on midwifery. He writes in the preface to the *Diseases*:

This work, prepared at the request of many of my pupils, presents the results of my observations and reflections on the diseases peculiar to women. These diseases may be traced to the effects of irritation and of sedation in the different tissues and organs of the economy, especially of the uterine system. The causes of such disturbances are exceedingly diversified; but, so much depends on displacements of the uterus, that it was thought advisable to devote a separate part to their consideration, especially as the consequences and treatment of such accidents are still the subjects of much professional discussion . . . .

The work is dedicated to Charles Delucena Meigs (1792–1869). It consists of three major parts: "Diseases of irritation"; "Displacements of the

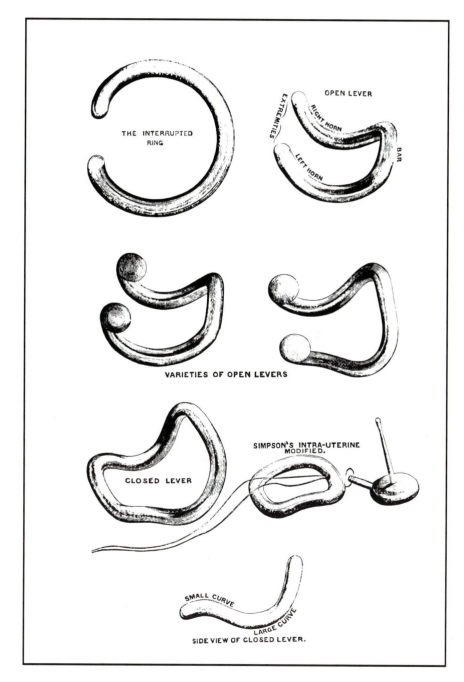

Fig. 104. (GY9) A wide variety of lever pessaries used for uterine displacements are depicted by Hodge (page 331).

uterus"; and "Diseases of sedation." In chapter 5 Hodge provides a lengthy description of his well-known pessary. There are no plates, although numerous illustrations are included. A revised second edition was published in 1868.

GY10. **WILLIAM HEATH BYFORD** (1817–90). *A treatise on the chronic inflammation and displacement of the unimpregnated uterus.* 215pp. Philadelphia: Lindsay & Blakiston, 1864.

Byford was a founder of the American Gynecological Society. Known primarily as a gynecologist, he received his M.D. from the Medical College of Ohio in 1845 and was on the faculty of the Chicago Medical College from 1859 to 1879. He performed the first ovariotomy in Chicago in 1861. The *Treatise* was the first textbook of gynecology in the Midwest, and sold for $2.00. A second edition appeared in 1871. Byford writes in the preface:

> This work was originated in the honest conviction, that such a treatise is necessary. The junior members of the profession are called upon, soon as they commence practice, to prescribe for, and treat the ailments herein described. It could not well be otherwise, seeing that the uterus is so frequently diseased. I need not inform them, or their older brethren, of the want of definite instruction on these subjects in ordinary treatises on Diseases of Women; and the consequent great differences of opinion prevailing among medical men everywhere in reference to them. It is with the hope of in some slight degree supplying this want, and aiding to correct these differences, that I have undertaken the task of furnishing a monograph . . . .

There are fourteen chapters, including "General considerations"; "Sympathetic accompaniments of uterine disease"; "Local symptoms"; "Etiology"; "Prognosis"; "Complications of inflammation of cervix"; "Position of inflammation"; "Progress and terminations"; "Diagnosis"; "General treatment"; "Local treatment"; "Nitrate of silver and its substitutes"; "Treatment of submucous inflammation"; and "Displacements, their philosophy and treatment." The appendix contains detailed descriptions of six cases of uterine pathology. Among Byford's other books is *A treatise on the theory and practice of obstetrics* (New York: William Wood, 1870). (See GY11.)

GY11. **WILLIAM HEATH BYFORD** (1817–90). *The practice of medicine and surgery, applied to the diseases and accidents incident to women.* 566pp. Philadelphia: Lindsay & Blakiston, 1865.

As professor of obstetrics and diseases of women and children at Chicago Medical College, Byford played a major role in founding the Hospital for Women and Children in Chicago. From 1870 to 1890 he served on the gynecology faculty of Rush Medical College. This volume was written " . . . to furnish the student and junior members of the profession a concise, yet sufficiently complete, practical, and reliable treatise to meet their wants in everyday practice . . . . " There are thirty chapters, covering topics such as "Accidents of the labia and perineum"; "Vaginitis"; "Cancer of the uterus"; "Ovarian tumors"; and "Diseases of the breasts." The work is a massive compendium of facts, but is mini-

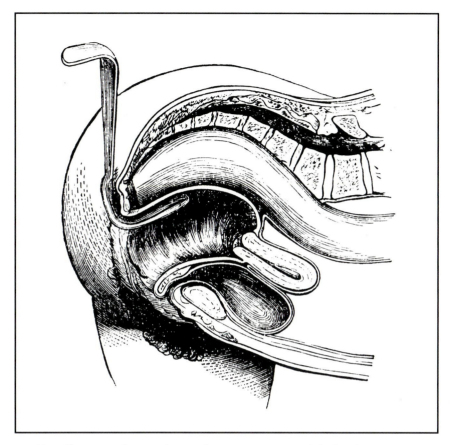

Fig. 105. (GY12) Sims demonstrates placement of his double duckbill vaginal speculum in this wood engraving, figure 3 on page 12.

mally illustrated. Further editions were published in 1867, 1881, and 1888. (See also GY10.)

GY12. **JAMES MARION SIMS** (1813–83). *Clinical notes on uterine surgery; with special reference to the management of the sterile condition.* 401pp. New York: William Wood, 1866.[G-M 6057]

One of America's premier surgeon-gynecologists of the nineteenth century, Sims received his M.D. from Jefferson Medical College in 1835. He served as president of the American Medical Association in 1876 and of the American Gynecological Society in 1880. Sims was also instrumental in founding the Women's Hospital in New York. For numerous reasons, the Sims family settled in Europe for varying periods of time, and the *Notes* was written during a sojourn in London. The work has an interesting history. It was originally serialized in *Lancet* in 1864–65. The articles engendered a great deal of debate within the medical community, and when the work finally appeared in book form it was met by a storm of controversy. Recognized for its forceful style, it presented an abundance of bold and original thought. However, critics inveighed against its casual and fragmentary nature, its complete absence of system, and, above all, its frank presentation of subjects previously considered taboo. As Seale Harris writes in *Women's surgeon, the life story of J. Marion Sims* (New York: Macmillan, 1950, pages 243–52):

> The aspect of the work which excited the most heated condemnation
> was Sim's forthright account of a number of experiments he had con-

ducted in the field of artificial and instrumental impregnation of the human female. His reports of his methods and stratagems and of the results he had achieved were as strictly factual and unsensational as he could make them, but the very fact that he dared to experiment at all in such forbidden territory and to publish his findings was enough to arouse some of his readers to shocked indignation. That a supposedly reputable medical man should stoop to such practices, they protested, was incredible! Particularly distressing to the sensibilities of certain critics was his account of the way he had found it necessary in some instances to visit sterile married couples in their bedrooms and to apply there various measures (including, occasionally, etherization of the wife) to overcome the obstacles preventing conception . . . . That the book should have wielded such an influence is really amazing in view of the fact that it was only a fragmentary piece of work—notably unsystematic, dealing with but a limited range of diseases, and even containing occasional inaccuracies . . . . Yet, despite all its omissions and defects, *Uterine Surgery* contained a vast amount of practical information and of solid, highly germinal advice . . . . It provided above all a new and in most respects original method of uterine investigation, making it possible to determine morbid conditions with an ease and precision which a few years since would have seemed not only marvellous but incredible . . . .

Writing in his autobiography, Sims notes (pages 329–30):

When I went abroad I thought I would occupy my leisure moments in writing my work on the Accidents of Parturition, and, as I knew I was to spend the summer at Baden-Baden, I took all my material, manuscript and drawings, for the purpose of writing the proposed book. About the middle of June, 1863, I began it. I had piles of manuscripts and piles of illustrations, and commenced classifying and arranging the material, working very hard for two days. The weather was excessively hot and exhausting, and at last I said to myself, "This work is too heavy; I am not equal to the task during such extremely hot weather. I will lay it aside until the autumn, and then I will set to work in earnest to write my great work," which I hoped and expected would send my name down to posterity. And then, said I, "Between now and October I will occupy my time in writing a pamphlet on the subject of sterility. I don't know a great deal about it, but I know more than anybody else, and I am sure a pamphlet on this subject will be welcomed by the profession everywhere." With this intention I dismissed the heavy work and commenced the lighter one of writing a pamphlet. I went on with the subject, and instead of its ending in a pamphlet form it became a book on all the diseases of women, leaving out the subjects of ovariotomy and the accidents of parturition, but embracing everything else in the department of gynecology. This book was entitled *Clinical Notes of Uterine Surgery*. It was so radical and revolutionary in all the methods adopted, and so startling in the results claimed in the treatment of many affections, that the profession did not at first readily accept its teachings, but in a few years it completely revolutionized the subject of gynaecology . . . . I have always said this book was a mere accident; that I never intended to write it. The book that I went to Baden-Baden to write has not yet been written.

The book was originally published by R. Hardwicke in London, with the American edition coming out a few months later. It was dedicated to Joseph F. Olliffe. Sims writes in the preface:

> In 1862, I voluntarily left my own country, on account of its political troubles. Our unfortunate civil war continued much longer than any of us anticipated. In consequence of this my residence abroad was prolonged far beyond my original intention. I therefore had time to look over my note-books, and to cull such facts as illustrate the method of treating Uterine Disease at the Woman's Hospital. Having an innate horror of writing, I have not tried to make a book; on the contrary, I have simply related in detail my various operations, and given the history of cases . . . .

There were eight chapters: "Conception occurs only during menstrual life"; "Menstruation should be such as to show a healthy condition of the uterine cavity"; "The os and cervix uteri should be sufficiently open, not only to permit the free exit of the menstrual flow, but also to admit the ingress of the spermatozoa"; "The cervix uteri should be of proper size, form, and density"; "The uterus should be in a normal position, i.e., neither anteverted nor retroverted to any great degree"; "The vagina must be capable of receiving and retaining the spermatic fluid"; "For conception, semen with living spermatozoa should be deposited in the vagina at the proper time"; and "The secretions of the cervix and vagina should not poison or kill the spermatozoa." On pages 16–18 there is an extensive description of Sims's duck-bill speculum. There are no plates, but the work contains 142 relatively crude wood engravings. This was the only edition. (See also GS44.)

GY13. **THOMAS ADDIS EMMET** (1828–1919). *Vesico-vaginal fistula from parturition and other causes: with cases of recto-vaginal fistula.* 250pp. New York: William Wood, 1868.[G-M 6058]

One of the founders of modern gynecology, Emmet received his M.D. from Jefferson Medical College in 1850. He never held an academic post, but, after associating with James Marion Sims (1813–83), he became surgeon-in-chief at the New York State Woman's Hospital. Among his best-known contributions to medical literature include work on the treatment of dysmenorrhoea and sterility resulting from anteflexion of the uterus [G-M 6055], surgical repair of lacerations of the cervix [G-M 6059], vaginal cystotomy for chronic cystitis [G-M 6063], and a technique for perineorrhaphy [G-M 6078]. In his autobiography, *Incidents of my life, professional-literary-social with services in the cause of Ireland* (New York: G. P. Putnam's Sons, 1911), Emmet writes (page 231):

> In 1868 I published my first medical work on *Vesico-vaginal Fistula from Parturition and Other Causes*, and this work established my reputation as a surgeon. For this book I received my first recognition on being made a member of the Berlin Obstetrical Society, and shortly after I was elected a member of the Medical Society of Norway. Since that time I have been made a member of every society in the world to which I could have any claim, with the single exception of the Obstetrical Society of London . . . .

Emmet dedicated this work to Sims and the lady managers of the Woman's Hospital. He explains in the preface:

> The material presented to the profession in this form was collected with a view of furnishing, through the pages of the *American Journal of the Medical Sciences*, a simple record of interesting cases . . . . It was soon apparent, however, that this could not be sufficiently condensed, within the allotted space of a journal, to do justice to the subject . . . . I have endeavored to illustrate, in as concise a manner as possible, the various difficulties which I have met with in operating for these injuries . . . .

The eighteen chapters, which present a comprehensive and valuable account of the management of vesico-vaginal fistula based on Sims's techniques, include "Instruments necessary for the operation"; "Vesico-vaginal fistulae, with laceration of the cervix uteri"; "Fistulae involving the upper portion of the vagina"; "Fistulae confined to the upper portion of the base of the bladder"; "Formation of a new urethra by aid of plastic surgery"; and "Vesico and recto-vaginal fistulae not resulting from parturition." There are thirty-four rather rudimentary engravings but no plates. There was only one edition. James Pratt Marr describes Emmet's work in his *Pioneer surgeons of the Woman's Hospital* (Philadelphia: F. A. Davis, 1957, pages 84–85):

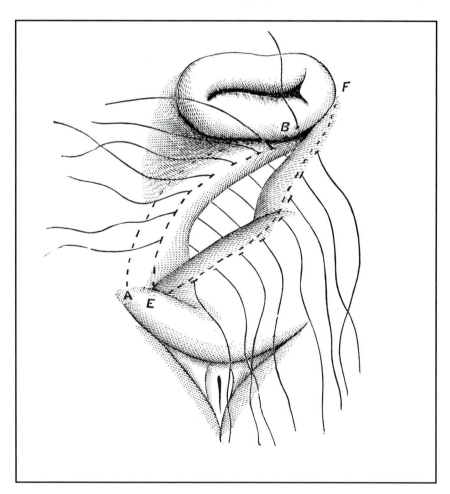

Fig. 106. (GY13) Case 34 from Emmet's monograph concerned a fistula involving the base of the bladder. This engraving on page 105 depicts the cicatrix and suture placement. Interestingly, the patient was three months pregnant when the operation was performed.

Emmet's volume gives a minutely detailed account of 273 patients suffering from vaginal fistula who had undergone operation prior to October 1867—a number which grew to 600 by the turn of the century .... It is interesting to note that of the 273 cases reported, five were considered inoperable—not because of the extent of injury but because the patient's excessive obesity made a proper exposure of the operating field impossible. Another patient was considered inoperable because a nervous irritability prevented her from assuming the knee-chest position for an adequate length of time. Quite possibly the use of anesthesia might have permitted her to be successfully treated but ether anesthesia was not given routinely at the Woman's Hospital until the late sixties. One group was discharged as inoperable because of "disorderly conduct." Emmet stated that more than 58 per cent of the vesico-vaginal fistula cases were poor immigrants from England, Scotland and Ireland. Usually within a year of their arrival they landed at the Woman's Hospital for reconstructive surgery.

Emmet was a renowned genealogist and Irish patriot, and based on these interests he wrote the following books: *The Emmet family with some incidents relating to Irish history and a biographical sketch of Prof. John Patten Emmet, M.D., and other members* (New York: private printing, 1898), the two-volume *Ireland under English rule, or a plea for the plaintiff* (New York: G. P. Putnam's Sons, 1903), and the two-volume *Memoir of Thomas Addis and Robert Emmet with their ancestors and immediate family* (New York: Emmet Press, 1915). (See also GY23.)

GY14. **THEODORE GAILLARD THOMAS** (1831–1903). *A practical treatise on the diseases of women*. 625pp. Philadelphia: Henry C. Lea, 1868. [G-M 6060]

Born on Edisto Island, Charleston, South Carolina, Thomas received his M.D. from the Medical College of his native state in 1852. After interning at Bellevue Hospital and studying in Paris and Dublin, he began practice in New York City. In 1863, Thomas was appointed professor of obstetrics and the diseases of women and children at the College of Physicians and Surgeons. Nine years later he became attending surgeon at the Women's Hospital. His most important work was the *Treatise*, considered the outstanding work on the subject in its day. He is also remembered for articles in medical journals on the first vaginal ovariotomy [G-M 6061], the use of gastro-elytrotomy as a substitute for cesarean section [G-M 6239], and a chapter on obstetrics and gynecology that he contributed to Edward Hammond Clarke's (1820–77) *A century of American medicine, 1776–1876* (Philadelphia: Henry C. Lea, 1876) [G-M 6586]. Having purposefully and methodically narrowed the field of his professional work in order to devote his entire time to gynecology, Thomas soon realized that the records of its progress were scattered through a mass of monographs, journals, and transactions of medical societies. For this reason, he was convinced of the need for a textbook to suit the student that would also serve as a reference book for the busy practitioner. The volume contains forty-five chapters and 219 illustrations. Among the surgical topics are "Rupture of the perineum" (chapter 5); "Fistulae of the female genital organs" (chapter 10); "Amputation

Fig. 107. (GY14) Thomas's work
had few original illustrations.
This original example, figure
125 on page 313, demonstrates
various degrees of retroversion
of the uterus.

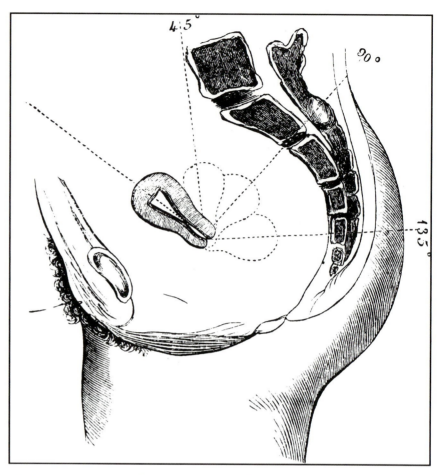

of the neck of the uterus" (chapter 40); and "Ovariotomy" (chapter 43).
James P. Marr writes in *Pioneer surgeons of the Woman's Hospital* (Philadelphia: F. A. Davis, 1957, pages 128–29):

> This work, the most complete and systematic treatise by an American
> author up to that time, preceded Emmet's textbook by 11 years. The
> text was translated into French, German, Italian, Spanish and Chinese
> and went through 6 editions and sold 60,000 copies, spreading Thomas'
> fame far and wide. Once when visiting a medical bookshop in Berlin,
> Thomas asked for some works on gynecology. The proprietor handed
> him a book which he declared not only the best in the shop, but the
> best of its kind ever published. Thomas found in his hand a translation
> of his own treatise. *A Practical Treatise* contains an excellent historical
> summary of gynecology from ancient times, which is unfortunately
> marred by a number of erroneous names and dates. The chapter on
> anatomy is ably written with special reference to the function of the
> perineal body and the necessity of restoring its integrity following even
> an incomplete rupture. Thomas states that in New York City it was a
> greater surgical catastrophe to rupture the perineum than to fracture a
> long bone.

Later editions were published in 1869, 1872, 1874, 1880, and 1891.
Thomas's other book is *Abortion and its treatment, from the standpoint of
practical experience* (New York: D. Appleton, 1890).

GY15. **REUBEN LUDLAM** (1831–99). *Lectures, clinical and didactic, on the diseases of women.* 112pp. Chicago: C. S. Halsey,1870.

Ludlam was professor of obstetrics and the diseases of women and children at Hahnemann Medical College of Chicago. He was president of the American Institute of Homeopathy in 1869. His *Lectures* was used in all the homeopathic colleges as the recognized authority on this subject. Ludlam writes in the preface: "The following lectures are the substance of those delivered by the author in the college and hospital in which he has served in the capacity of a teacher for many years . . . . " The first edition consisted of only 112 pages and was labeled "Part 1." Within two years, the book was enlarged to 612 pages and included thirty-four lectures covering a wide range of topics but with few illustrations. The second part was never separately published, but appeared within the second edition. This edition included an interesting chapter (No. 25) on the "Efficacy of uterine surgery versus uterine therapeutics." Gynecologic surgery is also discussed as the treatment for uterine fibroids. Other topics discussed include "Spinal irritation with amenorrhoea"; "Vomiting and convulsions"; and "Vaginismus." The work went through further editions in 1872, 1877, 1879, 1881, and 1888. Ludlum's other medical book is *A course of clinical lectures on diphtheria* (Chicago: C. S. Halsey, 1863).

GY16. **GEORGE HERBERT TAYLOR** (1821–96). *Diseases of women: their causes, prevention, and radical cure.* 318pp. Philadelphia: G. Maclean, 1871.

Taylor was best known for proselytizing the Swedish mechano-movement cure in America. *Diseases of Women* represents the first use of mechano-movement principles in the treatment of gynecologic problems. Taylor writes in the preface:

> Many excellent treatises on pelvic pathology and therapeutics are already before the medical profession and the public; yet there are principles involved in these subjects which no previous works discuss or even indicate. I am not aware of any treatise in which the causes even of the ordinary affections of the pelvic contents are distinctly pointed out, nor of any in which the complete cure of these affections is shown to depend on the removal of their causes. I know of no work which maintains the practicability of correcting the faulty position of the pelvic contents by strengthening their natural supports; none in which the possibility of removing pelvic hyperemia and its consequences by restoring the natural motions of the dominant parts are ever referred to, much less demonstrated . . . . Women are everywhere suffering from want of acquaintance with the physical laws of their being. No age or station is exempt. The need of the services of the physician is, to a large extent, due to inattention to and ignorance of principles easily understood and practiced. To point out these principles, and to show how simple, natural and eminently practical they are, has been my purpose . . . .

The twenty chapters include "The pelvic contents have no exceptional tendency to disease"; "Influence of ordinary exercises on the health of the pelvic contents"; "Instrumental support of the uterus"; "Methods of employing gravitation as an aid in restoring the position of the pelvic contents"; "Kneading the abdomen—combination of kneading, with muscular action and gravitation"; and "Morbid emotion—hysteria." A substantial glossary of medical terms appears at the end of the book. (See also GS123.)

GY17. **EDWIN NESBIT CHAPMAN** (1819–88). *Hysterology: a treatise, descriptive and clinical, on the diseases and the displacements of the uterus.* 504pp. New York: William Wood, 1872.

A graduate of Yale College in 1842 and of Jefferson Medical College in 1845, Chapman settled in Brooklyn immediately after graduation. He served as professor of obstetrics, diseases of women and children and clinical midwifery at Long Island College Hospital until 1868, when he resigned his duties at the dispensary and began private practice. Chapman defines the subject of this work in the preface:

> The body of the work is a reproduction of my lectures . . . being designed for the first as well as the second course students . . . . I have ventured to coin a new word, hysterology, as a more distinctive title of a monograph on uterine disease than gynecology, that, embracing all the diseases peculiar to the female, is too broad in its signification. The words vaginocele and rectocele are of a hybrid character, and would, except for the want of better and the common employment of a similar one, vaginismus, be quite inexcusable . . . .

The twelve chapters include a wealth of information plus numerous wood engravings. There was only one edition. Chapman's other medical

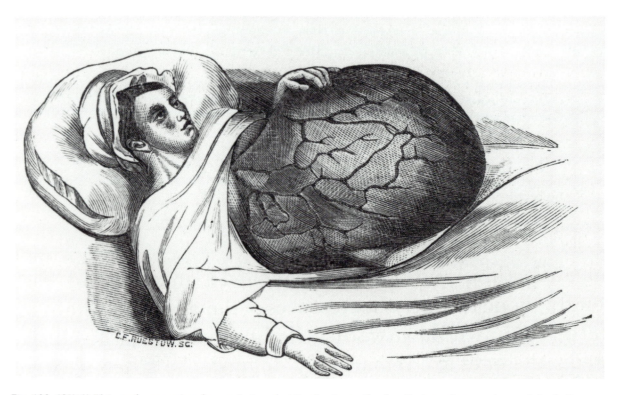

Fig. 108. (GY18) This crude engraving demonstrates what Peaslee terms the fourth stage of an ovarian cyst, including enlarged veins on the abdomen (figure 31 on page 111).

book is *Antagonism of alcohol and diphtheria* (Brooklyn: Union-Argus Steam Printing Establishment, 1878).

GY18. EDMUND RANDOLPH PEASLEE (1814–78) *Ovarian tumors; their pathology, diagnosis, and treatment, especially by ovariotomy.* 551pp. New York: D. Appleton, 1872.

One of the most illustrious men in American medicine, Peaslee matriculated at Dartmouth College and received his M.D. from Yale in 1840. He soon became associated with Dartmouth Medical College, an affiliation which lasted most of his life as a lecturer on various medical subjects. Always active in organized medicine, Peaslee was president of the American Gynecological Society in 1877.

This book was written while Peaslee was professor of gynecology at Dartmouth (the first professorship of gynecology at an accredited medical school in the United States) and simultaneously attending surgeon at the Woman's Hospital in New York. *Ovarian tumors* was considered his crowning literary achievement. It was dedicated to Ephraim McDowell (1771–1830), "the father of ovariotomy," and to Thomas Spencer Wells (1818–97), "the greatest of ovariotomists." It is an interesting volume which combines painstaking historical research, good diagnostic teaching, a prudent and practical guide to medical and surgical treatment, and a sound discussion of pathology. Peaslee absolutely establishes the claim of McDowell to be the first ovariotomist and likewise that the first successful ovariotomy took place in America. There is an exhaustive bibliography of works related to ovariotomy on pages vii-xv. The preface describes the scope of the book:

> The following work was undertaken from a conviction that a practical treatise, in the English language, upon the subjects of which it treats, is greatly needed. While several writers have published their individual experience, more or less extensive, as ovariotomists, no work has appeared of broader scope, which proposes to cover the whole ground, so far as is practicable, within the limits of a single volume . . . .

There are fifty-six illustrations but no plates. The eighteen chapters are divided into two parts: "Normal anatomy, pathology and treatment of ovarian tumors—excepting by ovariotomy" and "Ovariotomy—its history, statistics, indications, prognosis, operative methods, and after-treatment." This was the only edition. Peaslee's other book is *Human histology in its relation to descriptive anatomy, physiology, and pathology* (Philadelphia: Blanchard & Lea, 1857).

GY19. DAVID HAYES AGNEW (1818–92). *Lacerations of the female perineum; and vesico-vaginal fistula; their history and treatment.* 141pp. Philadelphia: Lindsay & Blakiston, 1873.

Agnew was professor of surgery at the University of Pennsylvania when this volume was published. The contents of the work had already appeared in the *Pennsylvania Hospital reports* in 1865 and the *Medical and surgical reporter* in 1867. Because Agnew constantly received requests for copies of these papers, he decided to collate them in book form so they could be widely distributed. There are numerous illustrations but no plates. The book is difficult reading because it lacks a table of contents and a detailed index. (See also GS88.)

GY20. **WASHINGTON LEMUEL ATLEE** (1808–78) *General and differential diagnosis of ovarian tumors, with specific references to the operation of ovariotomy; and occasional pathological and therapeutical considerations.* 482pp. Philadelphia: J. B. Lippincott, 1873.

Atlee, together with his brother John Light Atlee (1799–1885), established the operation for ovariotomy in the United States. Active in medical organization at the county, state, and national levels, he was a founding member of the American Gynecological Society, and vice-president of the American Medical Association (1875). Atlee graduated from Jefferson Medical College in 1829 and practiced medicine in Pennsylvania throughout his life. His major contributions to medical literature include a table of all known operations of ovariotomy from 1701 to 1851 [G-M 6038], a study of the surgical removal of uterine fibroids for which he was awarded a prize by a medical society [G-M 6039], and the description of an operation for vesico-vaginal fistula [G-M 6047]. John Light Atlee performed the first successful double oophorectomy [G-M 6034]. Atlee writes in the preface to *Ovarian tumors*:

> In offering this volume to the members of the medical profession, the author is merely responding to a call long and repeatedly made by numerous friends throughout the United States . . . . The book is a mere transcript of his own clinical experience, recorded at the moment of examination, and comprises the result of observations continuously pursued since the year 1843 . . . .

The book consists of two sections: "General diagnosis of ovarian tumors" and "Differential diagnosis." The work discusss 149 case histories, and Atlee points out that

> . . . the cases frequently reveal errors committed by the author. He has purposely drawn from his early experience, at a time when he was most liable to err, in order to illustrate step by step the progressive advancement of knowledge in the diagnosis of abdominal tumors, and to show that the observer in this, as in other forms of disease, must necessarily be educated by repeated observations before he can be qualified as an expert . . . . Mistakes teach most valuable lessons, and, when discovered, are not likely to be repeated. Hence, in medicine, they should be recorded for the benefit both of science and of humanity . . . .

There are thirty-nine illustrations but no plates. This is Atlee's only medical book, and was the only edition.

GY21. **ALEXANDER JOHNSTON CHALMERS SKENE** (1837–1900). *Diseases of the bladder and urethra in women.* 374pp. New York: William Wood, 1878.

Skene was professor of the diseases of women at Long Island College Hospital when this volume was published. A pioneer gynecologist, he was a founding member of the American Gynecological Society. He was also associate editor of the *Archives of medicine, The American medical digest*, and the *New York gynecological and obstetrical journal*. He is best remembered for his description of the urethral glands [G-M 1225].

Skene's *Diseases* was " . . . originally intended for use in the college class room, and designed to embody only those things which the student and general practitioner require to know on the subject, in order to meet the demands of everyday practice." Skene wrote the work while engaged in practice because he " . . . became impressed with the fact that although numerous valuable publications existed on vesico-vaginal fistula, medical literature, in the English language at least, contained no systematic work on the many other diseases and functional anomalies of the bladder and urethra . . . . " Among the eight lectures in the book are "Anatomy of the bladder and urethra"; "Functional and organic diseases of the bladder"; "Cystitis"; "Neoplasms, cysts, tubercle, and carcinoma of the bladder"; "Diseases of the female urethra"; and "Dilatations and dislocations of the urethra." There are no plates and few illustrations. Lectures 7 and 8 contain the earliest descriptions of Skene's glands, their pathological conditions, and treatment. This was the only edition. Among Skene's other books are *Education and culture as related to the health and diseases of women* (Detroit: G. S. Davis, 1889). (See also GS187, GY33, and GY51.)

GY22. **ANSON L. CLARK** (?–?): *A treatise on the medical and surgical diseases of women.* 410pp. Chicago: Jansen & McClurg, 1879.

An eclectic physician, Clark was professor of obstetrics and diseases of women and of clinical gynecology at Bennett Medical College in Chicago. An associate editor of the *Chicago medical times*, he notes in the preface:

> Custom demands that a book should be announced by a preface. This is often made the vehicle by which the author announces to his readers his excuses for this public appearance. Having no excuses to offer, it may be proper to here state some of the reasons which have led to the production of this volume . . . . In these pages I have endeavored to as briefly and succinctly as possible state the known points of value in connection with each subject treated, avoiding upon the one hand a prolixity and extenuation of detail through which the busy practitioner has no time to follow, and upon the other hand, a brevity which would leave the matter incomplete. Having for nearly a score of years been so busily engaged in practice, that I have scarcely known a day of recreation, I have learned to appreciate the value of time.

The twenty-five chapters discuss such topics as "Rupture of the perineum"; "Genital fistulae"; "Metritis"; "Cancer of the uterus"; "Pelvic and ovarian tumors"; "Sterility"; "Pelvic cellulitis"; "Nervous disease"; and "Dyspareunia." Chapter 25 is interesting because it uses only metric weights and measures. Clark wrote no other medical books and his *Treatise* had only one edition.

GY23. **THOMAS ADDIS EMMET** (1828–1919). *The principles and practice of gynaecology.* 855pp. Philadelphia: Henry C. Lea, 1879.

Emmet was surgeon at the Woman's Hospital of New York when he published this most important textbook. Described as the first thoroughly scientific, comprehensive book on this subject in English, it was a condensed record of Emmet's large clinical practice. The work was dedicated to Emmet's father, John Patten Emmet (?–1842), professor of chemistry at the University of Virginia. Emmet writes in the preface:

> This work is essentially a clinical digest. It includes the results of my individual experience, and aims to represent the actual state of gynae-cological science and art . . . . In attempting to ascertain and formulate the laws which apply to diseases, and to analyze the results of treatment, I have compressed numerous histories and facts into a number of statistical tables, which present, in brief space, information that hundreds of pages would scarcely have sufficed to contain in detail. Their parallel, it is believed, is not to be found in the whole range of gynaecological literature . . . . For two continuous years they kept me occupied in hours not required for professional work, and to the minutest detail they have been prepared by myself, for I felt that their value rested on their accuracy, which I could not have vouched for if their compilation had been committed to others . . . .

The forty-three chapters include discussions of "Surgical instruments and appliances" (chapter 3); "Surgical treatment of fibrous growths of the uterus" (chapter 29); "Vesico- and recto-vaginal fistula" (chapter 31); "Conditions complicating the operation of ovariotomy" (chapter 41); and "General details in ovariotomy and abdominal ovariotomy" (chapters 42 and 43). The book contains sixty-two statistical tables which are scattered throughout the text. There are 130 illustrations but no plates. Subsequent editions were published in 1880 and 1884. (See also GY13.)

GY24. **WILLIAM GOODELL** (1829–94). *Lessons in gynecology.* 1,380pp. Philadelphia: D. G. Brinton, 1879.

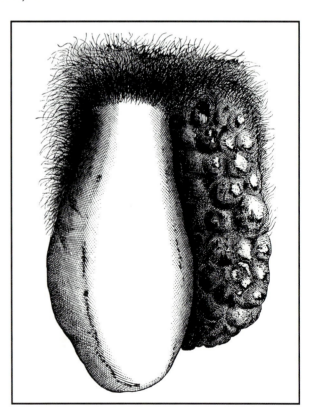

Fig. 109. (GY23) In this graphic wood engraving, figure 102 on page 593, Emmet demonstrates elephantiasis of the labium and hypertrophied clitoris in a 25-year-old patient.

Born on the island of Malta to missionary parents, Goodell graduated from Jefferson Medical College in 1854. In 1865, he was named physician-in-charge of the Preston Retreat, a gynecologic hospital in Philadelphia. In 1874, Goodell was appointed professor of clinical gynecology at the University of Pennsylvania. *Lessons* was his only book. He notes in his preface that "this book is not a treatise upon the diseases of women, but mainly the outcome of clinical and of didactic lectures delivered to the advanced students of the Medical Department of the University of Pennsylvania . . . . " There are twenty-nine lessons, including "Fistulae of the female genital organs"; "Ovariotomy by abdominal section"; "Vaginal ovariotomy"; and "The relation which faulty closet-accomodations (privies, earth-closets) bear to the diseases of women." There are eighty illustrations. Further editions were published in 1880, 1887, and a reprint of the third edition in 1890.

GY25. **WILLIAM BIDDLE ATKINSON** (1832–1909). *The therapeutics of gynecology and obstetrics, comprising the medical, dietetic, and hygienic treatment of diseases of women, as set forth by distinguished contemporary specialists.* 365pp. Philadelphia: D. G. Brinton, 1880.

Atkinson was one of American medicine's most famous biographers. He practiced obstetrics and gynecology in Philadelphia, and at the time he wrote the *Therapeutics* was lecturer on diseases of children at Jefferson Medical College and a physician in the department of obstetrics and diseases of women at Howard Hospital. An 1853 graduate of Jefferson, Atkinson later served as editor of the *Transactions of the American Medical Association* while he was permanent secretary of that organization. He notes in the preface:

> In compliance with the wish of the publisher, the editor of the present volume has carefully reviewed the material prepared for it and has added extensively from recent treatises, monographs, and journals . . . . In accordance with the plan preferred by the publisher, precise directions in the plans of treatment have been preserved, and the exact formulae presented whenever these could be obtained . . . . It has been deemed best to preface each chapter with a "Synopsis of diagnostic points," setting forth, in brief but clear forms, the distinctive signs and symptoms between the diseases considered in the chapter . . . .

Part 1, "Gynecological therapeutics," consists of three chapters: "Diseases of the ovaries, disorders of menstruation, and general diseases"; "Diseases of the uterus and its annexes"; and "Diseases of the vagina, urethra, and bladder." Part 2, "Obstetrical therapeutics," also has three chapters: "Disorders of pregnancy"; "Complications, disorders and sequelae of parturition"; and "Diseases of the mammary glands and of lactation." There are few illustrations. The volume was meant to serve as a companion piece to George H. Napheys's *Surgical therapeutics and medical therapeutics* (GS90). A second edition was published in 1881. Among Atkinson's other medical books are *Hints in the obstetric procedure* (Philadelphia: Collins, 1875) and *The physicians and surgeons of the United States* (Philadelphia: Charles Robson, 1878).

GY26. **MORTON MONROE EATON** (1839–89). *A treatise on the medical and surgical diseases of women, with their homeopathic treatment.* 782pp. New York: Boericke & Tafel, 1880.

Eaton was a homeopathic physician practicing in Cincinnati who specialized in obstetrics and gynecology. The preface gives his reasons for writing this text:

> First, because I have been for several years repeatedly urged to do so by prominent homeopathic physicians . . . . Secondly, because homeopathic colleges have been obliged to recommend, and homeopathic physicians and students have been obliged to provide themselves with, allopathic works upon these diseases; thereby giving a certain amount of sanction to the treatment therein advocated . . . . Thirdly, because it seems time that homeopathists should have complete textbooks on all branches of medical education . . . . Fourthly, because the homeopathic physicians of Illinois and Ohio . . . have honored me with their confidence, and shown their respect by giving me prominence in regard to these diseases, and because I have had a large experience in their treatment for over twenty years, in hospital and private practice . . . .

There are seventy chapters, including "Ovariotomy" (chapter 25); "Femoral hernia, inguinal hernia, labial hernia, vaginal hernia, and hydrocele" (chapter 34); "Fistulae" (chapter 46); "Tumors of the breast, cancer, and amputations of the breast" (chapter 61); and "Extirpation of the uterus—ablation of the uterus, hysterotomy, etc." (chapter 66). There are thirty-one plates with over 250 illustrations. This was the only edition. Among Eaton's other books are *Domestic practices for parents and nurses* (Cincinnati: M. M. Eaton, Jr., 1882).

GY27. **PAUL FORTUNATUS MUNDE** (1846–1902). *Minor surgical gynecology: a manual of uterine diagnosis and the lesser technicalities of a gynecological practice.* 381pp. New York: William Wood, 1880.

Born in Dresden, Germany, Munde came to the United States at an early age and graduated from Harvard Medical School in 1866. After spending several years of study in Europe, he returned to America and in 1874 assumed editorial responsibility for the *American journal of obstetrics*. One of the founding members of the American Gynecological Society, he eventually served as its president. When this volume was written, Munde was professor of gynecology at Dartmouth Medical College and physician for diseases of women in the Out-Door Department of Mt. Sinai Hospital in New York. This book is dedicated to Fordyce Barker (1818–91). Munde describes his approach in the preface:

> It is not a detailed account of larger operations which the general practitioner needs—these he can study up for special cases, when such occur to him, or he will probably transfer them to some specialist of whom there is nowadays no lack—but a knowledge of all the minute technicalities of local examination, digital and instrumental, and of the various manipulations and minor operations which he is liable to meet with every day. This information I have endeavored to supply in this book . . . . This work has thus almost involuntarily assumed the charac-

ter of a text-book . . . all references to literature and historical descriptions have, as a rule, been omitted . . . .

Part 1 discusses gynecologic examination, including instruments and couches. Part 2 consists of fifteen chapters and discusses minor gynecological manipulations and applications. There are 300 illustrations but no plates. The book is volume 28 in Wood's Library of Standard Medical Authors. A second edition was published in 1885. Among Munde's other books are *The diagnosis and treatment of obstetric cases by external (abdominal) examination and manipulation* (New York: William Wood, 1880) and *A sketch of the management of pregnancy, parturition and the puerperal state, normal and abnormal* (Detroit: G. S. Davis, 1887). (See also GY44.)

GY28. **SAMUEL JAMES DONALDSON** (?–?). *Contributions to practical gynecology. Part I. Practical observations upon uterine deflexions. Part II. Practical observations upon dysmenorrhoea.* 134pp. New York: Trows, 1882.

Donaldson was a surgeon in the gynecological wards at Ward's Island Hospital in New York. He spent most of his professional life in

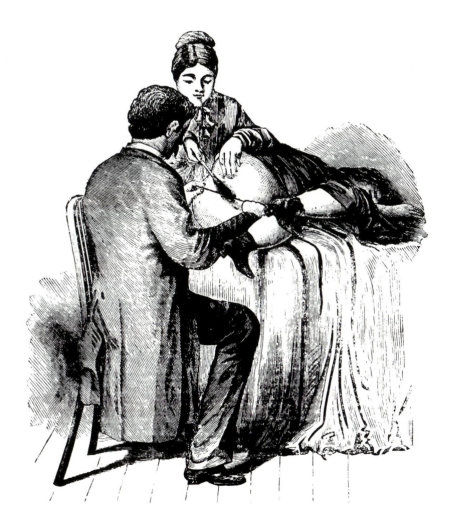

Fig. 110. (GY27) This illustration (number 53, page 75) shows the position of patient, nurse, and physician in examination using Sims's speculum.

New York. This book presents the substance of two essays which he read before the New York Medico-Chirurgical Society in April and May 1882. Donaldson never intended to publish the *Contributions*, but was encouraged to do so by "my professional brethren." He writes in the preface that "My chief desire has been to deal in as concise a manner as possible with fundamental practicalities only, and I have therefore avoided all obscure and elaborate speculation . . . . " There is no table of contents, making the volume difficult to read.

GY29. **HENRY JACQUES GARRIGUES** (1831–1913). *Diagnosis of ovarian cysts by means of the examination of their contents.* 112pp. New York: William Wood, 1882.

Garrigues was born in Copenhagen and graduated from that city's medical school in 1869, but eventually settled in New York. He is generally considered to have introduced antiseptic obstetrics in America. Garrigues was named obstetric surgeon at the Maternity Hospital and physician in the gynecologic department of the German Dispensary. He became a fellow of the American Gynecological Society in 1877 and served as vice-president in 1897. This was his first book, and it appeared in only one edition. It consists of seven chapters, including "Ovarian cysts"; "Non-ovarian cysts"; "Peritoneal fluids"; and "Tapping". There are few illustrations. Among his other books are *Practical guide in antiseptic midwifery in hospital and private practice* (Detroit: G. S. Davis, 1886), *A textbook of the science and art of obstetrics* (Philadelphia: J. B. Lippincott, 1902), and *Gynecology, medical and surgical* (Philadelphia: J. B. Lippincott, 1905). (See also GY46.)

GY30. **CHARLES HENRY MAY** (1861–1943). *Manual of the diseases of women, being a concise and systematic exposition of the theory and practice of gynaecology.* 357pp. Philadelphia: Lea Brothers, 1885.

May was known primarily as an ophthalmologist, but he was quite interested in gynecologic surgery early in his career. He had just completed a term as house physician at Mt. Sinai Hospital when this volume was published. May later became assistant to the chair of ophthalmology at the New York Polyclinic. This work is notable because he wrhen he was only twenty-three years old. He notes in the preface:

> . . . the author has aimed to give, in as concise a manner as possible, an exposition of the theories and practice of the diseases peculiar to women, which shall represent the accepted views in this modern science. These have been condensed, classified, and arranged so as to make the book a short and systematic treatise . . . . The author claims no originality for any of the statements embodied in the volume; it is chiefly a compilation . . . . Written at the request of the author's quiz classes, it is intended to aid the student, who after having carefully perused larger works, desires to review the subject; and it may also be useful to the practitioner who wishes to refresh his memory rapidly, but has not the time to consult larger works . . . .

The thirteen chapters include "Affections of the vulva"; "Perineal body"; "Vagina"; "Uterus"; "Fallopian tubes"; "Ovaries"; "Pelvic connective tissue"; "Disorders of menstruation"; and "Disorders of the reproductive

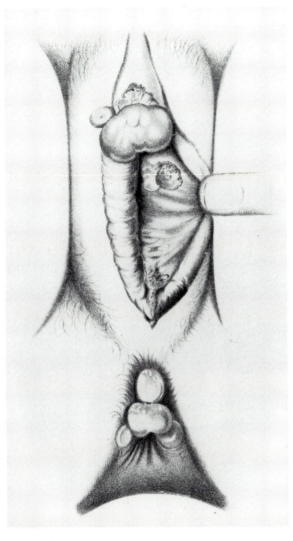

Fig. 111. (GY31) Mann demonstrates lupus hypertrophicus of what he terms fibroma diffusum. Originally thought of as a venereal disease, its true etiology is a form of cutaneous tuberculosis. The lithographers for this color plate (number 1, page 526 in volume 2) were T. Sinclair and Sons of Philadelphia.

function." The book was revised by Leonard Rau, and this version appeared as a second edition in 1890. Among May's other books are *An index of materia medica; with prescription writing, including practical exercises* (New York: William Wood, 1887) and *Manual of the diseases of the eye* (New York: William Wood, 1900).

GY31. **MATTHEW DARBYSHIRE MANN** (1845–1921). *A system of gynecology by American authors.* 2 vols., 789pp. and 1,180pp. Philadelphia: Lea Brothers, 1887-88.

The first American gynecologic textbook to be written by more than one author, the *System of gynecology* crystallized and successfully promulgated many newer techniques. Mann graduated from Yale in 1867 and from the College of Physicians and Surgeons of New York in 1871. From 1882 to 1910 he served as professor of obstetrics and gynecology at the University of Buffalo. A pioneer gynecologist, Mann was president of the American Gynecological Society in 1895. Because of his esteem in Buffalo medical circles, Mann served as chief surgeon in charge of William McKinley (1843–1901) following the assassination attempt on

Fig. 112. (GY33) Inflammation
of Skene's glands is depicted in
the top figure of this chromolithograph, figure 4 on page
886. The bottom figure depicts
an operation for prolapsus of
the bladder and urethra. R. L.
Dickinson made the original
drawings.

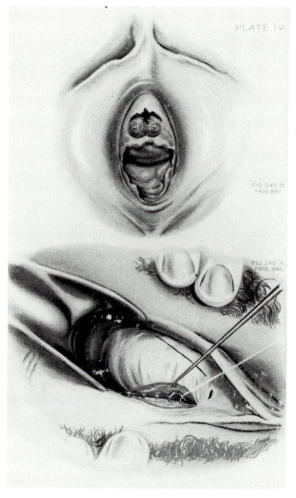

the president in 1901. Volume 1 of the work contains three color plates
and 201 engravings on wood. Among the contributors and their chapters were Edward W. Jenks (1833–1903), "Historical sketch of American
gynecology"; Henry J. Garrigues (1831–1913), "Development and
malformations of the female genitals"; Emilius C. Dudley (1850–1928),
"General considerations of gynecological surgery"; Alexander J. C. Skene
(1837–1900), "General therapeutics"; and Alphonso D. Rockwell (1840–
1908), "Electricity in gynecology." Volume 2 contains four color plates
and 361 wood engravings. Among the contributors to this volume were
T. Gaillard Thomas (1831–1903), "Extra-uterine gestation"; Samuel W.
Gross (1837–1889), "Tumors of the breast"; Roswell Park (1852–1914),
"Diseases of the breast other than tumors"; William T. Lusk (1838–1907),
"Malignant diseases of the uterus"; Howard A. Kelly (1858–1943),
"Injuries and lacerations of the perineum and pelvic floor"; and William
Goodell (1829–1894), "Treatment of ovarian and of extra-ovarian
tumors." The work appeared in only one edition. Mann's other book is
*A manual of prescription writing with a full explanation of the methods of
correctly writing prescriptions* (Philadelphia: G. P. Putnam's Sons, 1878).

GY32. **ALLEN CORSON COWPERTHWAITE** (1848–?). *A textbook of gynecology*. 533pp. Chicago: Gross & Delbridge, 1888.

A homeopathic physician, Cowperthwaite served as professor of materia medica and diseases of women in the Homeopathic Medical Department of the State University of Iowa. An 1869 graduate of Hahnemann Medical College in Philadelphia, Cowperthwaite was an influential figure in American homeopathy, having served as president of the American Institute of Homeopathy. He writes in the preface:

> During the past eleven years, I have seriously felt the need of a textbook for students that would be systematic in its arrangement, concise in its details, and cover the entire list of diseases comprehended by the term "gynecology," together with their homeopathic therapeutics. After long waiting in the hope that some one better qualified would assume the unenviable task of preparing such a work, I have, at the earnest solicitation of students and professional friends, taken it upon myself to make the attempt, and the present volume is the result of my labors. That I have presented nothing strikingly new or original is probably true, but I have endeavored to collate only from recognized authorities, and to include the very latest that is known regarding the pathology and treatment of gynecological diseases . . . .

The work contains sixty-four chapters, including six (Nos. 59–64) on breast diseases. Ovariotomy is discussed in chapter 45. The book has three appendices, including one on dry heat in the treatment of uterine disease (pages 520–22). There was only one edition. Among Cowperthwaite's other books are *Insanity in its medico-legal relations* (Philadelphia: J. M. Stoddart, 1876), *An elementary text-book of the materia medica* (Chicago: Duncan Brothers, 1880), and *A textbook on the practice of medicine* (Chicago: Halsey Brothers, 1901).

GY33. **ALEXANDER JOHNSTON CHALMERS SKENE** (1837–1900). *Treatise on the diseases of women*. 966pp. New York: D. Appleton, 1888.

Skene was a founder of the International Congress of Gynecology and Obstetrics and was honorary president at the Geneva Congress in 1896. He was professor of gynecology at Long Island College Hospital. The *Treatise* was his most important book and is dedicated to Thomas Keith (1827–95). Skene describes the plans of the work in his preface:

> This book was written for the purpose of bringing together the fully matured and essential facts in the science and art of gynecology, so arranged as to meet the requirements of the student of medicine, and be convenient to the practitioner for reference. In the plan adopted, the diseases peculiar to women are, as far as possible, divided into three classes. The first class comprises those which occur between birth and puberty; the second, those between puberty and the menopause; and the third, those which come after the menopause . . . .

The table of contents includes fifty-one chapters on a wide variety of topics. The last chapter (pages 929–50) provides an interesting commentary on the relation of insanity in women to gynecologic diseases. The book contains 251 engravings and nine chromolithographs. Further editions were published in 1893 and 1898. (See also GS187, GY21, and GY51.)

GY34. **GEORGE RINALDO SOUTHWICK** (1859–1930). *A practical manual of gynaecology.* 408pp. Boston: Otis Clapp & Sons, 1888.

At the time of this manual's publication Southwick was assistant professor of obstetrics at Boston University School of Medicine. The preface states:

> The author believes that uterine diseases are largely due to faults either of nutrition or of vascular or nervous supply, and, like other diseases, can be effectually and permanently cured by internal medication. In his practice and experience in teaching he has felt the need of a practical manual of gynaecology in which the general practitioner and student could readily find all the details of minor surgical gynaecology, diagnosis, local treatment, and therapeutics of uterine diseases. This book has been designed, therefore, as a safe and practical guide for these classes rather than for the specialist . . . .

The topics of the twenty-seven chapters include "Minor surgical gynaecology and the principles of local treatment"; "Malignant diseases of the sexual organs"; and "Tumors of the ovaries and broad ligaments." The book contains numerous figures and an extensive index (pages 401-08). A second edition was published in 1890. Among Southwick's other books are *A domestic handbook of the diseases of women and of midwifery* (Boston: Hygienic Publications, 1892).

GY35. **FRANCIS HENRY DAVENPORT** (1851–?). *Diseases of women: a manual of non-surgical gynecology.* 317pp. Philadelphia: Lea Brothers, 1889.

Davenport was assistant in gynecology at Harvard Medical School when he published this book. In writing it, Davenport notes in the preface that he had

> . . . two main objects: in the first place, to give the student clearly, but with considerable detail, the elementary principles of the methods of examination, and the simple forms of treatment of the most common diseases of the pelvic organs; and, in the second place, to help the busy general practitioner to understand and treat the gynecological cases which he meets with in the course of his everyday practice . . . . All surgical gynecology, except such simple procedures as demand no special skill, has been omitted, and the very rare affections which even the specialist seldom sees have also not been considered . . . .

There are fourteen chapters, including "Method of examination"; "Amenorrhoea"; "Scanty menstruation"; "Menorrhagia"; "Dysmenorrhoea"; "Displacements of the uterus"; "Chronic inflammatory conditions of the uterus"; "Common affections of the vulva and vagina"; "Tents, and their uses"; "Metrorrhagia"; "Diseases of the ovaries and tubes"; "Pelvic peritonitis and pelvic cellulitis"; and "Necessary instruments and appliances." There were numerous illustrations but no plates. Later editions appeared in 1892, 1898, and 1902.

GY35.1. **BENJAMIN FRANKLIN WEAVER** (1839–?). *Woman's guide to health: a treatise on the diseases of the female genital organs.* 114pp. Bucyrus, Ohio: private printing, 1889.

Weaver was a little-known general practitioner who lived in Ohio. This scarce monograph deals with medical gynecology and contains little information about operative procedures. Weaver also wrote numerous pamphlets describing ways that laypeople could use to make self-diagnoses of ordinary health problems. These pamphlets are summed up in his other book-length work, *The lightning doctor; a self diagnostician and practical doctor book for private families, students and physicians* (Akron: Saalfield Publishing, 1905).

GY36. **EDWIN BRADFORD CRAGIN** (1859–1918). *Essentials of gynaecology.* 192pp. Philadelphia: W. B. Saunders, 1890.

Cragin was one of New York's most respected gynecologists. He served as professor of gynecology and obstetrics at the College of Physicians and Surgeons from 1899 until his death. A graduate of Yale in 1882, he received his M.D. from the College of Physicians and Surgeons in New York in 1886. At the time this work was published, he was attending gynecologist at the Roosevelt Hospital. This volume is the tenth in Saunders's Question-Compends Series. It was available in cloth for $1.00 and interleaved for taking notes for $1.25. Cragin was frequently criticized for turning out so little scientific work during his professional life, although he did write a textbook on obstetrics. He writes in the preface to the *Essentials*, "No one appreciates more fully than the author the inadequacy of this little work for a thorough study of gynaecology. This has not been the aim. He only hopes that as a means of review and as a summary of the results of more extensive reading, the student may find the work of some value . . . . " The entire book is arranged in the form of questions and answers. There is an extensive table of contents. Fifty-eight illustrations are included, but no plates. Further editions were published in 1891, 1893, 1897, 1901, 1905, and 1907.

GY37. **ANDREW JACKSON HOWE** (1825–92). *Operative gynaecology.* 336pp. Cincinnati: Robert Clarke, 1890.

Howe was professor of surgery at the Eclectic Medical Institute in Cincinnati when this volume was published. There are fifteen sections: "Female genital organs"; "Diagnostics, antiseptics, and anaesthesia"; "Gynaecological apparatus"; "Uses of the uterine sound and vaginal speculum"; "Diseases of the external genitalia"; "Menstruation"; "Uterine diseases"; "Uterine displacements"; "Tumors of the uterus"; "Hysterectomy"; "Abdominotomy"; "Urinary diseases of the female"; "Rupture of the perinaeum"; "Hermaphroditism"; and "Treatment of puerperal mammae." In the preface, Howe makes several interesting comments about Listerism:

> I have not spoken in the highest terms of Listerism, from the fact that the scheme, as a whole, is not worthy the commendations that have been bestowed upon it. While it was deemed, at first, as the *sine qua non* of abdominal surgery, the earliest blows carbolic spray received were at the hands of the most skillful ovariotomists. It was found that the potent antiseptics were irritating and poisonous, so that less favorable results were attained than when no antiseptics were utilized. Cleanliness is the best aseptic . . . .

Pages 328–36 contain an extensive index. This was Howe's last major work and was published in only one edition. (See also GS84, OR25, and OP22.)

GY38. **EGBERT HENRY GRANDIN** (1855–?) and **JOSEPHUS H. GUNNING** (?–?). *Practical treatise on electricity in gynaecology.* 171pp. New York: William Wood, 1891.

At the time this monograph was written, Grandin was an obstetric surgeon at the New York Maternity Hospital and chairman of the section on obstetrics and gynecology of the New York Academy of Medicine. Gunning was an instructor in electro-therapeutics at the New York Post-Graduate Medical School and Hospital. This illustrated work consists of only six chapters: "General considerations and descriptions of apparatus"; "Routine uses of electricity"; "Electrolysis"; "Static, Franklinic, or frictional electricity"; "The treatment of malignant growths by the galvano-cautery"; and "Electricity in obstetrics." The use of electricity in all phases of American medicine was explored during the 1880s and 1890s. Among the major researchers was Alphonso David Rockwell (1840–1908), who wrote *The medical and surgical uses of electricity* (New York: William Wood, 1896); this book served as the preeminent text in this field. During the same period the American Electro-Therapeutic Association was formed and had its first annual meeting September 24–26, 1891, in Philadelphia. Grandin and Gunning note in the preface that their aim was

> . . . to present, as far as possible, an unbiased estimate of the value of electricity in the treatment of the diseases peculiar to women. The agent is considered, not from the standpoint of a specific, but as a valuable adjuvant to routine therapeutic methods. Whatever positive assertion may be found in the work is the outcome of ample and prolonged study and experience . . . .

It is of interest that the authors thank William J. Morton (1846–1920) for his help in explaining the use of static induced current (GS172).

GY38.1. **HENRY MORRIS** (?–?): *A compend of gynaecology.* 178pp. Philadelphia: P. Blakiston & Son, 1891.

This volume is the seventh in Blakiston's Quiz-Compends Series. It was available in cloth for $1.00 or interleaved for taking notes for $1.25. It contains forty-five illustrations. Morris had previously served as a demonstrator of obstetrics and diseases of women and children at Jefferson Medical College. He writes in the preface:

> This little book is written to redeem a promise, too long delayed in its fulfillment, which was made by the author to his students and to the publishers some years ago . . . and consists to a great extent of the course of instruction which he gave . . . He has endeavored to make the portion of the work which deals with "gynaecological examinations" as practical as possible, in the hope that it may prove useful to the beginner, and to the physician who from want of constant practice in gynaecology, may, when called upon to make an examination, be at a loss as to the best methods of procedure, or puzzled as to the significance

of what is found. The latter portion of the book is intended as an epitome of the diseases of women rather than a treatise on the subject, and it is hoped may be of use to the student . . . .

Among the chapters are "Diseases of the external genitalia, internal genitalia, and uterus"; "Uterine neoplasms"; "Lacerations of the cervix"; "Diseases of the oviducts and ovaries"; and "Diseases of the pelvic peritoneum and connective tissue." There was only one edition.

GY39. **G. W. BRATENAHL** (?–?) and **SINCLAIR TOUSEY** (1864–?). *Gynecology*. 221pp. Philadelphia: Lea Brothers, 1892.

Part of Lea's Student Quiz Series, this volume was available for $1.00. Bratenahl was an assistant in gynecology at the Vanderbilt Clinic in New York, while Tousey was assistant surgeon in the outpatient department of Roosevelt Hospital. The book is arranged in the form of questions and answers and contains seventeen chapters. Among them are "The perineal body and pelvic floor"; "Neoplasms of the uterus"; "Diseases of the ovaries"; "Extra-uterine pregnancy"; "Diseases of the pelvic peritoneum and fascia"; and "Electricity in gynecology." This was the only edition. Tousey's other book is *Medical electricity and röntgen rays with chapters on phototherapy and radium* (Philadelphia: W. B. Saunders, 1910).

GY40. **AUGUSTIN H. GOELET** (1854–1910). *The electro-therapeutics of gynaecology*. 3 vols. Detroit: G. S. Davis, 1892.

Goelet was one of the earliest to experiment with the use of electricity in medicine. He was vice-president of the American Electro-Therapeutic Association and editor of the *Archives of gynaecology, obstetrics and paediatrics* when this work was published. Goelet maintained a practice in New York, where most of his research was performed. The first volume deals with electro-physics and electro-physiology. Its five chapters are "Electro-physics"; "Galvanic current"; "Faradic current"; "Static electricity and its currents"; and "Apparatus." The second volume covers electro-therapeutics. Goelet makes note of his research in the preface:

> The necessity for a practical guide for the application of electricity to gynaecology, according to the modern and most approved methods of Apostoli and his followers, was so forcibly urged upon me by many who have read my various contributions to the journals that I was persuaded to undertake the task, the outcome of which is the present work . . . . It has been my aim to simplify the electro-physics so that it can be understood by anyone, no matter how limited his previous knowledge of the subject may be . . . . The chapter on apparatus contains a description of only such instruments as I have had a personal acquaintance with, either directly or indirectly, which explains why those of my own design predominate . . . . In the part devoted to electro-therapeutics, I have endeavored to present succinctly an outline of a personal clinical experience, which, I must say, has been abundantly satisfactory . . . . In confining the text to the subject under consideration, I would not be misunderstood as advocating the electrical treatment to the exclusion of other measures and remedies of unquestioned value.

This was the only edition. Goelet's other book is *The technique of surgical-gynecology, devoted exclusively to a description of the technique of gynecological operations* (New York: International Journal of Surgery, 1900).

GY41. **CHARLES H. BUSHONG** (?–?). *Modern gynecology: a treatise on diseases of women.* 380pp. New York: E. B. Treat, 1893.

An assistant gynecologist at the Demilt Dispensary and an attending physician at the Northern Dispensary in New York, Bushong received his medical education and training in that city. This volume deals mainly with nonsurgical gynecology. It was the only book that Bushong wrote, but was received well enough to justify publication of an expanded second edition in 1898. The work has numerous illustrations.

GY42. **FRANKLIN HENRY MARTIN** (1857–1935). *Electricity in diseases of women and obstetrics.* 278pp. Chicago: W. T. Keener, 1893.

Martin played a key role in several aspects of American surgery—most notably as the driving force behind the founding of the American College of Surgeons. Born in Ixonia, Wisconsin, Martin received his M.D. from Chicago Medical College (now Northwestern University) in 1880. He practiced obstetrics and gynecology in Chicago for his entire professional life.

Martin was among the first surgeons in the United States to practice aseptic surgery. He also devised a method to reduce the mortality in operations for uterine fibroids by devising a procedure for tying off the uterine arteries to cause atrophy of the fibroid. He founded and edited the monthly journal *Surgery, gynecology and obstetrics*, to which he later added the *International abstract of surgery*. After organizing the Clinical Congress of Surgeons of North America in 1910, Martin merged the organization three years later into the American College of Surgeons. During World War I, he served on the Council of National Defense and was a member of the General Medical Board, which oversaw the mobilization of physicians, surgeons and dentists. In 1919, Martin was president of the American Gynecological Society, and later helped edit the *American journal of obstetrics and gynecology*. *Electricity* was written when he was professor of gynecology at the Post-Graduate Medical School and attending surgeon at the Woman's Hospital. Martin notes in the preface:

> This book has been written as a text-book for students and practitioners of medicine. The author's ideal of a textbook is one which considers each subject of which it treats from its primaries to the arrangement of primaries into principles, and finally to the practical applications of such principles to the subject in hand; this evolution must be accomplished without traveling too fast for the beginner or too slow for the advanced . . . . Fully one-third of this book is occupied with presenting the primaries of electricity, of arranging these primary facts into laws, of developing these known laws into principles which may be depended upon to accomplish results . . . . Another third of the book is occupied with illustrations and apparatus . . . . The remaining third

of the book deals in the application of the principles laid down in the earlier portions to the practical treatment of diseased conditions . . .

The thirty-nine chapters include "Employment of incandescent street wire current for therapeutic purposes" (pages 88–93); "Apostoli's treatment of fibroids" (pages 124–28); "Galvanism for cancer" (pages 204–08); and "Galvano-cautery surgery in gynecology" (pages 249–70). There are numerous illustrations. Martin describes the writing of this work in the first volume of his two-volume autobiography *The joy of living* (Garden City: Doubleday & Doran, 1933, pages 257-58):

> At about this time (1884), there were occasional references in French literature to Georges Apostoli's use of electricity in the treatment of fibroid tumors of the uterus. Looking for any clue that promised relief in these cases, I began a systematic study of Apostoli's methods, and was led immediately into an investigation of electricity as it was then known: the static machine with its great glass plates and the sparks it produced; the galvanic current, a continuous current produced by piles and simple batteries arranged in series; and the faradic current, an alternating current of induced electricity, which stimulated the skin surfaces and contracted muscles when applied to nerve centers. The dynamo was only a curious plaything; and Edison's electric incandescent light was in the early stages of its development. As I proceeded with my study, I obtained an understanding of Ohm's law, the relation of resistance to voltage, and the resulting electric current or ampere strength. The increasing number of articles pertaining to this new science spurred me on to a hasty crystallization and systematization of my own knowledge into outline chapters, which several years later formed the basis of a textbook, entitled "Electricity in Gynecology." My investigation revealed that electricity, intelligently-applied, would check hemorrhage, especially in cases of tumors of the uterus which expanded the interior membranous surface from which bleeding occurred. As a large percentage of the cases I had observed were of that character, it was manifest that great relief could be afforded if hemorrhage could be controlled . . . .

There was only one edition of this monograph. Among Martin's other books are *A treatise on gynecology* (Chicago: Cleveland Press, 1903), *South America from a surgeon's point of view* (New York: Fleming H. Revell, 1922), *Gorgas, a biography* (Chicago: 1924), and *Australia and New Zealand, a monograph* (Chicago: 1924). His two-volume autobiography was also published as a single volume with the title *Fifty years of medicine and surgery* (Chicago: Surgical Publishing, 1934).

GY43. **JOHN MONTGOMERY BALDY** (1860–1934). *An American textbook of gynecology, medical and surgical.* 713pp. Philadelphia: W. B. Saunders, 1894.

Baldy was editor of this textbook and at the time of its publication served as professor of gynecology at Philadelphia Polyclinic. He is perhaps best remembered for having performed the first gastrectomy in America [G-M 3518]. In addition, he is credited with modifying John C. Webster's (1863–1950) method of treating retrodisplacement of the uterus [G-M 6116].

This textbook is part of The American Text-Book Series published by Saunders. This series became one of that company's most successful publishing ventures. Included in the series are *Applied therapeutics* by James C. Wilson (1847–1934), *Diseases of children* by Louis Starr (1849–1925) and Thompson S. Westcott (1862-?), *Diseases of the eye, ear, nose, and throat* by George E. de Schweinitz (1858–1938) and Burton Alexander Randall (1858–1932) (OT70), *Genito-urinary and skin diseases* by Lemuel Bolton Bangs (1842–1914) (GU39), *Legal medicine and toxicology* by Frederick Peterson (1859–1938) and Walter Haines, *Obstetrics* by Richard C. Norris (1863–?) and Robert L. Dickinson (1861–1950), *Pathology* by John Guiteras and David Riesman, *Physiology* by William H. Howell (1860–1945), *Surgery* by William W. Keen (1837–1932) and J. William White (1850–1916) (GS154), and *The theory and practice of medicine* by William Pepper (1843–98).

Baldy's book was available in cloth for $6.00 and in sheepskin or half morocco for $7.00, but was sold by subscription only. Other contributors to the work included a who's who of American gynecologists: Henry T. Byford (1853–?), Edwin B. Cragin (1859–1918), James H. Etheridge , William Goodell (1829–94), Howard A. Kelly (1858–1943), Florian Krug, E. E. Montgomery (1849–1927), William R. Pryor (1858–1904), and George Tuttle (1866–?). Unlike modern textbooks, the work does not indicate the authors of individual chapters, because, according to Baldy,

> this work embodies as nearly as possible the combined opinions of all the authors, although it is to be understood that each individual author must be free from absolute responsibility for any particular statement: especially is this so for the reason that the Editor has endeavored by adding to and subtracting from the text to render it as uniform in its statements as possible . . . .

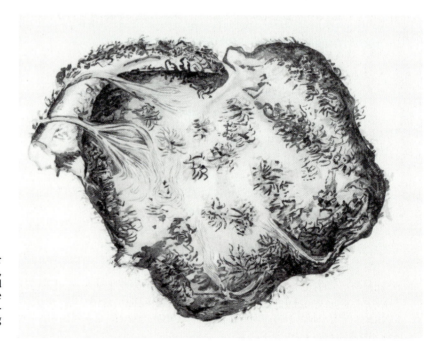

Fig. 113. (GY43) This color plate, figure 30 on page 458, demonstrates a pyosalpinx and ovarian abscess showing the remnants of universal adhesions. This particular drawing was original to Baldy.

The eighteen chapters include topics such as "Sterility"; "Lacerations of the soft parts"; "Genital fistulae"; "Malignant diseases of the female genitalia"; "Uterine neoplasms"; "Pelvic inflammation"; "Ectopic gestation"; and "After-treatment in gynecological operations." This last chapter (pages 660–87) is unique in American gynecologic literature because for the first time post-operative complications (i.e., vomiting, flatulence, hemorrhage, shock, and sepsis) are discussed and their treatment summarized. There are 360 illustrations and thirty-seven colored and halftone plates. A second edition was published in 1898.

GY44. PAUL FORTUNATUS MUNDE (1846–1902). *A report of the gynecological service of Mount Sinai Hospital, New York, for the twelve years from January 1st, 1883, to December 31st, 1894.* 116pp. New York: William Wood, 1894.

Munde became gynecologist at Mt. Sinai in 1881. He performed most of his clinical work there, but also worked at St. Elizabeth's and the Italian Hospital in New York. The *Report* was initially published in the October-December 1895 number of the *American journal of obstetrics.* There was a demand for its publication in book form, and some minor modifications were made to accomplish this. The work contains forty-eight illustrations and a number of remarkable tables detailing cases of gynecologic disease and their results. There was no separate gynecologic department at Mt. Sinai before 1877. In this respect the hospital did not differ from the majority of others in the United States. For this reason this volume is an important work because it provides a look at one of the earliest gynecologic services in this country and describes its day-to-day administration and professional results. Unfortunately, the monograph contains no table of contents or index, making it difficult to peruse. (See also GY27.)

GY45. JAMES CRAVEN WOOD (1858–?). *A textbook of gynecology.* 858pp. Philadelphia: Boericke & Tafel, 1894.

Wood was professor of gynecology at Cleveland Medical College after having served for eight years as professor of obstetrics and the diseases of women and children in the University of Michigan's Homeopathic Department. A well-known homeopathic gynecologist, he was previously president of the Homeopathic Medical Society of the State of Michigan. Wood explains his views on the ideal form of a textbook in the preface:

> When, four years ago, the publishers of this volume requested me to write a text-book on gynecology, I consented to undertake the task only after receiving assurances from them that their views were in entire harmony with my own, regarding the field to be covered by such a work. An ideal text-book, according to my conception, was one which should not only embody in concise form for the specialist the most advanced teachings of the American and European schools of gynecology, but should present these teachings in such a way as to enable the student of medicine and the non-specialist to obtain at least an intelligent knowledge of the subject without exhaustive research . . . .

The most interesting part of the work is the illustrations, about which Wood comments:

> I cannot but feel that the profession will appreciate the large number of illustrations from the Museum of the Royal College of Surgeons, London. I am not aware that any American specialist has before utilized that splendid pathological collection for this purpose. All of the photographs of these specimens, as well as photographs and drawings obtained from my own cases, were taken under my personal supervision.

There are fifty-two chapters covering a wide range of topics, including "Electricity in gynecology" (pages 152-69); "Antisepsis in gynecology" (pages 170–83); "Ovariotomy" (pages 702-36); and "Lacerations and injuries of the perineum and pelvic floor" (pages 815–46). Illustrative cases are indexed on pages xiv-xvii. There are two plates and 206 figures. A second edition was published in 1898.

GY46. **HENRY JACQUES GARRIGUES** (1831–1913). *A text-book of the diseases of women*. 390pp. Philadelphia: W. B. Saunders, 1894.

Garrigues served as professor of obstetrics at New York Post-Graduate Medical School and Hospital when he published this volume. He notes in this book's preface:

> In writing this book I have first had in view the large class of physicians who have not had the advantage of hospital training, and who go to a post-graduate school in order to learn gynecology. They can only stay a short time, and they want a full but concise exposition . . . . Secondly, I have tried to satisfy the requirements of that much larger class who would like to go to such an establishment, but who find it impossible to leave their practice . . . . Finally, I think the book will be found useful by undergraduates studying in medical colleges . . . . This being a book for general practitioners and students, I have omitted all references to the historical development by which gynecology has attained its present stage, as well as all reports of special cases . . . .

The book is divided into general and special divisions. The former consists of eight parts: "Development of the female genitals"; "Anatomy of the female pelvic organs"; "Physiology"; "Etiology in general"; "Examination in general"; "Treatment in general"; "Abnormal menstruation and metrorrhagia"; and "Leucorrhea." The special division discusses diseases of the "Vulva"; "Perineum"; "Vagina"; "Uterus"; "Fallopian tubes"; "Ovaries"; and "Pelvis." The book also contains an interesting appendix on sterility and one of the first discussions of sexual therapy for lack of orgasm (page 659). The work is well illustrated with 310 engravings and color plates. It was originally available in an octavo clothbound volume for $4.00 or in sheepskin or half morocco for $5.00. A second edition was published in 1897. (See also GY29.)

GY47. **FRED BYRON ROBINSON** (1854–1910). *Landmarks in gynecology*. 2 vols. Detroit: G. S. Davis, 1894.

Robinson practiced in Chicago, where he was professor of gynecology at the Chicago Post-Graduate School. He is not well known but was nevertheless an influential surgeon, having been an early experimenter in surgical research. Robinson was among the first American surgeons to perform extensive animal studies. However, this two-volume work, unlike his other books, contains little in the way of experimental protocols. Instead, as Robinson notes in the preface:

> The following pages contain an abstract of some of my lectures during the past three years. I have divided the subject into prominent "Landmarks," for convenience of teaching and for the purpose of impressing upon practitioners the chief features in gynaecology. The "Landmarks" which I consider of chief importance are: (1) anatomy; (2) menstruation; (3) labor; (4) abortion; (5) gonorrhoea; (6) tumors. Probability is the rule of life, and it is safe to say that in one of these landmarks will be found the disease from which the patient suffers. This classification calls attention to the significant clinical events in the life of a woman . . . . Much of the material . . . has been gleaned from personal work in dissections, from autopsies, and from clinical work in gynaecological and abdominal surgery. I claim, therefore, to present in this little book some original views and new classifications—the result of much personal labor . . . .

A second edition was published as a single volume in 1901. (See also GS149.)

GY48. HENRY TURMAN BYFORD (1853-?): *Manual of gynecology.* 488pp. Philadelphia: P. Blakiston & Son, 1895.

The son of William Heath Byford (1817-90), Byford was professor of gynecology and clinical gynecology at the College of Physicians and Surgeons of Chicago and professor of clinical gynecology at the Woman's Medical School of Northwestern University. The work contains 234 illustrations, many of which were original to Byford. The preface explains the purpose of the book:

> It has been the endeavor of the author of this book to supply the student with a manual of gynecology complete enough for study or reference in his college course as well as a guide to him during his first years of practice. It is also intended as an adequate exposition of the subject to the older general practitioner, who recognizes the impropriety of an attempt on his part to manage the more complicated cases, or perform the more difficult operations belonging to gynecology . . . .

The book is divided into ten parts: "Diagnosis and treatment"; "Development and anomalies of development"; "Functional and nervous diseases"; "Traumatic lesions of the genital tract"; "Displacements"; "Inflammatory lesions"; "Genital tuberculosis"; "Malignant diseases"; "Tumors of the female genital organs"; and "Ectopic pregnancy, pelvic hematocele, and pelvic hematoma." Further editions were published in 1897 and 1903.

GY49. JOHN MARIE KEATING (1852–93) and HENRY CLARK COE (1856–1940). *Clinical gynaecology, medical and surgical by eminent American teachers.* 904pp. Philadelphia: J. B. Lippincott, 1895.

This work assigns responsibility for the opinions expressed in the chapters to their individual authors for the first time in an American gynecologic text. Keating died during the planning stages of the book, and Coe, who was professor of gynecology at New York Polyclinic, carried out his plans and wishes as far as possible. Keating is best remembered as a pediatrician, although early in his career he was gynecologist at St. Joseph's Hospital in Philadelphia. Active in medical politics, Keating served as editor of the *Archives of pediatrics* and as president of the American Pediatric Society. Among his other books are *The mother's guide in the management and feeding of infants* (Philadelphia: Henry C. Lea's Son, 1881), *Practical lessons in nursing* (Philadelphia: J. B. Lippincott, 1887), *Diseases of the heart and circulation in infancy and adolescence* (Philadelphia: P. Blakiston & Son, 1888), the five-volume *Cyclopaedia of the diseases of children, medical and surgical* (Philadelphia: J. B. Lippincott, 1889–99), *How to examine for life insurance* (Philadelphia: P. Blakiston & Son, 1890), *Saunders's pocket medical lexicon, being a dictionary of words and terms used in medicine and surgery* (Philadelphia: W. B. Saunders, 1890), and *A new pronouncing dictionary of medicine, being a voluminous and exhaustive hand-book of medical and surgical terminology* (Philadelphia: W. B. Saunders, 1892). In the preface Coe explains his part in the work:

> The impulse which has been given to the clinical teaching of medicine and surgery during the past ten years by the establishment of numerous post-graduate schools throughout the country has been communicated to recent text-books, in which the practical has largely superseded the theoretical. The practitioner at the present day is not only keenly alive to the fact that immense advances have been made in medicine since his student days, but is filled with the laudable ambition to keep abreast of them. To enable him to do this, information must be imparted to him in a clear, concise, and more or less dogmatic form. This is the object aimed at in the present volume, which represents the combined experience of a number of clinical teachers selected by the former editor as men who, while disposed to be conservative, were none the less progressive and free from hobbies . . . . The editor takes this occasion to fulfil a promise made to the late Dr. Keating. It was the latter's expressed wish, when he recognized the fact that he would be unable to complete this work, that he should not be held responsible for any views contained in it regarding the destruction of the living foetus which might appear to be contrary to the tenets of the Catholic Church . . . .

Among the nineteen chapters are "Gynaecological technique" by Hunter Robb (1863–1940); "Traumatic lesions of the vulva, vagina, and cervix" by Matthew D. Mann (1845–1921); "Genital tuberculosis" by J. Whitridge Williams (1866–1931); "Inflammatory lesions of the pelvic peritoneum and connective tissue" by Henry T. Byford (1853–?); "Displacements of the uterus" by Paul F. Munde (1846–1902); "Ectopic pregnancy" by William T. Lusk (1838–1907); and "Diseases of the female breast" by Dudley P. Allen (1852–1915). This was the only edition.

GY50. **JOHN WESLEY LONG** (1859–1926). *Syllabus of gynecology, based on the American text-book of gynecology.* 133pp. Philadelphia: W. B. Saunders, 1895.

As professor of gynecology at the Medical College of Virginia and gynecologist at the medical school's hospital, Long was quite prominent in gynecology in the South. Long explains in his preface that he wrote the *Syllabus* for three reasons:

> ... first, to be used as lecture notes; secondly, to enable the student more intelligently to follow and remember the lectures; and finally, as a convenient reference for practitioners. This Syllabus is based upon the American Text-Book of Gynecology, because I believe this work reflects the most advanced gynecological thought and work. In writing the Syllabus I have not only adopted the classifications and endorsed the principles enunciated, but I have endeavored also to conform to the phraseology of the Text-Book, so that the reader may more readily understand the subject under consideration when reading these notes. At the same time I have not hesitated to differ from, or to add to, the Text-Book whenever in my judgment it was best to do so....

The book was available interleaved for $1.00. There was only one edition.

GY51. **ALEXANDER JOHNSTON CHALMERS SKENE** (1837–1900): *Medical gynecology, a treatise on the diseases of women from the standpoint of the physician.* 529pp. New York: D. Appleton, 1895.

Skene writes in the preface that

> ... the growth of gynecology in recent times has been phenomenal, especially in the direction of surgery.... It appears in medical literature that surgery has been more assiduously cultivated than medicine. This may have induced some to push the surgical treatment of diseases of women to extremes, and in some degree to neglect medicine.... The popularity of the author's contributions to gynecological surgery in the past raises the hope that this work may meet with an equally favorable reception.

The volume is arranged in three parts: Part I. deals with "The primary differentiation of sex, development and growth during early life, and the conditions favorable to the evolution of normal organization and the attainment of a healthful puberty..."; Part II. treats "The characteristics of sex, the adaptation of structure to function, the predisposition to particular diseases, and the causes of certain affections peculiar to women..."; Part III. discusses "The menopause, or the transition from active functional life toward advanced years, and then the diseases of the latter period...."

The book has a total of forty-two chapters and twenty-four figures, but no plates. There were no further editions. (See also GS187, GY21, and GY33.)

GY52. **CHARLES BINGHAM PENROSE** (1862–1925). *Syllabus of the lectures on gynecology.* 149pp. Philadelphia: W. F. Fell, 1896.

Penrose is best known as the eponymous inventor of a cigarette drain composed of rubber tubing containing a length of absorbent gauze. He was professor of gynecology at the University of Pennsylvania, having graduated from Harvard College in 1881 and received both an M.D. and Ph.D. from the University of Pennsylvania in 1884; he retired from active practice in 1899. The *Syllabus* is quite scarce, its publication having been arranged by William A. N. Dorland (1864–1956) solely for the use of students in the graduating class of the university where Penrose taught. His lectures were compiled to serve as a guidebook to enable students to follow the course more readily. The volume includes a detailed index but has no table of contents. No illustrations were used. This was the only edition. (See also GY54.)

GY53. **WILLIAM HUGHES WELLS** (1859–1919). *A compend of gynecology.* 262pp. Philadelphia: P. Blakiston's Son, 1896.

An 1891 graduate of Jefferson Medical College, Wells was adjunct professor of obstetrics and diseases of infancy at Philadelphia Polyclinic. He had previously served as assistant demonstrator of clinical obstetrics at Jefferson. The *Compend* was the seventh in Blakiston's Quiz Compend Series. It cost eighty cents; an interleaved version for taking notes was available for $1.25. There were over 150 illustrations. Wells writes in the preface:

> In placing this little book before the medical profession, the author is fully aware of there being little that is original in its pages; however, a number of years' experience as demonstrator and quizmaster have convinced him that, notwithstanding the necessary lengthening of college courses and the more thorough division of teaching caused by the immense progress in the medical sciences, there is still a demand among students for a book which will be a condensation of the best teachings of the present day, and with this object in view this little book has been written . . . .

The table of contents lists seventeen major subjects, including antisepsis in gynecology. Further editions were published in 1899, 1903, and 1910. Among Wells's other books is a *Manual of the diseases of children* (Philadelphia: P. Blakiston's Son, 1898,) written with John M. Taylor (1855–?).

GY54. **CHARLES BINGHAM PENROSE** (1862–1925). *A textbook of diseases of women.* 529pp. Philadelphia: W. B. Saunders, 1897.

This *Textbook* is important because in it Penrose provides the first description of the drain that he devised and that now bears his name (pages 463–67). The Penrose drain was the most popular and most widely used drain of its time, and remains popular even today. Penrose explains in the preface that

> I have written this book for the medical student. I have attempted to present the best teaching of modern gynecology, untrammelled by antiquated theories or methods of treatment. I have, in most instances, recommended but one plan of treatment for each disease, hoping in this way to avoid confusing the student or the physician who consults the book for practical guidance. I have, as a rule, omitted all facts of anatomy, physiology, and pathology which may be found in the general text-books upon these subjects . . . .

The book consists of forty-three chapters and is profusely illustrated. Chapters 39–43 are devoted to the techniques of gynecological operations and treatment after celiotomy. The work was well received, and further editions appeared in 1897, 1899, 1901, 1904 and 1908. (See also GY52.)

GY55. **EMILIUS CLARK DUDLEY** (1850–1928). *Diseases of women; a treatise on the principles and practice of gynecology.* 637pp. Philadelphia: Lea Brothers, 1898.

A well-known gynecologist, Dudley was professor of gynecology at Northwestern University Medical School when this work was published. There are 422 illustrations, of which 47 are in color, and two color plates. The preface explains why the large number of illustrations was used:

> This book is designed to be a practical treatise on gynecology, for the use of practitioners and students; to contain the most approved precepts in principles and practice; and to exclude whatever is not founded in pathology or carefully observed experience . . . . In order to give clearness and brevity to the text, and to bring out important distinctions with force, illustrations in an unusual number, and largely-from original drawings, have been introduced . . . .

The volume is divided into five parts: "General principles"; "Inflammations"; "Tumors, tubal pregnancy, and malformations"; "Traumatisms"; and "Displacements of the uterus and other pelvic organs, massage." Further editions appeared in 1899, 1902, 1904, and 1908. Among Dudley's other books is *Gynecology* (Chicago: Yearbook Publishers, 1902).

GY56. **HOWARD ATWOOD KELLY** (1858–1943). *Operative gynecology.* 2 vols., 563pp. and 557pp. New York: D. Appleton, 1898. [G-M 6108]

A major figure in the development of gynecological and abdominal surgery, Kelly established the field of gynecology as distinct from that of obstetrics. He received his M.D. from the University of Pennsylvania in 1882. By 1889, Kelly had advanced to the position of professor of obstetrics at Pennsylvania. In that year he moved to Baltimore, where he began his lengthy association with the Johns Hopkins Hospital and School of Medicine. Although considered a gynecologist, Kelly also devised many new techniques for the diagnosis and treatment of kidney and bladder disease. Among his more prominent contributions to medical literature are works on the design of various rectal and vesical specula [G-M 3526]; the introduction of aeroscopic examination of the female bladder and catheterization of the ureters [G-M 4187]; a method of uretero-ureteral anastomosis including the use of the catheter as a temporary ureteral splint [G-M 4188]; the use of wax on a bladder catheter tip so that it registers any pressure from sharp stones, thus providing an important means of diagnosing calculi [G-M 4295]; hysterorrhaphy [G-M 6086]; and the removal of pelvic inflammatory masses by the abdomen after bisection of the uterus [G-M 6109]. *Operative gynecology* was important for a number of reasons. Not only did these volumes proclaim to the world Kelly's leadership in gynecology, but they introduced to medical circles the images by Max Brödel (1870–1941) that revolutionized medical illustration. The work contained twenty-four plates and over 550 original illustrations. It was dedicated to Robert P. Harris (1822-99). Kelly writes in the preface:

> My aim in writing this book has been to place in the hands of the many friends who have from time to time visited me and followed my work, a convenient summary of the various gynecological operations I have

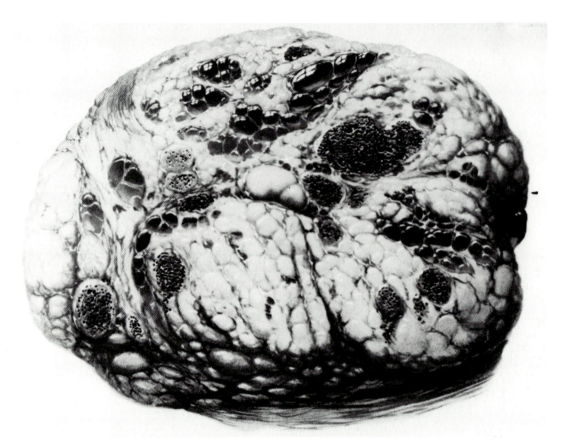

Fig. 114. (GY56) A magnificent color plate by Max Brödel, figure 20 on page 382 in volume 2, shows an angiomyoma of the uterus with cystic degeneration. I. Prang of Boston was the lithographer.

found best in my own practice. It is far from my purpose to present a digest of the literature of the subject, or even to describe all the important operations; if I had set out to do this, the book would never have been written in the midst of the pressing practical duties of my work. Gynecology is so young a science, and many of its surgical procedures are as yet so incompletely developed, that I think the best service a gynecologist can render his specialty is to record accurately his own experience . . . . I have few claims to originality to urge, and these are, I think, clearly set forth in the text . . . .

Volume 1 contains nineteen chapters, including "Sepsis, asepsis, and antisepsis in hospitals"; "Bacteriology"; "Anesthesia"; and "Principles involved in plastic operations." The second volume consists of chapters 20–38. Among the topics are "General principles and complications common to abdominal operations"; "Complications arising after abdominal operations"; "Ovariotomy"; "The radical cure of hernia"; and "The conduct of autopsies." Audrey W. Davis describes the genesis of this book in her biography of Kelly, *Dr. Kelly of Hopkins* (Baltimore: The Johns Hopkins Press, 1959, pages 113–15):

Shortly after his arrival in Baltimore, Kelly determined to write an operative gynecology. Having made this decision, he became concerned about the illustrations. He considered those with which he was familiar extremely poor, rather coarse, and utterly lacking in depth . . . . In talking over his quandary with Professor Franklin P. Mall one day, Kelly asked Mall if he knew a good artist to illustrate the proposed work. It so happened that Mall did; he highly recommended Max Broedel, then working for Ludwig in Germany. Dr. Kelly at once wrote to Broedel, inviting him to join the gynecological staff. It took a lot of correspondence and the lapse of several years to gain his consent and to make the necessary arrangements, but at last, in 1894, Broedel arrived in Baltimore . . . . Four years after Broedel began work at the Hopkins, Kelly's two-volume *Operative Gynecology* appeared . . . . Those who had previously been hampered by the wretched old woodcuts handed down through the decades realized at a glance what Broedel had effected by his totally new conception of the presentation of surgery in pictures so vivid that the whole world was led first to admire and then to copy them . . . .

A second edition of this work was published in 1899–1900. Kelly wrote numerous other medical works, some of which Brödel also illustrated. They include *The vermiform appendix and its diseases* (Philadelphia: W. B. Saunders, 1905) [G-M 3571], written with Elizabeth Hurdon (1869–1941); the two-volume *Gynecology and abdominal surgery* (Philadelphia: W. B. Saunders, 1907), coauthored with Charles P. Noble (1863–1935); *Medical gynecology* (New York: D. Appleton, 1908); *Myomata of the uterus* (Philadelphia: W. B. Saunders, 1909), written with Thomas S. Cullen (1868–1953); *Diseases of the kidney, ureters, and bladder* (Philadelphia: W. B. Saunders, 1914), with F. R. Burnham; and *Electrosurgery* (Philadelphia: W. B. Saunders, 1932), with Ward E. Grant. Another interesting work is *The stereo clinics* (1908–1915), comprising eighty-four sections of stereograms depicting gynecological operations photographed throughout the United States. Kelly was also a medical historian of major repute and wrote *Walter Reed and yellow fever* (New York: McClure & Phillips, 1906), *Some American medical botanists* (Troy: Southworth, 1914), the two-volume *Cyclopedia of American medical biography, comprising the lives of eminent deceased physicians and surgeons from 1610–1910* (Philadelphia: W. B. Saunders, 1912), and *A dictionary of American medical biography, lives of eminent physicians of the United States and Canada, from the earliest times* (New York: D. Appleton, 1928) [G-M 6728] in collaboration with Walter L. Burrage (1860–1935). Kelly's other books included *Snakes of Maryland* (1936) and *A scientific man and the Bible* (1925).

VI. UROLOGY

GU1. **ALEXANDER HODGDON STEVENS** (1789–1869). *Lectures on lithotomy.* 93pp. New York: Adlard & Saunders, 1838.

Stevens attended Yale College and received his M.D. from the University of Pennsylvania in 1811. He practiced in New York from 1819 to 1839 and was a surgeon at New York Hospital. The lectures were delivered in December 1837 at New York Hospital, although Stevens was professor of clinical surgery at the College of Physicians and Surgeons. There is no table of contents and only a limited index, which makes the volume difficult to peruse. The first lecture discusses varying types of lithotomies and provides a great deal of statistical information from European sources. Like many American surgeons of the time, Stevens had studied extensively abroad and much that he learned was incorporated into this text. He is best remembered for having served as the second president of the American Medical Association in 1848. There were no other editions.

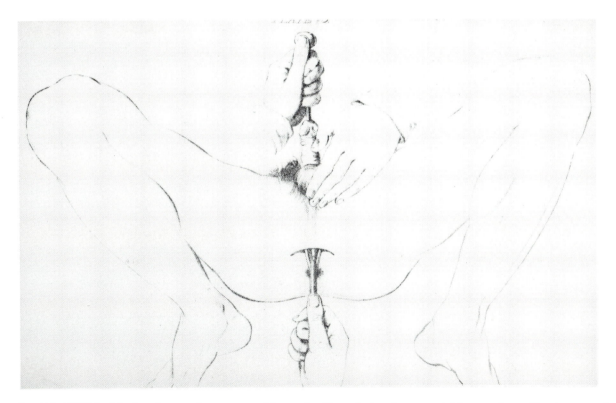

Fig. 115. (GU1) In this plate Stevens demonstrates "the mode of introducing the prostatic bisector, directed by the grooved staff from the bottom of the external wound through the prostate gland, into the bladder."

GU2. **EDWARD H. DIXON** (1808–80). *A treatise on diseases of the sexual organs; adapted to popular and professional readings, and the exposition of quackery, professional and otherwise.* 260pp. New York: W. Taylor, 1846.

From 1849 to 1864, Dixon published *The scalpel*, a quarterly journal which satirically exposed the foibles and abuses of medicine and domestic life. In the forty-seven volumes of this journal are numerous essays detailing day-to-day life in New York City and daily occurrences in the practice of a surgeon.

Dixon's *Treatise* went through seven editions within two years. The first part consists of fifteen chapters, most of which discuss syphilis, its symptoms, and their treatment. The second part deals with gonorrhea and comprises sixteen chapters. However, the majority of these chapters also deal with topics other than gonorrhea, including "Strictures of the urethra"; "Circumcision" (as Dixon notes, an "admirable custom of the Jews"); "Swellings and other enlargements of the testicle"; "Malignant or cancerous diseases of the testicle"; "Varicocele"; "Cancer of the penis"; and "Spermatorrhea." Chapter 16 describes the "Morbid developments and surgical treatment of onanism or masturbation." Text-books of the period frequently considered masturbation a disease, although they typically contradicted one another in their efforts to describe exactly what symptoms this particular disease caused. Dixon writes in a most intriguing preface:

> The writer of these pages is unwilling to subject himself to the aspersion which will probably follow their appearance, without an explanation of the motives that induced him to prepare them; and as those who censure often doubt the statements of such as incur their animadversion, he hopes by the nature and distinctness of an avowal rarely made by authors, as well as the internal evidence of the book itself, to obtain full credit for what he is about to say. In the first place then, the motive is self-interest . . . . A diversified practice of fifteen years' duration, with a minute and comprehensive knowledge of the medical policy of the day, has entirely convinced him that the most effective causes are operating, to break down the slender barrier hitherto existing, between the accomplished surgeon and the vilest empyric. This has long rested on a foundation as feeble as the public intelligence on medical subjects, and the only wonder is, that it has so long withstood the onslaught: the late act of the legislature is the legitimate sequence of its own miserable policy, in granting to colleges monopolies to teach, or rather to huckster diplomas. The profession is now open to all:—yes, so far as the fostering care of that great "caterer and dry nurse of the state," an American legislature can extend its maternal arms, the most profound of our number may enter the lists for public favor, with his boot black. This kind protection of the public health, was absolutely a necessary appendage to their previous enlightened act; for these colleges, alas for poor human-ity, have been animated with such persevering zeal for the numerical, not the intellectual strength of their graduates, (upon the yearly number of whom the subsistence of many of their professors entirely depends,) that the country is flooded by men totally destitute

either by education or habits of philosophic thought, for the profession to which they have so unhappily been admitted . . . .

(See also GY2.)

GU3. **HOMER BOSTWICK** (?–1862). *A treatise on the nature and treatment of seminal diseases, impotency, and other kindred affections: with practical directions for the management and removal of the cause producing them; together with hints to young men.* 251pp. New York: Burgess & Stringer, 1847.

Bostwick was a surgeon who practiced in New York and an early specialist in genitourinary problems. He comments in the preface:

> This book is the result of much thought and extended observation. Many works upon the same subject have been written and gazetted to the world, the aim of which seems to have been to picture in the gloomiest colors the most frightful symptoms of this peculiar class of diseases, without holding out one ray of hope or word of consolation to the afflicted. The reader will discover in these pages quite a different motive on the part of the author. Instead of trying to alarm and excite the fears of patients, he has been enabled to exhibit the most abundant evidence that complaints of this nature are susceptible of being cured . . . . From what I have just said—with the intelligent reader from his own conclusions—it will readily be perceived that to be cured of such disorders, no policy can be more suicidal than for patients either to rely upon themselves, or upon the ignorant quacks and the vile nostrums so eloquently advertised and puffed in the newspapers of the day. These imposters, who make such high pretensions, know just as little of the malady as the persons do who apply to them; and it is the bold and extraordinary effrontery with which such charlatans show themselves before the public, that enables them to delude the unwary victim, and swindle him of his last dollar; and, what is far worse, greatly aggravate his disease.

The *Treatise* contains nine chapters with seven plates. There is an interesting appendix on pages 239–51, which contains various prescriptions to treat seminal diseases. A second edition with thirteen plates was pub-lished in 1848. Among Bostwick's other books is *An inquiry into the cause of natural death, or death from old age* (New York: Stringer & Townsend, 1851). (See also GU4.)

GU4. **HOMER BOSTWICK** (?–1862). *A complete practical work on the nature and treatment of venereal diseases, and other affections of the genito-urinary organs of the male and female.* 348pp. New York: Burgess & Stringer, 1848.

Bostwick was a New York surgeon who specialized in genitourinary diseases. This rather scarce but important book is beautifully illustrated with thirty-seven colored plates and numerous other wood engravings. Chapters 1 and 2 detail the anatomy of the male and female genitals. The next eighteen chapters deal with the symptoms and treatment of venereal diseases. Included are detailed descriptions of primary (chancre and bubo), secondary, and tertiary syphilis. Chapter 21 discusses "Gleet"; chapters 22–24, "Stricture of the urethra"; chapter 25, "False passages"; chapter 26, "Infiltration of urine, abscess and fistulae"; chapters 27 and 28, "Hydrocele, circocele and varicocele"; and the final chapter, "Disease of the prostate gland." Bostwick notes in the preface:

> There are no maladies to which the human family is liable, of deeper importance, either in a medical or moral point of view, than those arising from impure sexual intercourse. With their moral bearings, in a work of this nature, we properly can have nothing to do. As medical men, it is our business to look at disease merely as it affects life and health; and our efforts are directed, not to the reformation of man's vicious propensities, but to the mitigation of his bodily sufferings . . . . Quackery has profited by the neglect that venereal diseases have experienced, and it is notorious that pretenders have secured a large share of such practice. It is time for the profession to free itself from this reproach. The welfare of society is as deeply concerned in this, as it can possibly be with any other disease that afflicts the human family. Entertaining such opinions, I resolved to present to my medical brethren a book, which will, I trust, afford every facility for becoming intimately acquainted not only with the mode of treating this class of diseases, but for knowing their exact appearance when they occur. Such a work I believe is still wanted . . . . This undertaking has been to me one of considerable labor. Every author

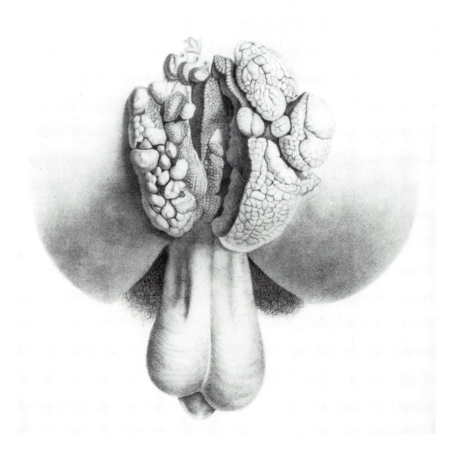

Fig. 116. (GU4) This magnificent colored plate, figure 12 on page 154, drawn from nature by Frances Michelin, shows polymorphous vegetations in the area of the anus. Boswick was uncertain of their true cause and related it to syphilis. In modern terminology, they are called "condyloma acuminatum."

of any pretension I have examined, and whatever I have found useful has been incorporated in the following pages. My aim has been to make not a theoretical, but a practical book . . .

(See also GU3.)

GU5. **SAMUEL DAVID GROSS** (1805–84). *A practical treatise on the disease and injuries of the urinary bladder, the prostate gland, and the urethra.* 726pp. Philadelphia: Blanchard & Lea, 1851.

In this, the first American textbook to provide a systematic approach to genitourinary diseases, Gross lists himself as professor of surgery at the University of Louisville. In reality, the book was written while he occupied the chair of surgery at the University of the City of New York in 1850–51. Gross notes in the preface:

> While every other organ of the body has had its expounder and monographist, it is a singular fact that no systematic treatise has yet appeared, in the English language, on the maladies of the structures in question, especially those of the bladder, which are so common and so important, both in their pathological and practical relations. There has not yet been an attempt made on the part of any American writer to supply this deficiency; and it is no disparagement to the foreign works which have been republished in this country to assert, that, valuable as in many respects they are, they are far in arrear of the existing state of the science to which they relate . . . .

The book comprises three major parts, which include forty-two chapters. The 106 illustrations are black-and-white engravings. There are no plates. Gross describes his work on this book in his *Autobiography* (volume 1, pages 93–94):

> On my way from New York to Louisville I left with Blanchard & Lea of Philadelphia the manuscript of a work entitled *A Practical Treatise on the*

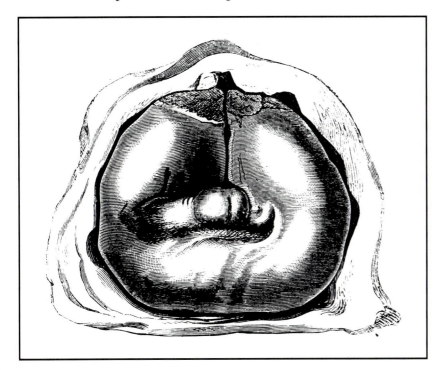

Fig. 117. (GU5) This wood engraving, figure 85 on page 563, from Gross's collection, demonstrates hypertrophy of the prostate and consequent impediment to normal urination.

Diseases, Injuries and Malformations of the Urinary Bladder, the Prostate Gland, and the Urethra, which was published by that firm in 1851. Such a work had long been needed, and it was at once accepted as an authority upon the subject of which it treated. The only monographs on these affections, of any importance, in the English language, were those of Sir Benjamin C. Brodie and Mr. William Coulson, two comparatively meagre productions, deficient in completeness and unsatisfactory, although valuable, especially the first. The object of my work was to present in a systematic and connected form, a full and comprehensive account of the diseases and injuries of the organs in question. The materials had been long accumulating upon my hands, and not less than three years were finally spent in arranging them for publication. The original design was to issue a separate volume of plates, of the size of nature, as a companion to the book; but it was soon discovered that this would so much enhance the expense as to place the work beyond the reach of many of those for whose benefit it was more particularly prepared. It was illustrated by upwards of one hundred engravings on wood, of which nearly one-half were expressly made for it. A second edition, greatly enlarged and improved, was issued in 1855. It formed a closely-printed octavo volume of nine hundred and twenty-five pages, illustrated by one hundred and eighty-four woodcuts, and comprised, along with my personal experience, a digest of the existing state of the science. In an appendix of twenty-nine closely-printed pages is the first and only attempt ever made by any writer, as far as I am aware, to furnish a complete account of the prevalence of stone in the bladder and of calculous disorders in the United States, Canada, Nova Scotia, Europe, and other countries . . . A new edition of this work has just been— September, 1876—issued under the able editorship of my son, Dr. S. W. Gross. He has rewritten much of the work, has introduced much new matter, and has thus produced a valuable treatise, fully up to the existing state of the science . . . .

(See also GS16, GS19, GS34, GS46, GS49, and OR2.)

GU6. **ALBAN GILPIN GOLDSMITH** (1795–1876). *Diseases of the genitourinary organs.* 96pp. New York: Wiley & Halsted, 1857.

An interesting figure in American surgical history, Goldsmith (whose name had been changed from Smith by an act of the New York legislature in 1839) never received an M.D. Instead, he took private lessons under Ephraim McDowell (1771–1830) and attended private medical lectures given by Joseph Parrish (1779–1840). Because of Goldsmith's early association with McDowell, he is believed to have been present at the first ovariotomy in 1809, and is known to have performed the third ovariotomy in the United States (1823). In 1833 Goldsmith was appointed professor of surgery at the Medical College of Ohio, but was not reappointed four years later when the faculty was reorganized. Shortly thereafter, the regents of the College of Physicians and Surgeons of New York offered him the chair of surgery, which he accepted. However, his academic career in New York was short-lived. He resigned after only two years at the college and remained in private practice in New York for the rest of his life. *Diseases* was the only book Goldsmith wrote. He writes in the introduction:

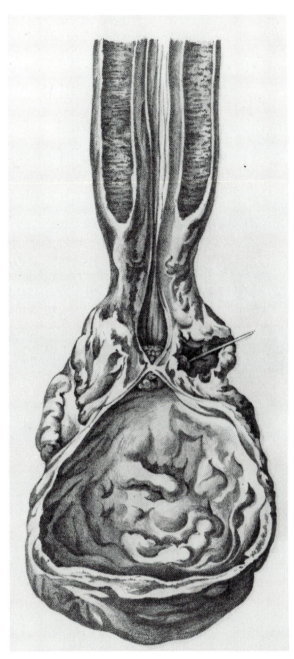

Fig. 118. (GU6) Goldsmith shows a chronically impacted calculus in the neck of the bladder, which ultimately led to creation of a stricture at the site. The specimen in this lithographic plate (number 4, page 36) was from the author's own pathology collection.

I have been so often solicited to publish the results of my experience in diseases of the genito-urinary organs, that I have concluded to put forth this little volume, as a beginning; simply detailing a few of the facts that have come under my observation, and the inferences that I have thought could be rationally drawn from them . . . . I have not written this book either for profit or reputation, as I have lived long enough to know that they are both "bubbles." . . .

There are four colored lithographs and five other woodcuts. The contents include "Gonorrhea (local disease; symptoms; pathology and treatment; extends to the bladder; swelled testicle, or epididimitis; gonorrheal rheumatism; and, popular remedies)"; "Stricture of the urethra (spasmodic; valvular; indurated or permanent stricture; introduction of the catheter; and, treatment of stricture)"; "Fistula in the perineum"; "Lithotripsy"; and "Seminal weakness." This was the only edition.

GU6.1. WILLIAM WALLACE MORLAND (1818–76). *Diseases of the urinary organs; a compendium of their diagnosis, pathology, and treatment.* 579pp. Philadelphia: Blanchard & Lea, 1858.

Morland was an attending surgeon at the Central Office of the Boston Dispensary when this volume was published. He graduated from Dartmouth College in 1838 and received his M.D. from Harvard Medical School in 1841. In 1855, in association with Francis Minot (1821–99), he succeeded Jerome Van Crowningshield Smith (1800–79) as editor of the *Boston medical and surgical journal* (the direct predecessor of today's *New England journal of medicine*). Morland remained in this position until 1860. The *Diseases* mainly comprises two Boylston Prize- winning essays from 1855 to 1857. There are two parts: "Diagnosis" and "Pathology and treatment." The work does not contain any plates. The twelve chapters deal almost entirely with the kidneys, ureters, and bladder or urethra. The sexual organs are little mentioned. Numerous references to surgical therapy are found, including rupture (page 323) and wounds of the bladder (page 356), vesical fistulae (page 359), and treatment of vesical calculus (pages 408–46). An extensive appendix (pages 513–61) contains discussions of several interesting surgical cases. There was just one ed-ition. Morland wrote only one other book, a Fiske Fund Prize Essay entitled *The morbid effects of the retention in the blood of the elements of the urinary secretions* (Philadelphia: Blanchard & Lea, 1861).

GU7. FREEMAN JOSIAH BUMSTEAD (1826–79). *The pathology and treatment of venereal diseases: including the results of recent investigations upon the subject.* 686pp. Philadelphia: Blanchard & Lea, 1861.

Bumstead graduated from Williams College and in 1851 received his M.D. from Harvard Medical School. He shortly thereafter traveled to Europe, where he spent a few months studying venereal diseases in Paris. Upon his return, he moved to New York and was eventually appointed lecturer on venereal diseases at the College of Physicians and Surgeons and surgeon at St Luke's Hospital. It was at this time that he wrote the *Pathology*. His reputation increased tremendously, and in 1867 Bumstead was promoted to professor of that specialty. He writes in the preface:

> The object in the preparation of this work has been to furnish the student with a full and comprehensive treatise upon venereal diseases, and the practitioner with a plain and practical guide to their treatment. In carrying out this design, theoretical discussions have been made subordinate to practical details; and, in the belief that the success of treatment depends quite as much upon the manner of its execution as upon the general principles upon which it is based, no minutiae, calculated to assist the surgeon or benefit the patient, have been regarded as unworthy of notice . . . .

The work is divided into two parts: "Gonorrhea and its complications" and "The chancroid, its complications, and syphilis." The book contains numerous woodcuts but no plates. Revised editions were published in 1864, 1870, 1879, and 1883. The latter two were coauthored with Robert W. Taylor (1842–1908). In 1900 a sixth edition was brought out under the sole authorship of Taylor entitled *A practical treatise on genito-urinary and venereal diseases and syphilis*. A final edition was published in 1904.

GU8. **JOHN WILLIAMS SEVERIN GOULEY** (1832–1920). *Diseases of the urinary organs: including stricture of the urethra, affections of the prostate, and stone in the bladder*. 368pp. New York: William Wood, 1873.

Gouley was one of America's earliest and most renowned genito-urinary specialists. He received his M.D. from the College of Physicians and Surgeons in New York in 1853. Most of his professional life was spent in that city, where in 1866 he was named professor of clinical surgery and genitourinary diseases in the medical department of the University of the City of New York. From 1876 to his retirement, he was professor of diseases of the genitourinary system. The two-volume *History of urology* (Baltimore: Williams & Wilkins, 1933), prepared under the auspices of the American Urological Association, notes his contributions to urology (volume 1, pages 72–73):

> The domain of urology at that time was bounded on the north by the seminal vesicles. What it consisted in may be learned from *Diseases of the Urinary Organs Including Stricture of the Urethra, Affections of the Prostate and Stone in the Bladder*. The author, John W. S. Gouley . . . . had been an assistant to Dr. Van Buren but had left his office largely because of a difference of opinion as to which of them was inventor of the tunnelled catheter. Gouley long outlived his master but remained always the typical old style clinical urethral specialist . . . . He has the honor of being the first distinguished urologist whose temperament excluded him from membership in the American Association of Genito-Urinary Surgeons, and the still greater honor of having produced in 1873 this volume which is in the strictest sense a treatise on urology. It opens with a discussion of urethral stricture covering seven chapters. The endoscope of Dr. Fisher of Boston (1824) is mentioned, as well as the urethroscopes of Desormeaux, Cruise and Otis, though it does not appear that Dr. Gouley used them. Such complications as "extravasation of urine," rupture of the bladder, ureteritis, pyelitis, hydronephrosis and pyonephrosis are commented upon. Next come chapters on "Traumatic Lesions of the Urethra," "Retention of Urine" (from stricture), "Rupture of the Urethra," "Urethral Fistulae" and "Rupture of the Bladder." Two chapters are then devoted to the prostate, covering prostatitis, prostatorrhea, and hypertrophy. The last three chapters are devoted to bladder stones. No mention is made of congenital abnormalities (excepting stricture at the meatus), tuberculosis or tumor. With the exception of the twelve lines devoted to the renal complications of urethral stricture, no notice is taken of diseases of the kidney. Tabetic bladder paralysis, at this time generally called "reflex urinary paralysis," is ascribed to phimosis or to congenital-stricture. Naturally bacteria are not among the dramatis personae that appear upon this stage . . . . A curious re-version to primitive methods is the chapter on "Treatment of Stricture by Division . . . . "

Fig. 119. (GU8) A gunshot wound to the shaft of the penis during the Civil War necessitated amputation with resultant fistula formation in the perineum. This illustration, figure 49 on page 179, shows the healing seven years later. Gouley states that "he urinated but three or four times a day, and had no bladder complication . . . but was troubled with inordinate sexual desires . . . the fellow had the effrontery to contract the marital tie, but his bride ran away on the next day."

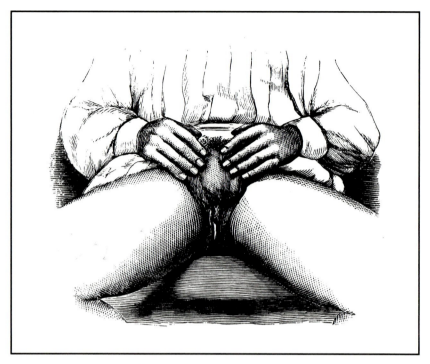

The volume contains 103 wood engravings and as written in the preface, "This work is based on lectures given at Bellevue Hospital, and in the medical department of the University of the City of New York, and embodies the results of the author's experience in private practice and in the public institutions . . . He has endeavored to write a handy-book on the pathogeny, clinical history, and treatment of some of the graver surgical diseases of the male urinary organs . . . . "

Among Gouley's other books are *Diseases of man: data of their nomenclature, classification & genesis* (New York: J. H. Vail, 1888), *Conference on the moral philosophy of medicine* (New York: Rebman, 1906), and *Surgery of genito-urinary organs* (New York: Rebman, 1907). (See also GU25.)

GU9. **WILLIAM HOLME VAN BUREN** (1819–83) and **EDWARD LAWRENCE KEYES** (1843–1924). *A practical treatise on the surgical diseases of the genito-urinary organs, including syphilis.* 672pp. New York: D. Appleton, 1874.

One of New York's most renowned surgeons, Van Buren was professor of the principles of surgery, diseases of the genito-urinary system and clinical surgery at Bellevue Hospital Medical College. Keyes graduated from Yale in 1863 and received his M.D. from the University of the City of New York in 1866. At the time this volume was published, he was professor of dermatology at Bellevue Hospital Medical College and surgeon at the Charity Hospital's venereal division. Keyes was a pioneer in American dermatology and urology, having taught the first course in dermatology in the United States in 1870 and establishing the first ward in America for genitourinary patients at Bellevue in 1875. He also founded and served as first president of the American Association of Genito-Urinary Surgeons in 1887. Keyes introduced the technique of administering continued small doses of mercury in treating syphilis in 1877, a method which became the standard treatment for over twenty years. The American Urological Association's *History of urology* gives the following account of Van Buren and Keyes (volume 1, pages 76–78):

> In 1874, the year after the publication of Gouley's book, appeared a volume which though by no means exclusively a treatise on urology was destined to exert enormous influence upon the urological practice of the ensuing generation . . . . The scope of Van Buren's and Keyes' volume was very much wider than that of Gouley's and the strictly urological portions of it far more evenly balanced from the modern point of view. The book rests on an anatomical basis, each section opening with a few paragraphs on anatomy followed by anomalies, etc. Stone and stricture still dominate. Out of about 300 pages devoted to urology, 68 are devoted to stricture and 98 to bladder stone. Yet the ureters have at least the dignity of a chapter three-quarters of a page in length . . . . The authors of this volume though united by no bond of blood or marriage, stood in the devoted relation to each other of father and son. The elder was dignified in carriage, slow in discourse, entirely urbane . . . . The junior author . . . for five years struggled with this volume, of which he boasted that the preface and the chapters on stone were written by Van Buren and the rest by himself, and read aloud to the elder author on winter evenings until sleep overtook the sage, whereupon the pace was quickened. But the substance of all that was not dermatology or venereal diseases in this volume is manifestly based upon the surgical experience of the senior author . . . .

Part 1 ("Diseases of the genito-urinary organs") is divided into twenty-eight chapters and contains over forty plates. Part 2 ("Chancroid and syphilis") comprises thirteen chapters. It was originally available in cloth for $5.00 or sheepskin for $6.00. The book was thoroughly revised and rewritten by Keyes in 1888 (GU20). Among Keyes's other medical books are *The tonic treatment of syphilis* (New York: D. Appleton, 1877); *Some fallacies concerning syphilis* (Detroit: G. S. Davis, 1890); *Venereal diseases; their complications and sequelae* (New York: William Wood, 1900), written jointly with Charles H. Chetwood (1866–?); and *Diseases of the genito-urinary organs* (New York: D. Appleton, 1910). (See also GS60, GS119, CR6, and GU12.)

GU10. **JOHN KING** (1813–93). *Urological dictionary: containing an explanation of numerous technical terms; the qualitative and quantitative methods employed in urinary investigations; the chemical characters, and microscopical appearances of the normal and abnormal elements of urine, and their clinical indications.* 266pp. Cincinnati: Wilstach & Baldwin, 1878.

King was one of America's best-known eclectic physicians. He received his medical education at the Reformed Medical College of the City of New York, where he graduated in 1838. He had a rather peripatetic career, but eventually settled in Cincinnati where he held the chair of obstetrics and diseases of women and children at the Eclectic Medical Institute after 1851. In 1878 he served as president of the

National Eclectic Medical Association. He is best remembered for the pioneering work he performed as a pharmacologist, having introduced several medicinal resins. The *Dictionary* contains thirty-nine woodcuts but no plates. Its most interesting feature is its twenty-seven tables meant "to aid the investigator in effecting rapid calculations during his observations," which are located throughout the text and in a special index. Although the work is not a surgical text per se, King notes in the preface that

> the capability of examining urine to assist in the diagnosis, prognosis, and therapeutics of disease, as manifested by the numerous works that have already appeared upon the subject, is recognized at this day as an important and necessary acquisition to medical practice,—one which no physician who values his professional standing can afford to ignore or neglect. The present Dictionary, while it lays no claim to erudition, nor to originality, is designed as a *multum in parvo* to the physician and the chemist, affording information concerning urinary technicalities and urinary investigations together with their clinical importance, that is not to be found in any one book yet published, and which, it is hoped, will prove instructive and useful . . . .

There is no table of contents. This was the only edition. Among King's other books are *The American eclectic dispensatory* (Cincinnati: Moore, Wilstach & Keys, 1852), *American eclectic obstetrics* (Cincinnati: Moore, Wilstach & Keys, 1855), *The American family physician; or, domestic guide to health* (Cincinnati: Longley Brothers, 1857), *Women; their diseases and their treatment* (Cincinnati: Longley Brothers, 1858), *The microscopist's companion; a popular manual of practical microscopy* (Cincinnati: Rickey & Mallory, 1859), and *The causes, symptoms, diagnosis, pathology, and treatment of chronic diseases* (Cincinnati: Medical Publishing, 1870).

GU11. **FESSENDEN NOTT OTIS** (1825–1900). *Stricture of the male urethra, its radical cure.* 352pp. New York: G. P. Putnam's Sons, 1878.

Otis graduated from Union College in 1849 and received his M.D. from the New York Medical College in 1852. He was in private practice in New York from 1862 to 1871. From 1871 to 1890 he served as professor of genitourinary and venereal diseases at the College of Physicians and Surgeons. Otis is best remembered as the first to use local anaesthesia in urology [G-M 4179]. The volume consists of seventeen chapters, including "Chronic urethral discharges" "Strictures of large calibre"; "Dilating urethrotomy"; "Urethrotomy, external and internal"; "Van Buren and Keyes on urethral calibre"; "Cure of perineal fistula"; "Errors of English and French schools"; "Relations of gleet to stricture"; and "Strictures of small calibres." The final chapter is most notable for a table detailing 136 operative cases of stricture. It is said that this book was so well received that for the next ten years every obscure urinary disorder from renal tuberculosis to urinary paralysis was treated by radical cure of a supposed urethral stricture. A second edition was published in 1880. Among Otis's other books are *Clinical lectures on the physiological pathology and treatment of syphilis; together with a fasciculus of classroom lessons covering the initiatory period* (New York: G. P. Putnam's Sons, 1881). (See also GU17 and GU21.)

GU12. **EDWARD LAWRENCE KEYES** (1843–1924). *The venereal diseases, including strictures of the male urethra.* 348pp. New York: William Wood, 1880.

Keyes was professor of dermatology and adjunct professor of surgery at Bellevue Hospital Medical College. This volume is No. 65 in Wood's Library of Standard Medical Authors. Keyes dedicated the book to William Van Buren (1819–83). Keyes outlines some of his views in the preface:

> This volume is designed by the publishers to be one of a series addressed to the general medical practitioner. My aim has, therefore, been to present the various venereal diseases as clearly as possible, avoiding such unnecessary refinement upon theoretical and mooted points as would be apt to lead to confusion or to error. Practical utility, as well as what I believe to be sound doctrine, has been kept constantly in view, and no effort has been made to display a long list of remedies . . . . I have opposed the views of those gentlemen who are throwing confusion in the way of the general practitioner by trying to break down the distinctions between the initial lesion of true syphilis, and chancroid; and who teach that chancroid may be derived from the products of the syphilitic early or late lesions. I have also taken issue with the experimenters who claim to prevent syphilis by excising the initial lesion, on the ground that something more than induration in a sore is necessary in order to prove it to be a syphilitic chancre . . . . Finally, I have raised my voice, for what it may be worth, in protest against the views of the new school in urethral pathology, which seems to claim that every natural undulation in the tissues of the pendulous urethra is a stricture fit for cutting, and that all the ills of the genitourinary passages may be accounted for by

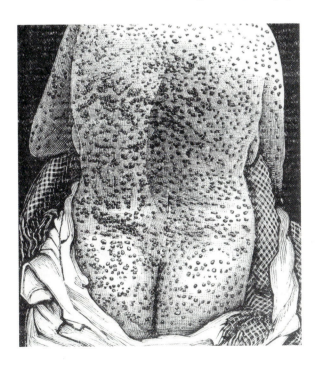

Fig. 120. (GU12) The illustrations in Keyes's work were wood engravings. This engraving, figure 10 on page 158, details generalized tubercular syphilis.

the existence of these undulations, and, usually, made to disappear when the latter are cut . . . .

The book had three parts: "Chancroid"; "Syphilis"; and "Gonorrhoea." There are no plates, but the book does contain forty-one wood engravings. There were no other editions. (See also GU9 and GU20.)

GU13. **SAMUEL WEISSELL GROSS** (1837–89). *A practical treatise on impotence, sterility, and allied disorders of the male sexual organs.* 174pp. Philadelphia: Henry C. Lea's Sons, 1881.

At the time this volume was written, Gross was lecturer on venereal and genitourinary diseases and clinical surgery at Jefferson Medical College. One of the foremost surgeons of his day, he believed that instead of relying on pressure alone to combat hemorrhaging, as was usually done, veins should be ligated as arteries were. He was also a vigorous early proponent of antiseptic surgery. Gross writes in the preface:

> My aim has been to supply in a compact form practical and strictly scientific information, especially adapted to the wants of the general practitioner, in regard to a class of common and grave disorders, upon the correction of which so much of human happiness depends . . . . I find that, with few exceptions, the woman alone commands attention in unfruitful marriages. The importance of examining the husband before subjecting the wife to operation will be appreciated when I state that he is, as a rule, at fault in at least one instance in every six.

There are only four chapters: "Impotence"; "Sterility"; "Spermatorrhoea"; and "Prostatorrhoea." The book has no plates but sixteen illustrations. It was available in cloth for $1.50. Further editions were published in 1883 and 1887. (See also GS97.)

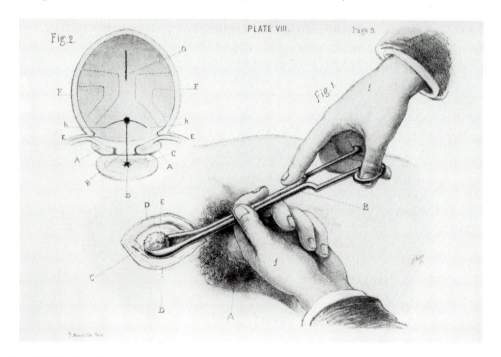

Fig. 121. (GU15) This chromolithograph plate, figure 8 on page 91, portrays Helmuth's method of extracting a bladder stone through an abdominal incision. H. Faber drew the plate and F. Moras of Philadelphia was lithographer.

GU14. **ALEXANDER W. STEIN** (1841–97). *A study of tumors of the bladder, with original contributions and drawings.* 94pp. New York: William Wood, 1881.

Born in Hungary, Stein received his M.D. from the University of the City of New York in 1867. He was professor of visceral anatomy and physiology at New York College of Dentistry from 1868 to 1875 and concurrently served as professor of comparative histology and physiology at New York College of Veterinary Surgery. He notes in the preface:

> . . . I began an inquiry as to the exact status of the literature upon tumors of the bladder. Although our subject required considerable research, having to seek chiefly in medical journals for the information, the field explored proved full of interest and replete with valuable information. I have endeavored to make this monograph as complete as possible in every practical detail bearing on the nature, symptomatology, diagnosis, and treatment of the diseases of which it treats . . . .

The contents include a detailed bibliography of bladder tumors; "Classification of tumors"; "Symptomatology"; "Diagnosis"; "Duration and prognosis"; and "Treatment." There are twelve drawings but no plates. This was the only edition.

GU15. **WILLIAM TOD HELMUTH** (1833–1902). *Suprapubic lithotomy; the high operation for stone-epicystotomy-hypogastric lithotomy (the high apparatus).* 93pp. New York: Boericke & Tafel, 1882.

Helmuth was one of the leading homeopathic surgeons in America from the 1860s until his death. He was a founder of the Homeopathic Medical College of Missouri and in 1867 served as president of the American Institute of Homeopathy. He was a vigorous defender of antiseptic and aseptic surgical procedures and in 1876 performed one of the earliest antiseptic operations in the United States (an ovariotomy). Helmuth's *Lithotomy* is a beautifully illustrated work containing eight lithographic plates and numerous wood engravings. At the time of its publication he was professor of surgery at New York Homeopathic Medical College. Helmuth comments on several procedures in his preface:

> In these days, when the entire surgical world is so deeply interested in Bigelow's litholapaxy, or, as it should be named, "the American method of lithotrity," it would appear almost inappropriate to call attention to any form of lithotomy, especially to that one, which, in the estimation of many surgeons, is the most unreliable, and only to be performed under most peculiar circumstances. So convinced, however, is the author of these pages that epicystotomy will, before many years have passed, receive a high place among all the cutting operations for stone in the bladder, especially in those cases in which litholapaxy is inappropriate, that this essay is offered to the profession . . . .

There are only five chapters, with the last demonstrating the method of epicystotomy and its aftertreatment. There was only one edition. (See also GS36.)

GU16. **EDWARD CARROLL FRANKLIN** (1822–85). *A manual of venereal diseases; being a condensed description of those affections and their homeopathic treatment.* 111pp. Chicago: Gross & Delbridge, 1883.

A professor of surgery in the homeopathic department of the University of Michigan, Franklin has been forgotten by American surgical historians. However, he was quite influential in his day because of his massive literary output. This short work consists of six chapters: "History of venereal diseases"; "Gonorrhoea and other diseases"; "Chancroid"; "Syphilis"; and two chapters on "Constitutional syphilis." Franklin discusses homeopathic theories of syphilis in the preface:

> This compendium of venereal diseases has been prepared for the use of practitioners and students of medicine, as a summary only of the recent investigations and advance views touching the various sequelae that follow in the train of these contagious disorders, and to lay before the profession the knowledge of the present day gained by the use of comparatively small doses of medicine in their treatment. Believing in the "dualistic theory" that the origin of the exciting virus which produces the local contagious ulcer, differs from that which develops true syphilis, the terms *chancroid* and *syphilis* are used to designate these two essentially distinct conditions. It is not intended that this little treatise shall take the place of the larger works on venereal diseases, but that it shall be a useful guide and a ready reference to the general practitioner . . . . As such it is committed to the profession, trusting that humanity may be benefited by its teachings, and that homeopathy may receive the proper credit due it in the more successful treatment of these affections by attenuated medicines, which our brethren of the allopathic school are slowly and grudgingly adopting.

This was Franklin's last textbook; he died less than eighteen months after its publication. (See also GS65, GS107, GS108, and OR35.)

GU17. **FESSENDEN NOTT OTIS** (1825–1900). *Practical clinical lessons on syphilis and the genitourinary diseases.* 2 volumes in one, 590pp. New York: Bermingham, 1883.

One of America's premier surgeons, Otis was fourth president of the American Association of Genito-Urinary Surgeons in 1890. This work is a massive compendium, with volume 1 devoted to syphilis and chancroid and volume 2 discussing gonorrhea and its sequelae. At the time of its publication, Otis was clinical professor of genitourinary diseases at the College of Physicians and Surgeons in New York. His preface explains the origin of this work:

> For a number of years it has been my custom, to distribute, from time to time, to the students of the College of Physicians and Surgeons, short papers, of a few pages each, which were entitled "Class-room Lessons." In these I endeavored to embody important principles, in the study of syphilis and the genito-urinary diseases. The lessons were intended to prevent errors, arising from inattention, or from misunderstanding of the statements made during the lectures. This was rendered especially necessary, from the fact that my own views, on certain important points, differed, essentially, from those embodied in the text-books in general use. In the first place, on the subject of syphilis: I had been

unable to accept the statements of all authorities, that it was a mysterious, instantaneous, poisoning of the organism, in defiance of all known physiological and pathological laws . . . . In the second place: early in my clinical teaching, I had found myself unable to accept the conventional views, held by authorities on many important points in genito-urinary diseases. Especially as to the nature and treatment of gonorrhea and urethral stricture and the normal urethral calibre . . . .

Volume 1 consists of thirty lessons describing all manifestations of syphilis and their treatments. Lessons 31–62 in volume 2 deal with gonorrhea. The remaining twenty-three lessons touch on various topics and use numerous case presentations. There are no plates, although the work is heavily illustrated. (See also GU11 and GU21.)

GU18. **WILLIAM THOMAS BELFIELD** (1856–1929). *Diseases of the urinary and male sexual organs.* 351pp. New York: William Wood, 1884.

Belfield was born in St. Louis and graduated from Rush Medical College in 1878. Considered the outstanding urologist in Chicago, he is reported to have been among the first in America to demonstrate the tubercle bacillus and the gonococcus. He was also a leader in teaching bacteriology. At the time this work was published, Belfield was pathologist at Cook County Hospital and surgeon in the genitourinary department at the Central Dispensary. He performed the first suprapubic prostatectomy in the United States in 1886 and introduced cystoscopy to the Midwest. Belfield writes in the preface:

When the preparation of this volume was undertaken, it was the author's hope to present a resume of current knowledge of the topics herein discussed, with comments suggested by personal observation and experience. In the execution of this plan he has been seriously embarrassed by the brevity of the period allotted for the work, which has permitted no opportunity for a minute scrutiny of pertinent literature, for a careful revision of the text, nor for the addition of a bibliography. Yet, as the patience of the publishers has been already severely tried by the author's unavoidable tardiness, he prefers to submit the original draft of the book, incomplete and crude as it may seem, rather than to postpone still further the appearance of a volume long since due . . . . Convinced that a lack of care and thoroughness in the investigations of patients is responsible for many failures in the management of urinary and genital disorders especially, the author has endeavored to present fully the necessity and the means for diagnosis as an essential preliminary to treatment . . . .

Diseases of the urinary organs are discussed in nineteen chapters, and those of the male sexual organ in chapters 20–23. Like most of the other books in Wood's Library of Standard Medical Authors (of which this is volume 90), there are no plates and only twenty-four wood engravings. Among Belfield's other medical books are *On the relations of microorganisms to disease* (New York: Trow, 1883) and *The practical home physician; a popular guide for the management of household disease* (Chicago: Western, 1884), cowritten with Henry M. Lyman (1835–1904), Christian Fenger (1840–1902), and H. Webster Jones.

GU19. **HENRY O. WALKER** (1843–1912). *The treatment of diseases of the bladder, prostate, and urethra.* Detroit: G. S. Davis, 1887.

Walker was a graduate of Albion College and received his M.D. from Bellevue Hospital Medical College in 1867. He returned to his home city of Detroit, where he soon began to specialize in diseases of the genitourinary organs and the rectum. His only academic post was professor of diseases of genitourinary ograns and rectum at Detroit Medical College. This small volume was part of Series III of Davis's Physicians' Leisure Library. It was available paperbound for twenty-five cents or in cloth for fifty cents. The book is now extremely scarce.

GU20. **EDWARD LAWRENCE KEYES** (1843–1924). *The surgical diseases of the genito-urinary organs, including syphilis.* 704pp. New York: D. Appleton, 1888.

This volume was a revision of Van Buren and Keyes's previous book on the same subjects (GU9). However, Keyes completely rewrote it following Van Buren's death, and it is thus essentially a new work. At the time of its publication, Keyes was professor of genitourinary surgery, syphilology, and dermatology at Bellevue Hospital Medical College. He notes in the preface:

> Time and surgical advance have destroyed in great part the value of the original treatise upon which this revision is founded, making it an unsafe guide as a textbook upon certain subjects. The original book for which my dear old master and myself were mutually responsible was issued in 1874, and since that date until the present time has received no material alteration. The whole subject of litholapaxy has had its birth since that date; suprapubic cystotomy has been restored to a new life; the surgery of the kidney has been constructed anew, and radical changes have been introduced into the surgery of the tunica vaginalis

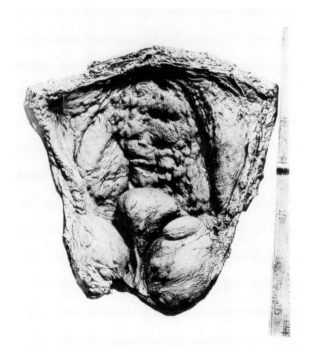

Fig. 122. (GU22) Watson made extensive use of photogravure plates in his work. This particular one (number 8, page 61) demonstrates hypertrophy of the lateral and median lobes of the prostate.

and that relating to the treatment of varicocele . . . . to bring the book up to date, therefore, it became necessary to recast it entirely, and the publishers have found it expedient to destroy the old stereotyped plates and to set up the entire book anew in type . . . . I have missed the kindly counsel and the mature judgment of my friend and teacher, without which the original of this work would not have been written. His absence from this revision is to be deplored; but I feel justified in making the revision because there appears to be a demand for it, and because all the text of the original work came from my pen except chapters XIV, XV, XVI, and XVII on stone. One of these chapters I have left unchanged, out of respect to my former partner; the others have been rewritten. The book as it stands is an honest exhibit of my views upon all the subjects considered.

There are twenty-eight chapters in part 1, "Diseases of the genito-urinary organs" and thirteen in part 2, "Chancroid and syphilis." Revised editions of this book were published in 1903 and 1905. These printings were written with Keyes's son, Edward Loughborough Keyes (1873–?), also a well-known urologist. He in turn wrote the following textbooks: *Syphilis* (New York: D. Appleton, 1908) and *Disease of the genito-urinary organs considered from a medical and surgical standpoint, including a description of gonorrhea in the female and conditions peculiar to the female urinary organs* (New York: D. Appleton, 1910). (See also GU9 and GU12.)

GU21. **FESSENDEN NOTT OTIS** (1825–1900). *The male urethra, its diseases and reflexes.* 86pp. Detroit: G. S. Davis, 1888.

Otis was clinical professor of genitourinary diseases at the College of Physician and Surgeons in New York. This small volume was part of Series IV of Davis's Physicians' Leisure Library. The table of contents (pages v-viii) is rather extensive and includes Halsted's method of treating gonorrhea (page 65) and his irrigation apparatus (page 66). Other interesting topics include the cure of gleet by division of meatus (page 78) and a retrojection apparatus for treatment of gonorrhea (page 64). This was the only edition. (See also GU11 and GU17.)

GU22. **FRANCIS SEDGWICK WATSON** (1853–1942). *The operative treatment of the hypertrophied prostate.* 167pp. Boston: Cupples & Hurd, 1888.

Watson was one of the premier urologists in Boston. At the time this work was published he was surgeon to outpatients at Boston City Hospital and instructor in minor surgery and the surgery of the urinary organs at Harvard Medical School. Watson was to remain associated with these two institutions for the remainder of his professional life. He is best remembered for having performed the first median perineal prostatectomy in 1889 [G-M 4266]. He was elected to membership in the American Association of Genito-Urinary Surgeons in 1887, the second year of its existence. This monograph was delivered as a paper before that association when it met as part of the first triennial meeting of the Congress of American Physicians and Surgeons in Washington, D.C., in 1888. Watson explains the reasons for this work in his preface:

In the study of this subject I was led to two conclusions, viz., that in spite of the meagreness of many clinical reports of cases, there was nevertheless sufficient material from reliable observers to be of value if collated; and furthermore, that the profession is performing radical operations upon the hypertrophied prostate with greatly increasing frequency, but without having established any rational groundwork for the practice to rest upon. Further investigation led me to the belief that it was a simple matter to supply such a groundwork. And in the hope of furthering this subject, the investigation and its results are offered together with some additional suggestions as to technique.

The contents include a rather substantial bibliography, and chapters such as "Enumeration of surgical methods"; "Status of contemporary surgical opinion"; "Absence of rationale in surgical treatment"; "Principal objects of this work"; "Anatomical data"; "Inferences derived from their study"; "Clinical data"; "Immediate and remote results of operations"; "Author's cases and instruments"; and "Conclusions, and additional notes on one or two points of technique." It was illustrated with a number of lithographic plates. This was the only edition. Other books by Watson include the two-volume *Disease and surgery of the genitourinary system* (Philadelphia: Lea & Febiger, 1908), written with John J. Cunningham; *A day with the specialists; or, cured at last; a tragic farcelet* (New York: Grafton, 1910); and a privately printed autobiography, *A bundle of memories* (Boston: 1910–11).

GU23. **HAL C. WYMAN** (1852–1908). *Diseases of the bladder and prostate.* 132pp. Detroit: G. S. Davis, 1891.

Wyman was one of the earliest surgeons to perform basic science research. He served as professor of surgery at the Michigan College of Medicine and Surgery in Detroit. The preface explains his purpose:

These pages have been written for the purpose of getting together the best ideas concerning the injuries and diseases of the bladder and prostate, to enable the writer to do better work for the sufferers from a class of very painful and dangerous infirmities. If his fellow practitioners find after reading them any material which will kindle enthusiasm for the same studies, he will feel amply repaid for the time devoted to writing.

The book has no table of contents and only a limited index, which makes it difficult to read. (See also GS136.)

GU24. **CHARLES HOWARD CHETWOOD** (1866–?). *Genito-urinary and venereal diseases.* 178pp. Philadelphia: Lea Brothers, 1892.

Chetwood practiced in New York, where he was visiting surgeon at Demilt Dispensary's department of surgery and genitourinary diseases. This volume is part of Lea's Students' Quiz Series and was available for $1.00; an interleaved version for taking notes cost $1.25. The book was designed primarily as a quiz-compend, and Chetwood notes in the preface: ". . . the method which the author has endeavored to follow is to present the various subjects by questions which would be apt to arise in the mind of the student and practitioner, and to form the answers in a conversational and descriptive manner, avoiding terse summaries . . . . "
The topics include "Anatomy and physiology"; "Syphilis"; "Chancroid";

"Disease of the male urethra"; "Gonorrhea"; "Diseases of the penis and adjacent parts"; "Cutaneous affections"; "Prostate gland"; "Bladder"; "Ureters"; "Kidney"; and "Testicle and cord." There was only one edition. Chetwood's other book, *Venereal diseases; their complications and sequelae*, was coauthored with Edward Lawrence Keyes (1843–1924) (New York: William Wood, 1900).

GU25. **JOHN WILLIAMS SEVERIN GOULEY** (1832–1920). *Diseases of the urinary apparatus; phlegmasic affections*. 342pp. New York: D. Appleton, 1892.

Gouley lists himself as "surgeon to Bellevue Hospital." This treatise was actually

> ... twelve lectures, principally on phlegmasic affections of the urinary apparatus, constituting the first part of a series, delivered during the autumn of 1891, and published in the *New York Medical Journal* ... revised [and] republished in this form as a contribution to the pathology and treatment of a class of diseases the gravity and frequency of which render them worthy of the closest study. The views expressed in these conferences are based upon long observation of morbid processes, frequent comparison of the effects of different means of cure, and careful examination of foreign and American works on adrology. Owing to the almost incessant advances in patho-histology, bio-chemics, and therapeutics, many of the conclusions herein stated may be regarded as only provisional.

Section 1 consists of three chapters dealing with general considerations. Special considerations are discussed in section 2 in chapters 4–12. There is a rather lengthy (pages 309–33) discourse concerning retention of urine from prostatic obstruction in elderly men, and its nature, diagnosis, and management. There were no other editions. (See also GU8.)

GU26. **GEORGE FRANK LYDSTON** (1858–1923). *Varicocele and its treatment*. 126pp. Chicago: W. T. Keener, 1892.

The author of innumerable texts, Lydston was an outstanding Chicago urologist who, because of sociopolitical considerations, was never allowed to become a member of the Chicago Urological Society. He received his M.D. in 1879 from Bellevue Hospital Medical College. Lydston moved to Chicago in 1882 and remained there for the rest of his professional career. In 1891 he was named professor of the surgical diseases of the genitourinary organs and venereal diseases at Chicago College of Physicians and Surgeons and surgeon-in-chief of the genitourinary and venereal department at West Side Dispensary. With numerous illustrations, this monograph was Lydston's first book-length work. He writes in the preface that " ... an attempt has been made to present in a concise and at the same time in a comprehensive manner a review of the subject of varicocele and its treatment .... [but] no attempt has been made to consume paper by verbose padding, the salient points being kept in view .... " The eight chapters are quite detailed, with operative treatment found in chapter 7. The final chapter contains an extensive bibliography on varicocele. Among Lydston's other books are *Addresses and essays* (Louisville: Renz & Henry, 1891); *Over the hookah;*

the tales of a talkative doctor (Chicago: F. Klein, 1896), *Panama and the Sierras; a doctor's wander days* (Chicago: Riverton, 1900), *The diseases of society (the vice and crime problem)* (Philadelphia: J. B. Lippincott, 1904), and *Impotence and sterility: with aberrations of the sexual function and sex-gland implantation* (Chicago, 1917). (See also GU27, GU28, and GU45.)

GU27. **GEORGE FRANK LYDSTON** (1858–1923). *Gonorrhoea and urethritis.* 216pp. Detroit: G. S. Davis, 1892.

Lydston was not only interested in genitourinary and venereal diseases but also served as lecturer on criminal anthropology at Union Law School. His work on criminal sociology dealt with forensic and degenerative factors from a broad critical viewpoint. In *Gonorrhoea* he writes that he " . . . has taken the liberty of reiterating the views upon the evolution of gonorrhoea which were originally published in an essay several years ago. Aside from this indulgence in more or less speculative theorizing, the work will, it is hoped, be found to be distinctively practical." There is no table of contents, but an extensive index appears on pages 209–16. There are few illustrations. This was the only edition. (See also GU26, GU28, and GU45.)

GU28. **GEORGE FRANK LYDSTON** (1858–1923). *Stricture of the urethra.* 334pp. Chicago: W. T. Keener, 1893.

Lydston was attending surgeon at Cook County Hospital as well as professor of the surgical diseases of the genitourinary organs and syphilology at the Chicago College of Physicians and Surgeons. He notes in the preface to this impressive and scarce work that

> this volume comprises essentially a series of classroom lectures upon urethral stricture. No attempt has been made to fill the work with rubbish from the literary dead lumber room, or to introduce innovations, more startling and misguided than practical. The genito-urinary specialist, or to use a more modern term, the andrologist, may find that a great deal of old straw has been threshed over, but the general practitioner and students—for whom the book is especially designed—may find a few grains of practicality not hitherto presented in a readily assimilable form . . . .

There are seven full-page color plates and eighty-five woodcuts. The book contains thirteen chapters; chapter 12 is of particular interest because it concerns the use of electrolysis for urethral stricture. (See also GU26, GS27, and GU45.)

GU29. **PRINCE ALBERT MORROW** (1846–1913), ed. *A system of genitourinary diseases, syphilology and dermatology.* 3 volumes. New York: D. Appleton, 1893–94.

The book was the first American textbook on genitourinary diseases to have multiple authors. Morrow was clinical professor of genitourinary diseases at the University of the City of New York and also surgeon at Charity Hospital. He received his M.D. from the University Medical College of New York in 1873. In 1898 he was named clinical professor of genitourinary diseases at University-Bellevue Hospital Medical College. A prolific writer, Morrow edited the *Journal of cutaneous and venereal diseases* from 1882 to 1892. He writes in the preface to the *System's* first volume:

> The genius of modern medical literature is clearly in the direction of division of labor and associated effort. The marked favor with which the numerous "Systems" and "Cyclopedias" which have appeared in recent years have been received by the profession would seem to show that the composite treatise represents the ideal method of bookmaking. In fact, cooperation is the essential condition of thoroughness and completeness in a work covering a wide range of subjects. The field of research in every department of medicine has grown so large that it is hardly possible for any one individual to carefully sift from the mass of new material accumulated by the great body of workers the facts and opinions which represent a distinct advance in our knowledge, and have a definite and permanent value . . . . The editor has enlisted the cooperation of distinguished specialists, each of whom has been selected for his special fitness to write on the subject assigned, and which has been, as far as practicable, the subject of his choice . . . . The authors are responsible for the views expressed in their respective articles, and to them is due the credit for whatever value the work may possess . . . .

Among the authors and their topics in volume 1 ("Genito-urinary diseases") are George Woolsey (1861–?), "Anatomy and physiology of the genitourinary organs"; Ramon Guiteras (1859–1917), "Diseases of the penis"; George Emerson Brewer (1861–1939), "Acute urethritis-gonorrhea"; Hermann Klotz (1844–?), "Endoscopy"; Frank Hartley, "Gonorrheal rheumatism"; James P. Tuttle (1857–1913), "Gonorrhea of the rectum, nose, mouth, ear, umbilicus, and axilla"; J. William White (1850–1916), "Stricture of the urethra"; W. T. Belfield (1856–1929), "Diseases of the prostate"; Joseph D. Bryant (1845–1914), "The functional disorders of micturition"; Eugene Fuller (1858–1930), "Diagnostic significance of pathological modifications in the urine"; Willy Meyer (1858–?), "Cystoscopy"; Samuel Alexander, "Cystitis"; George Ryerson Fowler (1846–1906), "Injuries and diseases of the bladder"; Alexander Stein (1841–97), "Rupture of the bladder"; Francis Sedgwick Watson (1853–1942), "Tumors of the bladder"; Arthur T. Cabot (1852–1912), "Stone in the bladder, prostate, urethra, and ureters"; Lewis A. Stimson (1844–1917), "Surgical diseases of the kidney"; John P. Bryson, "Tuberculosis uro-genitalis"; John A. Wyeth (1845–1922), "Hydrocele and spermatocele"; and Edward L. Keyes (1843–1924), "Varicocele".

Volume 2 ("Syphilology") includes chapters by W. R. Townsend on "Syphilitic affections of the bones"; John N. Mackenzie, "Syphilis of the upper air-passages, including the nose, pharynx, larynx, trachea, and bronchi"; W. T. Councilman (1854–1933), "Visceral syphilis"; Bernard Sachs, "Syphilis of the nervous system"; Charles Stedman Bull (1844–1911), "Syphilis of the eye and its appendages"; and Edward Martin (1859–1938), "Chancroid." There are numerous color plates and illustrations throughout all three volumes. Morrow's other books consist of *Venereal memoranda* (New York: William Wood, 1885), *Drug eruptions: a clinical study of the irritants of drugs upon the skin* (New York: William Wood, 1887), *Atlas of skin and venereal diseases* (New

York: William Wood, 1888–89), and *Social diseases and marriage, social prophylaxis* (New York: Lea Brothers, 1904).

GU30. **BUKK G. CARLETON** (1856–1914). *A manual of genito-urinary and venereal diseases.* 315pp. New York: Boericke, Runyon & Ernesty, 1895.

Carleton was a homeopath who was genitourinary surgeon and specialist at the Metropolitan Hospital in New York. He received his medical education at the New York Homeopathic College and graduated in 1876. In 1902 he was elected professor of genitourinary surgery at his alma mater. The *Manual* was his first book and is said to have been the best selling special work by a homeopathic surgeon, perhaps because it was the first homeopathic work published on urology. It was originally available in cloth for $3.00 or half morocco for $4.00. The thirty-nine chapters cover a wide range of subject matter. Included are special sections on "Venereal diseases of the eye" by Charles Deady and "Vesical calculus and external urethrotomy" by William Francis Honan. A reprint of the first edition appeared in 1901. This was the first homeopathic work issued by Boericke, Runyon & Ernesty. Among Carleton's other books are *Symptomatic index of the homeopathic materia medica in urological diseases* (New York: Boericke & Tafel, 1903) and *A treatise on urological and venereal diseases* (Philadelphia: Boericke & Tafel, 1905). (See also GU40 and GU41.)

GU31. **EDWARD MARTIN** (1859–1938). *Impotence and sexual weakness in the male and female.* 102pp. Detroit: G. S. Davis, 1895.

Martin was surgeon at Howard Hospital and clinical professor of genitourinary surgery at the University of Pennsylvania. He later became one of the most prominent surgeons in Philadelphia. This small monograph contained four chapters: "Impotence and sexual weakness"; "Prostatorrhea"; "Involuntary seminal emissions"; and "Impotence of the female." A second edition was published in 1895. (See also GS134, GS142, GS147, and GU38.)

GU32. **EUGENE FULLER** (1858–1930). *Disorders of the male sexual organs.* 241pp. Philadelphia: Lea Brothers, 1895.

Fuller was a graduate of Harvard Medical School, but practiced for most of his life in New York. At the time this volume was published he was an instructor in genitourinary and venereal diseases at New York Post-Graduate Medical School. Fuller is best remembered for having been the first to accomplish the removal of both intravesical and intraurethral enlargements of the prostate by the process of suprapubic enucleation [G-M 4263]. From 1885 to 1895, he was associated with Edward L. Keyes (1843–1924). The *Disorders* was a product of their large clinical practice, and according to the American Urological Association's *History of urology,* (volume 1, page 80) "was the most strikingly original work that New York urology produced during the latter part of the nineteenth century." Fuller comments in the preface:

Considering the importance of a properly regulated sexual function to the happiness and well-being of man, it is remarkable that hitherto so little scientific study and attention should have been devoted to investigations upon that subject . . . . The rich harvest reaped by advertising mediums and quacks in this department is in great measure due to the unsatisfactory manner in which these cases are handled by the regular profession . . . . My opinion is that trouble located in the sexual apparatus, and primarily, at least, largely independent of nervous conditions, is the chief cause of sexual disturbance in the male; and that the various neuroses and psychological prostaons stand in the order named as other causes . . . .

The seven chapters are "Anatomy"; "Physiology"; "Pathology"; "Clinical features"; "Differential diagnowelve l; "Treatment and pro compli170; and "Illustrative instances." There are only a few illustrations. Fuller's other book is *Disease of the genito-urinary system; a thorough treatise on urinary and sexual surgery* (New York: Macmillan, 1900).

GU33. **ROBERT WILLIAM TAYLOR** (1842–1908). *The pathology and treatment of venereal diseases.* 1,002pp. Philadelphia: Lea Brothers, 1895.

Taylor was born in England but came to America as a boy in 1850. He graduated from the College of Physicians and Surgeons in New York in 1868. He soon came under the influence of Freeman J. Bumstead (1826–79), and as a result turned his attention from general practice to the study of venereal and genitourinary diseases. At the time this volume was published, Taylor was clinical professor of venereal diseases at his alma mater and surgeon at Bellevue Hospital. He was a founding member and early president of the American Dermatological Association. The work is massive in scope. Taylor writes in the preface:

In preparing this volume the endeavor has been made to present the subjects herein considered on a level with our advanced knowledge of today. So vast is the mass of accumulated knowledge regarding venereal diseases, their sequelae, and allied conditions, that no one man's experience can cover the whole ground. Consequently, the author who would offer to the profession an acceptable textbook on these subjects must supplement his own studes and observation by the experiences of all observers whose works show inherent evidence of truth and progress, and he must deduce therefrom, in a thoroughly scientific and conservative spirit, the essential facts and the concrete knowledge thus far obtained . . . .

Part 1, "Gonorrhea and its complications" consists of forty-two chapters, and part 2, "Chancroid or soft chancre," consists of seven chapters. Syphilis is discussed in part 3 in thirty-eight chapters. The book contains 230 illustrations and seven color plates. There were no further editions. (See also OR31 and GU37.)

GU34. **ROBERT W. STEWART** (1853–?). *The diseases of the male urethra.* 221pp. New York: William Wood, 1896.

Stewart practiced in Pittsburgh, where he was an attending surgeon at Mercy Hospital. This work contains twenty-six chapters, most of which are devoted to forms of urethritis. Chapter 8 discusses urethral endoscopy, and chapter 9 treats urethral mensuration. Cowperitis and epididymitis are treated in chapters 17 and 19, respectively. Stewart comments in the preface:

> It may be justly asserted that in no part of the human frame does an accurate conception of its structure and functions have so important a bearing on the proper understanding of its diseases as in the urethra, and it may be said with equal justice that in no other part of the human frame have such erroneous anatomical and pathological views been so obstinately maintained . . . . It will be the object of the writer to place before the reader the diseases of the urethra, as viewed from the modern stand-point, promising, however, that those facts relating to the subject that are too well established to be open for discussion will be dwelt upon as briefly as is consistent with their proper elucidation . . . .

This book was the only one Stewart wrote.

GU35. **FRANCIS E. DOUGHTY** (1847–?). *A practical working handbook in the diagnosis and treatment of diseases of the genito-urinary system and syphilis.* 461pp. Philadelphia: Boericke & Tafel, 1897.

Doughty, an 1868 graduate of the College of Physicians and Surgeons of New York, served as professor of genitourinary diseases at the New York Homeopathic Medical College. This rather scarce book presents Doughty's lecture notes as transcribed and edited by George Parker Holden, one of his students, a circumstance that is explained in the preface:

> This little work originated through the solicitation of a number of the author's classmates, during his college days. Its beginning appeared in the Fall of 1893, in printed unbound leaves of 88 pages . . . . This little edition was quite rapidly disposed of to the students of the different classes, and attracting the attention now and then of an already-established physician, there came an entirely unexpected demand from this outside source . . . . These lectures were delivered from headings merely, and in an off-hand style . . . and it will be readily understood that this valuable characteristic, appropriate enough in the present circumstances, could not be retained in a more pretentious book which must need preserve a stricter literary and classical form . . . . Thus this little treatise is finally launched upon its perilous journey amidst the world's august and ponderous volumes constituting medical literature.

The chapter headings include "Diseases of the bladder and testicle"; "Hydrocele"; "Hematocele"; "Galactocele"; "Spermatocele"; "Varicocele"; "Chancroid, bubo, and syphilis"; "Notable cases of hermaphroditism, and of elephantiasis of scrotum and penis"; and "Sexual neuroses." This was the only edition.

GU36. **NICHOLAS SENN** (1844–1908). *Tuberculosis of the genito-urinary organs, male and female.* 317pp. Philadelphia: W. B. Saunders, 1897.

Senn, who performed early research in the surgical management of tuberculosis, was professor of the practice of surgery and clinical surgery at Rush Medical College. He writes in the preface:

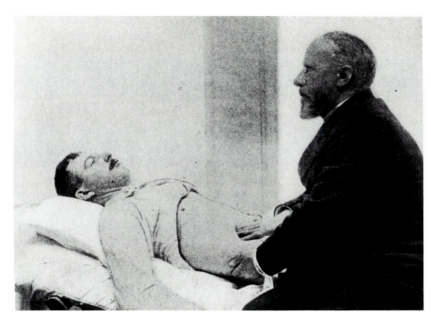

Fig. 123. (GU36) Senn had himself photographed while performing renal palpation (figure 25 on page 273).

> Tuberculosis of the male and female genito-urinary organs is such a frequent, distressing, and fatal affection that a special treatise on this subject at the present time appears to fill a gap in medical literature . . . . In the preparation of this book it has been the object of the author to place the available clinical material upon an etiologico-pathological basis . . . . The medical and surgical therapeutics of the affections of which this book treats are at this time not in a satisfactory state, but the opinions and views of surgeons of large experiences have been freely quoted, and in appropriate places the author has related the results of his own clinical observations.

Among the ten chapters are "Tuberculosis of the male genital organs"; "Testicle and epididymis"; "Female organs of generation"; "Vulva"; "Vagina"; "Uterus"; "Fallopian tubes"; "Ovary"; "Bladder"; and "Kidney." There are twenty-six illustrations with six color plates depicting histological structures. Of interest is the early use of clinical photographs in a urological textbook (figures 23, 25, 26). The book was available in cloth for $3.00. This was the only edition. (See also GS138, GS139, GS140, GS144, GS162, GS168, and OR49.)

GU37. **ROBERT WILLIAM TAYLOR** (1842–1908). *A practical treatise on sexual disorders of the male and female.* 451pp. Philadelphia: Lea Brothers, 1897.

Besides being a well-known clinical professor of venereal diseases at the College of Physicians and Surgeons (Columbia College) in New York, Taylor was an accomplished bibliophile. He collected one of the most valuable libraries on syphilology and dermatology in this country, with most of the rarer editions eventually being donated to the New York Academy of Medicine. Taylor describes his purpose in writing the book in the preface:

> The aim of the author of this volume has been to portray the various forms of sexual disorder in the male on the basis of advanced knowledge of the anatomy, physiology, and pathology of the various por-

tions of the sexual sphere. The failure of antecedent treatises on this subject to present to the reader clear cut and practical information on these disorders rests on the fact that symptoms of sexual debility—termed functional disturbances and sensory and motor neuroses—overmastered the minds of the writers, and, as a result, no completeness of description whatever was attained; but, on the contrary, unimportant points were unduly magnified, essential ones slurred over or wrongly presented, gross errors were made, and a standard of real pro-gress was not attained. Just so long as an author is biased by visionary theories and entrammelled by his study and descriptions of such symptoms as abnormal seminal losses, spermatorrhea, pollutions, sexual weakness and irritability, etc., he can be expected to produce an incomplete and unscientific treatise . . . . I venture to hope that this volume will prove a helpful manual to the general practitioner in the management of a very large group of cases which has heretofore been ill understood and even avoided by them.

The twenty-three chapters include "Nature and composition of the seminal fluid"; "Impotence"; "Azoospermatism"; "Masturbation and sexual excesses"; "Spermatorrhea"; "Sexual worry and hypochondriasis and sexual neurasthenia"; "Coitus reservatus vel interruptus"; "Withdrawal, or conjugal onanism"; "Priapism and sexual erethism"; "Sexual perversion"; and "Sterility in the female." There are seventy-three illustrations and eight plates in color and monotone. Further editions were published in 1900 and 1905. (See also OR31 and GU33.)

GU38. **JAMES WILLIAM WHITE** (1850–1916) and **EDWARD MARTIN** (1859–1938). *Genito-urinary surgery and venereal diseases*. 1,061pp. Philadelphia: J. B. Lippincott, 1897.

White graduated from the University of Pennsylvania Medical School in 1871. Initially appointed professor of genitourinary diseases at his alma mater, he was professor of clinical surgery when this volume was published. White later assumed the John Rhea Barton Chair of Surgery, which he held until 1911. Perhaps his most important claim to originality in surgical research was the concept that hypertrophy of the prostate could be cured by orchidectomy. This technique was widely utilized, although it eventually fell into disrepute. Martin was clinical professor of genitourinary diseases at the University of Pennsylvania. Agnes Repplier describes their collaboration in her *J. William White, M.D., a biography* (Boston: Houghton Mifflin, 1919, pages 88–89):

> In 1897 he published in collaboration with Dr. Edward Martin, a work on "Genito-Urinary Surgery and Venereal Diseases." It was an exhaustive and authoritative study, furnished with two hundred and forty-three illustrations, and seven coloured plates. The success which attended this volume . . . brought the doctor . . . sharply before the public eye . . . .

White and Martin write in the preface:

> In the preparation of this work we have endeavored to present clearly and with sufficient detail the generally accepted teachings of the day in regard to the pathology, symptomatology, diagnosis, and treatment of syphilis and genito-urinary diseases . . . . As it was our wish to make this

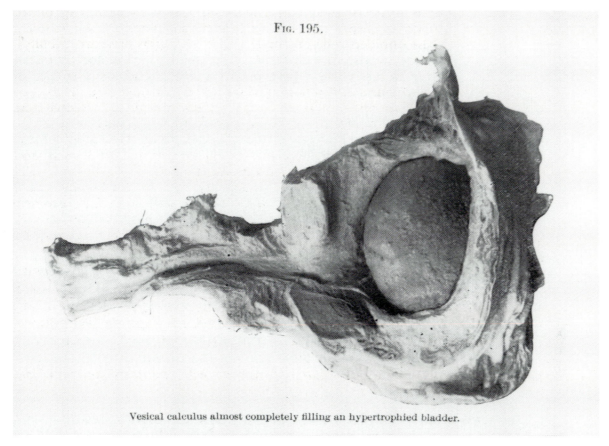

FIG. 195.

Vesical calculus almost completely filling an hypertrophied bladder.

Fig. 124. (GU38) White and Keys used this photograph (number 195, page 708) to demonstrate an enormous vesical calculus which had entirely filled a hypertrophied bladder.

> book one of practical use to the physician, much space has been devoted to symptomatology, diagnosis, and treatment. The pathological alterations characteristic of the diseases and injuries described have been briefly outlined, avoiding discussion of questions still unsettled. Historical considerations have been abbreviated as much as possible . . . .

There are twenty-nine chapters; chapter 27 ("Injuries and diseases of the prostate") presents White's theories on prostatic hypertrophy and treatment. Further editions were published in 1898, 1900, 1902, 1905, 1906, 1907, and 1910. (See also GS134, GS142, GS147, GS154, and GU31.)

GU39. **LEMUEL BOLTON BANGS** (1842–1914) and **WILLIAM AUGUSTUS HARDAWAY** (1850–1923). *An American textbook of genito-urinary diseases, syphilis and diseases of the skin.* 1,229pp. Philadelphia: W. B. Saunders, 1898.

Part of Saunders's American Text-Book Series, this comprehensive work was illustrated with 300 engravings and twenty full-page color plates. It was sold by subscription only for $7.00 in cloth or $8.00 in half morocco. Bangs was an 1872 graduate of the College of Physicians and Surgeons of New York and soon became associated with Fessenden Nott Otis (1825–1900). From 1889 to 1894 he was professor of genito-urinary diseases at the New York Post-Graduate Medical School and Hospital. At the time this volume was written, Bangs was consulting surgeon at St. Luke's Hospital in New York. Elected to membership in the American Association of Genito-Urinary Surgeons in 1887, he was the association's president in 1895. Hardaway was a well-known dermatologist from St. Louis who is best remembered for the first description of prurigo nodularis [G-M 4076]. When this book was published, he was professor of diseases of the skin and syphilis at Missouri Medical College. This book was a multiauthor work like the other books in this series. Among the contributors were G. Frank Lydston (1858–1923) on "Diseases of the male urethra"; B. Farquhar Curtis on "Diseases of the penis"; Eugene Fuller (1858–1930) on "Diseases of the testicle and its coverings, the cord, and the seminal vesicle"; Francis S. Watson (1853–1942) on "Vesical calculus"; Christian Fenger (1840–1902) on "Diseases of the ureter"; and John T. Bowen (1857–1941) on the "Physiology and anatomy of the skin." Among Hardaway's other books are *Essentials of vaccination; a compilation of facts relating to vaccine inoculation and its influence in the prevention of smallpox* (Chicago: Jansen & McClurg, 1882), *Manual of skin diseases, with special reference to diagnosis and treatment* (St. Louis: T. F. Lange, 1890), and *Handbook of cutaneous therapeutics, including section on the x-ray, high-frequency current and the minor surgery of the skin* (Philadelphia: Lea Brothers, 1907), authored with Joseph Grindon (1858–?).

GU40. **BUKK G. CARLETON** (1856–1914). *Medical and surgical diseases of the kidneys and ureters.* 253pp. New York: Boericke, Runyon & Ernesty, 1898.

This extremely elusive volume was designed as a companion piece to Carleton's *Genito-urinary and venereal diseases* (GU30). It thus completed coverage of uropoietic diseases. At the time it was published, Carleton was genitourinary surgeon and specialist at the Metropolitan Hospital in New York. One of America's most prolific authors on urological surgery, he nevertheless is an obscure figure in surgical history today. The volume was available in cloth for $2.75. It contains forty chapters. There are numerous illustrations and a small number of plates. A greatly revised edition containing thirty-three photomicrographs and six lucotype figures was published under the title *Uropoietic Diseases* in 1900 and again in 1902. (See also GU41.)

GU41. **BUKK G. CARLETON** (1856–1914). *A practical treatise on the sexual disorders of men.* 169pp. New York: Boericke, Runyon & Ernesty, 1898.

This work continues Carleton's series on uropoietic diseases. Carleton writes in the preface:

> The physical and mental manifestations of the sexual disorders of men have long been an unfailing source of profit to unscrupulous practitioners and charlatans, who, with their literature and advice, have often caused untold misery and almost irreparable damage. This class of ailments being so frequent and intractable the author believes that

a more complete understanding of them with their manifold complications and reflexes will lead to a better appreciation of their gravity. With this view in mind, this little volume is presented to the medical profession . . . .

There are twenty-one chapters, which provide a comprehensive look at the subject. No illustrations or plates are provided. A second edition appeared in 1900. (See also GU30 and GU40.)

GU42. **GEORGE MARQUET PHILLIPS** (1862–?).   *A handbook of genito-urinary surgery and venereal diseases.* 313pp. St. Louis: Shallcross & McCallum, 1898.

Phillips was professor of genitourinary surgery and venereal diseases at Barnes Medical College in St. Louis. He writes in the preface:

> This treatise is ventured in appreciation of the needs of the medical practitioner and those students of medicine who feel themselves unable, on account of the cost, or unwilling, on account of time, to devote themselves to the larger and more exhaustive works upon such matters . . . to be practical, and present all matters in their most comprehensive manner, has been aimed. The illustrations here produced are new, many being hand drawings by the celebrated histologist and artist, L. Crusius, M.D. (deceased) . . . .

The fourteen chapters include "Anatomy and physiology"; "Deformities"; "Urethral curve and irregularities"; "Urethral examination and diseases"; "Complications and gonorrhea"; "Diseases of the prostate"; "Chancroid"; "Diseases of the kidney"; "Stricture of the urethra"; "Stone in the bladder"; "Disturbances of urination"; "Tumors in the scrotum"; "Irregularities of testes"; and "Sexual disturbances." Many of the illustrations are halftone cuts. There were no further editions. Phillips's other book is *Prostatic hypertrophy from every surgical standpoint* (St. Louis: Ajod, 1903).

GU43. **KENT B. WAITE** (?–?). *A textbook of genito-urinary surgery.* 267pp. Cleveland: Privately printed, 1898.

Waite, the author of this extremely elusive text, was professor of genitourinary diseases and operative surgery at Cleveland University of Medicine and Surgery. He remains little known today because he was a homeopathic surgeon, and his only clinical affiliation was to Cleveland Homeopathic Hospital College. (This school later became part of Ohio State University Medical School in Columbus.) The text mainly presented Waite's personal views and was privately published in a limited printing.

GU44. **ELLWOOD R. KIRBY** (?–?). *Manual of genito-urinary diseases.* 143pp. Philadelphia: F. W. S. Langmaid, M.D., 1899.

Kirby was clinical professor of genitourinary diseases at the Medico-Chirurgical College in Philadelphia. He had formerly served as instructor of clinical surgery at the University of Pennsylvania. The volume contains nine chapters: "Kidney"; "Ureter"; "Bladder"; "Scrotum, cord and testicles"; "Prostate gland"; "Penis"; "Urethra"; "Chancroid"; and "Syphilis." Kirby notes in the preface:

> This little manual has been published in response to the repeated requests of the author's pupils, from notes used by him in teaching and quizzing. Effort has been made to present the matter briefly and clearly, therefore, authorities have not been cited nor cases quoted, and debatable points have been omitted. It is believed that the manual will be found abreast of the times and useful to those for whom it is intended.

This was the only edition. Among his other books is *Manual of surgery* (Philadelphia: F. W. S. Langmaid, 1900).

GU45. **GEORGE FRANK LYDSTON** (1858–1923): *The surgical diseases of the genito-urinary tract, venereal and sexual diseases.* 1,011pp. Philadelphia: F. A. Davis, 1899.

Lydston was known for his work on testicular transplantation, which he began in 1914; he claimed to have been the first to successfully perform such a procedure. Not content to write medical textbooks, Lydston turned to social commentary through various plays and other nonmedical writings. When this volume was published, he was serving as professor of the surgical diseases of the genitourinary organs and syphilology in the medical department of the State University of Illinois (the Chicago College of Physicians and Surgeons). Lydston writes in the preface:

> In view of the cordial manner in which my various contributions to the subjects embraced in this volume has been received by the profession, I have felt that the publication of a more comprehensive treatise hardly requires either apology or explanation. I have embraced the opportunity herein afforded me for airing a few heresies of my own, in juxtaposition with as much of the accepted and standard teachings as it is practicable to present in a work chiefly designed for the student and general practitioner rather than the specialist; but this may be pardoned. No attempt has been made to cover the literature of the various subjects comprised in this volume. The endeavor has been to give a practical survey of the field of genito-urinary and venereal disease, following as closely as practicable the plan of my course of lectures.

The book is illustrated with 235 engravings. There are ten parts divided into 43 chapters: "General principles of genito-urinary, sexual, and venereal pathology and therapeutics"; "Non-venereal diseases of the penis"; "Diseases of the urethra and gonorrhea"; "Chancroid and bubo and their complications"; "Syphilis"; "Diseases affecting sexual physiology"; "Diseases of the prostate and seminal vesicles"; "Urinary bladder"; "Surgical affections of the kidney and ureter"; and "Diseases of the testis and spermatic cord." A revised edition with seven colored plates was published in 1904. (See also GU26, GU27, and GU28.)

GU46. **ALONZO RICHARD MORGAN** (1830–?). *Repertory of the urinary organs and prostate gland, including condylomata.* 318pp. Philadelphia: Boericke & Tafel, 1899.

Morgan graduated from the Homeopathic Medical College in Philadelphia in 1852. He initially practiced in Syracuse, but accepted the chair of theory and practice of medicine at his alma mater in 1867. He resigned the following year to take a similar position at New York Medical College.

Due to failing health, he relinquished his professional duties in 1871 and moved to Waterbury, Connecticut. The preface explains the circumstances of this book and asserts Morgan's faith in homeopathy:

> Upon resuming active practice in 1890, after an enforced retirement of several years on account of prolonged ill health, I began gathering for my personal use all the indications to be found in existing repertories pertaining to the prostate gland . . . . After following this course for several months I found myself not unfrequently coming upon symptoms which I was unable to trace to any reliable source, and, therefore, undertook to verify the records by over-hauling the provings, a course which led me into a comparatively ungleaned field, so far, at least, as the harvest in this department had been garnered . . . and this consideration induced me to extend my field of observation so as to include the morbid phenomena of the whole urinary tract, from kidneys to meatus urinarius, together with the character and qualities of the urine and its sediments; the concomitants of micturition, also symptoms of the prostate gland, and, finally, condylomata; an accumulation of too much valuable material to be "hidden under a bushel . . . . "
> Homeopathy is either wholly and everlastingly true, or else it is a delusion and a fraud. Who shall judge? Shall it be the prejudiced individual who condemns without trial, or on who, after ample preparation and compliance with all necessary rules and regulations, arrives at an intelligent conclusion? Hahnemannians are sometimes charged with being exclusive, narrow and bigoted in their ideas of medical practice, because they really believe in the existence of an universal law of cure, and so believing, strive to follow it without deviation. How can an honest man do otherwise? Want of fidelity to principles by those claiming to be our faith has done more to discredit and retard the advancement of our cause than lack of success in curing the sick by its faithful exponents . . . We see upon referring to works on allopathic practice that their methods have been subject to continual changes, the charlatanism of one decade being not infrequently adopted as orthodox treatment the next. Standard allopathic authorities of but few years ago are today set aside ever by themselves as worthless, obsolete . . . While on the other hand, in contrast, we have the permanent and stable method of the faithful followers of Hahnemann, who today depend upon the identical works published by the author of homeopathy nearly one hundred years ago, reinforced by the observations and experiences of thousands of able and conscientious practitioners distributed throughout all quarters of the civilized world . . . .

There is no table of contents, but a limited index appears on page 314ff. The work is notable for the numerous tables providing homeopathic remedies for genitourinary diseases. There were no further editions.

VII. COLON AND RECTAL SURGERY

CR1. **GEORGE MacARTNEY BUSHE** (1793–1836). *A treatise on the malfomations, injuries, and diseases of the rectum and anus.* Text and separate atlas of 9 plates. 209pp. and 10pp. New York: French & Adlard, 1837.

Bushe was born in Ireland and received his medical training in Europe; he was brought to America in 1828 by the faculty of Rutgers Medical College in New Jersey to serve as professor of anatomy. He was widely regarded as an able surgeon and gave daily office lectures on surgery for almost three years. Unfortunately, he succumbed to tuberculosis immediately following the writing of this work. The book is an important but little-known text and is unique in the annals of American surgery since it is the only 19th-century surgical text with a separate atlas of plates, although this was a common European practice. The *Treatise* was dedicated to Joseph Skey, director of British military hospitals. Bushe writes in the advertisement for the book:

> Many years ago, I was induced to pay particular attention to the diseases of the rectum and anus, in consequence of their frequency, and the diversity of opinion which prevailed in relation to their nature and treatment. My opportunities for investigating them have been ample, and I may safely say, that I spared neither time, trouble, nor expense, in endeavouring to arrive at just conclusions. In the compilation of my researches, I have aimed at simplicity and conciseness, at the same time that I have been careful to omit nothing of importance . . . .

There are twenty-six chapters, including "Malformations of the rectum and anus"; "Neuralgia of the extremity of the rectum"; "Spasmodic contraction of the sphincter ani"; "Affections called hemorrhoidal"; "Itching of the anus"; "Excrescences about the anus"; "Stricture of the rectum"; and "Carcinomatous degeneration of the rectum." The atlas comprises nine lithographed plates; numbers 1–7 are hand-colored. In its time this book was considered among the ablest works on the subject in any language. This was the only edition.

CR2. **WILLIAM BODENHAMER** (1808–1905). *Practical observations on some of the diseases of the rectum, anus, and contiguous textures; giving their nature, seat, causes, symptoms, consequences, and prevention; especially addressed to the non-medical reader.* 255pp. Cincinnati: Privately printed, 1847.

A graduate of Worthington Medical College of Ohio University in 1839, Bodenhamer was America's first specialist in anal-rectal diseases. One of the most peripatetic of American surgeons, Bodenhamer states in a fascinating addenda that any patients who wish to visit him should know that he divides his time between Louisville and New Orleans in order to bring his medical advice to as many people as possible. According to the preface, Bodenhamer wrote the *Practical observations* for a non-medical audience:

> The object of the present work, is simply to call attention to a class of diseases, but imperfectly understood at the present day; by pointing out their location, their nature, their principal causes, their most prominent symptoms and their consequences; so as to enable those who are yet from their annoyance, to continue so, by avoiding their causes, and to encourage those who are laboring under any of them, by informing them that they can not only be treated but cured, by a new, safe, mild and scientific method . . . . It is not, however, the intention of the

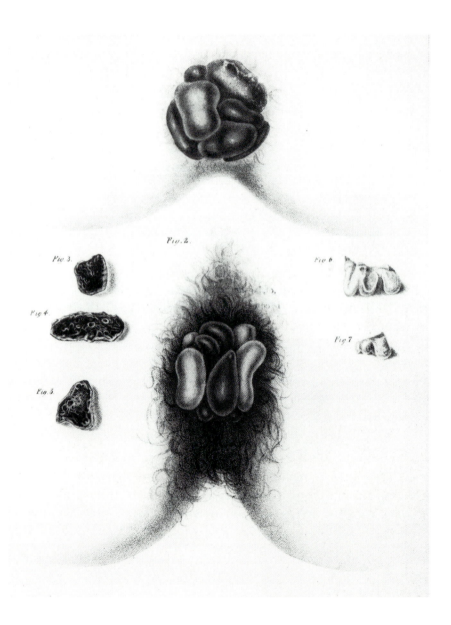

Fig. 125. (CR1) Bushe's color plates were drawn by Dr. Westmacott, and Buffords of New York served as the lithographer. This plate, figure 2 in the separate atlas, shows two views of internal hemorrhoids from a patient whom Bushe had operated on two years earlier.

author to give, in the present work, the peculiarities of his method; but he refers with pleasure to his triumphant success in the treatment of the diseases of the rectum and anus, as furnishing the most satisfactory and unanswerable evidence of its superior excellence. As the work is especially addressed to the unprofessional, it is as much as possible divested of the technicalities of the science, so that the non-medical reader can comprehend all that is important to be understood . . . .

Among the twenty-three chapters are "Statistics" (chapter 3); "Prolapsus ani" (chapter 9); "Excrescences of the anus" (chapter 13); "Neuralgia of the anus" (chapter 15); "Malignant degeneration of the rectum" (chapter 19); "Vaginal fistula" (chapter 21); and "Testimonials" (chapter 22). The most interesting aspect of the work is a five-page index with such entries as "Louis XIV, labored under fistula ani—his experiments"; "M. Felix received $30,000, for operating on the grand Monarque"; "Henry VIII is said to have died of fistula in ano"; "Death from procrastination"; and "Stricture of the rectum—the golden egg of quacks." A second edition appeared in 1855. (See also CR3, CR4, CR5, CR7, and CR11.)

CR3. **WILLIAM BODENHAMER** (1808–1905). *A practical treatise on the etiology, pathology, and treatment of the congenital malformations of the rectum and anus*. 368pp. New York: Samuel S. & William Wood, 1860.

> In the preface to his 1847 volume (CR2), Bodenhamer writes that
>
> > it may not be improper here to remark, that it is the design of the author, at no distant day, to present also to the medical profession, a practical work on those diseases, containing a plain statement of their seat, nature, cause, symptoms, and treatment. The work is to be illustrated by a number of colored plates, and exemplified by numerous cases.

He published his *Practical treatise* thirteen years later. It is a remarkable volume and is one of the major American works on anal-rectal conditions. It gathered for the first time into one book all the scattered studies from every nation with special reference to operative surgery. There were sixteen colored plates and 287 illustrative cases. Bodenhamer notes in the preface:

> No complete, systematic or practical work on the congenital malformations of the rectum and anus, has ever been published in this or any other country. The literature on this subject lies buried in undigested confusion in the various channels throughout the range of the science . . . . To remedy this serious evil and to fill this void, the author has endeavored to collect these scattered materials into one continuous whole, adding to them his own reflections and experience on the subject . . . .

The book comprises eleven chapters and includes an extensive bibliography (pages 17–36) and, most interestingly, a detailed description of abdominal artificial anus (pages 295-348). This remarkable early account of colostomy includes five pages devoted to the history of the operation. There was only one edition, which is quite scarce. (See also CR4, CR5, CR7, and CR11.)

CR4. **WILLIAM BODENHAMER** (1808–1905). *Practical observations on the etiology, pathology, diagnosis, and treatment of anal fissure.* 199pp. New York: William Wood, 1868.

Bodenhamer was practicing in New York when this work was published. Although he lists himself as professor of the diseases, injuries, and malformations of the rectum, anus, and genitourinary organs, he does not include the name of a medical school. Illustrated with sixteen simple drawings, *Practical observations* was the first work of its kind in America. Bodenhamer notes in the preface:

> The author's object in this work will be principally confined to the consideration of the diseases to which the term fissura ani really, truly, and legitimately belongs; and by so doing endeavor to remove some of the obscurities, the difficulties, and the confusion which surround it . . . . There is no complete and systematic treatise on the subject, and the disease is of exceedingly practical importance, in consequence of the great suffering to which it gives rise, and its frequent occurrence in our own country, and from the fact of its being not unfrequently overlooked, or confounded with some other diseases . . . . So far as the author's treatment of this disease is concerned, he has nothing new to offer in this work. It may be alleged by the learned and the experienced that, in treating such an apparently simple subject as anal fissure, the author has been too prolix, too diffuse; but let it be remembered that he has not written entirely nor even principally for these. "Doctis indoctisque scribimus." It is the great aim of the author to make that which is true, rather than that which is new, more generally known through all the ranks of the profession . . . .

Chapter 1 consists of an extensive history (pages 3–21) of anal fissure. Chapter 5 (section 3, pages 119–47) presents different methods of surgical treatment, including topical applications, cauterization, dilatation, incision of the mucous membrane, excision of the fissure, and complete division of the sphincters of the anus. The concluding chapter (chapter 6, pages 151–91) describes twenty-nine illustrative cases. An extensive bibliography of the subject appears on pages 192–99. (See also CR2, CR3, CR5, CR7, and CR11.)

CR5. **WILLIAM BODENHAMER** (1808–1905). *The physical exploration of the rectum; with an appendix on the ligation of haemorrhoidal tumours.* 54pp. New York: William Wood, 1870.

Bodenhamer writes in the preface that

> this little brochure does not profess to be anything more than an introduction to, or an outline of the subject, it nevertheless does not fail to include the most salient points. He therefore, trusts that sufficient has been presented to make it attractive and useful, especially to the student and junior practitioner, to whom, with its many defects, it is most respectfully addressed . . . .

There are four sections: "Introductory remarks"; "Anatomy of the rectum"; "Physical exploration"; and "Sounding the rectum." The book is illustrated by numerous drawings and includes a lengthy appendix (pages 43–54) describing the ligation of hemorrhoidal tumors. (See also CR2, CR3, CR4, CR7, and CR11.)

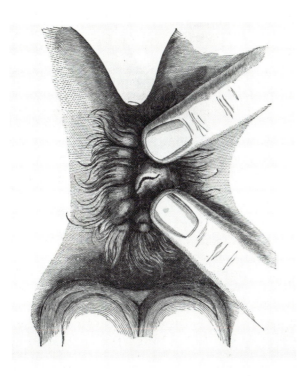

Fig. 126. (CR4) In this drawing (number 5, page 92) Boden-hamer demonstrates how an anal fissure can be located by placing a finger on each side of the lesion and pressing it out and down.

CR6. **WILLIAM HOLME VAN BUREN** (1819–83). *Lectures upon diseases of the rectum.* 164pp. New York: D. Appleton, 1870.

These lectures were delivered at Bellevue Hospital Medical College during the session of 1869–70. At that time, Van Buren was professor of the principles of surgery with diseases of the genitourinary organs at Bellevue. Although never considered a specialist in rectal pathology, Van Buren was such a well-known surgeon that his lectures, whatever their subject, commanded much respect. This small monograph contains eight lectures, including "Pruritus ani—erythema—herpes-chronic eczema—thread worm—haemorrhoids"; "Polypus—prolapsus ani—abscess"; "Fistula in ano"; "Fissure, or irritable ulcer"; "Stricture of the rectum"; "Cancer"; and "Diagnosis—means of exploration—neuralgia—atony—impacted feces—hygiene-special therapeutics." The book has neither illustrations nor index. (See also GS60, GS119, and GU9.)

CR7. **WILLIAM BODENHAMER** (1808–1905). *An essay on rectal medication.* 58pp. New York: William Wood, 1878.

This *Essay* comprises five sections: "General remarks"; "Methods of rectal medication"; "Rectal absorption"; "Recto-colonic products"; and "Resume." Bodenhamer printed the following explanatory note on the title page: "In the employment of an official therapeutic remedy, it is not only important and necessary to know in what case, in what dose, in what form, but also BY WHAT CHANNEL it should be administered." He goes on to remark in the preface:

> Rectal medication is a branch of medical inquiry, which, although not new, being coeval with clysters, will nevertheless be found by the student to be highly interesting, as well as generally and immediately useful. Indeed, the subject of the administration of medicines per anum

instead of per os, for the removal or the mitigation of diseases, besides those of the rectum itself, is of great importance. It is by no means as well understood as it should be, or as its merits demand, consequently it is well worthy of further investigation. Scarcely any attention has hitherto been paid to the rectum as an absorbing, or as a digesting organ, or to the nature of the chemical reactions which take place between the components of the remedy introduced into it, and the products in the form of secretions and excretions which are peculiar to, or are found in it . . . . The author has not, in the brief limits of this essay, given a complete disquisition of the several important principles involved in this subject; but he has, to the best of his ability, given an outline of them, with a view to stimulate inquiry and to evoke discussion. In it, however, the student will find sufficiently discussed, all the essential elements necessary to a thorough examination of the subject.

(See also CR2, CR3, CR4, CR5, and CR11.)

CR8. **ALEXANDER W. BRINKERHOFF** (?–1887). *Diseases of the rectum and new method of rectal treatment.* 266pp. Columbus: Privately printed, 1881.

This is one of the most intriguing of American surgical books, but, unfortunately, little information is available about its author. Brinkerhoff practiced in Upper Sandusky, Ohio, but was considered by most of the medical community to be both a nuisance and a quack. This elusive volume bears witness to some of his beliefs. It represents little more than a massive advertisement for the Brinkerhoff treatment of piles and other rectal and anal problems. As proof in point, the title page contains this claim:

> . . . an entirely new and almost absolutely painless method of treatment. The whole being a complete system of rectal treatment by means of newly invented and patented instruments, and lately discovered and patented medicines, perfected during more than three years of continuous and daily practice and the performing of more than thirty thousand operations without the loss of a single patient from treatment, or failure to cure a single case of piles.

There is an interesting table of contents (pages 263–66), including such topics as "What constitutes my system of rectal treatment" (pages 100–04); "Opinions of some who have used my system" (pages 156–66); "Certificates of testimonials from 22 individuals throughout the mid-West" (pages 201–19); "What composes my case of instruments and their pricelist" (page 220–22); and a list (pages 224–36) of many names of Brinkerhoff's patients together with their addresses. There are a few illustrations but no plates. (See also CR19.)

CR9. **CHARLES BOYD KELSEY** (1850–1917). *Diseases of the rectum and anus.* 299pp. New York: William Wood, 1882.

Kelsey was one of the pioneering rectal specialists in America. He received his M.D. from the College of Physicians and Surgeons in New York in 1873. This volume, which was number 92 in Wood's Library of Standard Medical Authors, was his first book. He lists himself as surgeon at St. Paul's Infirmary for diseases of the rectum and consulting surgeon for diseases of the rectum at Harlem Hospital. Kelsey writes in the preface:

> In preparing the following pages for publication, I have endeavored to condense into convenient form, for both student and practitioner, as great an amount as possible of practical information concerning diseases of the rectum and anus . . . . I have tried . . . to make it suitable for ready reference by student and practitioner, giving not only the results which have been reached by experiment and clinical experience, and which may be relied upon as the basis of practice, but in many questions marking out by foot-notes and references the way for any who may desire to go over for himself the ground which I have followed with no little difficulty . . . .

The fourteen chapters include "Practical points in anatomy and physiology"; "Congenital malformations of the rectum and anus"; "General rules regarding examinations, diagnosis, and operation"; "Inflammation of the rectum"; "Abscess and fistula"; "Haemorrhoids"; "Prolapse"; "Non-malignant growths"; "Non-malignant ulcerations"; "Non-malignant stricture"; "Cancer"; "Impacted feces and foreign bodies"; "Pruritus ani"; and "Spasm of the sphincter, neuralgia, wounds, rectal alimentation." The book has fifty-two wood engravings but no plates. (See also CR12, CR14, CR21, and CR22.)

CR10. **MORTIMER AYRES** (?–?). *Some of the diseases of the rectum and their homoeopathic and surgical treatment.* 78pp. Chicago: Duncan Brothers, 1884.

A little-known homeopathic physician, Ayres practiced in Rushville, Illinois. He describes his reason for writing this treatise in the preface:

> Having had occasion to treat many cases of diseases of the rectum, the author became possessed of some facts that enabled him to manage them with satisfaction. In time, he came to have quite a repute in his neighborhood for "curing piles." Some of his colleagues, learning of his success, urged him to write a treatise on the diseases of the rectum. To that he objected, but finally consented to write out a few ideas on some of the more common diseases of the rectum and their medical and surgical treatment. The author has endeavored to condense into a convenient form as great an amount as possible of practical information . . . . Those who look for this work to be a complete treatise on this subject will be disappointed. It expresses chiefly the results of his own experience . . . .

The eleven chapters include "Hygiene"; "Ulcers of the rectum"; "Fissure or irritable ulcer"; "Pruritus ani"; "Prolapsus"; "Polypus"; "Haemorrhoids or piles"; "Internal haemorrhoids"; "Abscess of the rectum"; "Fistula in ano"; and "Constipation." There are a few illustrations.

CR11. **WILLIAM BODENHAMER** (1808–1905). *A theoretical and practical treatise on the hemorrhoidal disease, giving its history, nature, cases, pathology, diagnosis, and treatment.* 297pp. New York: William Wood, 1884.

Bodenhamer was seventy-six years old when this comprehensive work was published. Some of the articles in this volume had been previously printed in the *New York medical record*. Bodenhamer describes the scope of this work in the preface:

> This treatise will be found to be a complete encyclopedia upon the subject of hemorrhoids, and is concluded by a copious literature of the subject, ranging from the remotest antiquity to the latest production of the day . . . . The author trusts that it will not be considered too wide a digression from the true scope of this treatise that so many topics have been introduced into it, which by some may be thought either to be wholly foreign to it, or to be now obsolete. The object, however, of entering so thoroughly and so lengthily into the subject has not been for the purpose of magnifying the hemorrhoidal disease, or of attaching to it an undue importance, but solely for the purpose of claiming for it that investigation and sober judgment which might result in bringing its practical treatment within the pale of rational principles, and of divesting it of much of the error, obscurity, and confusion which have been too long suffered to surround it, to the discredit and the detriment of medical science and to the encouragement of charlatanry . . . .

The thirteen chapters include "Hebraic history"; "Etymology and the application of the word hemorrhoids"; "Description and definition"; "Symptomatology"; "Etiology"; "Hemorrhoidal tumors"; "Hemorrhoidal flux"; "Differential diagnosis-prognosis"; "Consecutive accidents and complications of the hemorrhoidal disease"; "Are hemorrhoids salutary"; "Restoration of suppressed or retained hemorrhoids"; "Treatment"; and "Bibliography." This last chapter (pages 255-88) is significant because it provides an extensive review of the literature. The book contains two chromolithographic plates and thirty-one woodcuts. (See also CR2, CR3, CR4, CR5, and CR7.)

CR12. **CHARLES BOYD KELSEY** (1850–1917). *The pathology, diagnosis, and treatment of diseases of the rectum and anus.* 416pp. New York: William Wood, 1884.

Kelsey was in private practice in New York when he wrote this volume. The work had its basis in Kelsey's earlier volume on the same subject (CR9), but it

> . . . contains many changes, chiefly of such practical character as would naturally be suggested to a writer by the increased experience which comes from the daily practice of a specialty. The chapter on rectal hernia has been added entire, and many new illustrations . . . . My special aim has been to make the book a safe guide for the student and general practitioner, and to furnish, as far as possible in this way, that information which it is so difficult to acquire without the time and opportunity for special clinical study.

Pathology is over 110 pages longer than Kelsey's earlier work (CR9), and it has two color plates. They illustrate chancroids of the anus and hemorrhoids and proplasus. Further editions were published in 1890 and 1893. (See also CR14, CR21, and CR22.)

CR13. **J. WILLISTON WRIGHT** (?–?). *Lectures on diseases of the rectum.* 170pp. New York: Bermingham, 1884.

Wright was professor of surgery at the University of the City of New York. He notes in the preface that

> these lectures were delivered at the University . . . and subsequently published, from stenographer's notes, in the *Medical Gazette.* The demand for them soon exhausted the numbers of the journal in which they appeared, and owing to continued and repeated calls the publishers have deemed it advisable to present them in the present form.

The nine lectures include "Examination of the rectum"; "Abscess"; "Fistula in ano"; "Hemorrhoids"; "Pruritus ani"; "Fissure"; "Stricture"; "Polypus and prolapse"; and "Cancer of the rectum." Lecture 9 (page 150) is parti-cularly valuable for its description of operations of extirpation and colotomy. There are six rudimentary illustrations of instruments. No further editions were printed.

CR14. **CHARLES BOYD KELSEY** (1850–1917). *The diagnosis and treatment of haemorrhoids; with general rules as to the examination of rectal diseases.* 78pp. Detroit: G. S. Davis, 1887.

Part of Series II of Davis's Physicians' Leisure Library, the volume was available in paper for twenty-five cents and in cloth for fifty cents. Kelsey writes in the preface:

> Concerning this little book it is only necessary to say that it contains the results of my own experience with the various methods of curing hemorrhoids up to the present time. It is written solely for my fellow practitioners, and with the wish that they may find it a safe guide in practice. In it many of the questions which are constantly asked as to the value of different operations will be answered as far as I am able to do so.

The six chapters are "General rules for examination and diagnosis"; "Varieties of haemorrhoids"; "Treatment"; "Ligature"; "Injections"; and "Clamp." There are no plates. (See also CR9, CR12, CR21, and CR22.)

CR15. **EDMUND ANDREWS** (1824–1904) and **EDWARD WYLLYS ANDREWS** (1856–1927). *Rectal and anal surgery, with a description of the secret methods of the itinerants.* 111pp. Chicago: W. T. Keener, 1888.

Edmund and Edward Andrews were major surgical figures in Chicago for almost half a century; their book was the only nineteenth-century American surgical textbook to be coauthored by a father and his son. Edmund received his M.D. from the University of Michigan in 1852. Most of his professional career was spent at Chicago Medical College, and Northwestern University Medical School, where he was professor of clinical surgery. Among the first in the Midwest to use and promote Lister's antiseptic methods, he also pioneered the use of blood transfusions and is best remembered for advocating the use of an oxygen-nitrous oxide mixture as an anesthetic agent [G-M 5669]. Edward received his M.D. from Chicago Medical College in 1881. At the time this work was written he was adjunct professor of clinical surgery at his alma mater and surgeon at Mercy Hospital. Edward was vice-president of the American Surgical Association in 1924, and also helped found the American Association for Thoracic Surgery and the American College of Surgeons. In addition, he was one of the originators of the monthly journal *Surgery, gynecology and obstetrics*. The preface comments on the practices of itinerant "pile doctors":

> The untutored "pile doctors," alias the "itinerant rectal specialists," now traversing the country, have accomplished one good result. They have compelled physicians to give more attention to the neglected subject of rectal diseases. Hence, has arisen an urgent call for information on two points. 1. What are the best methods of diagnosis and treatment of these affections known to the regular profession? 2. What are the secret methods of the itinerants, and what is their value? To answer these questions this book is written. We have endeavored to condense into it the results of our own special investigations in this direction, and to give in a form at once compact, and yet sufficient for the guidance of practitioners, the established opinions and methods of the best men in America and Europe. To this we have added under each heading the secret methods and prescriptions of the irregulars, which we have been gathering up for several years past . . . .

There are ten chapters and thirty-seven figures. The book is fascinating reading for exposing the methods of nineteenth-century quacks and their foibles (page iv):

> They divided up the United States into districts, and sold local "rights" to practice the plan, after the manner of patent rights, each purchaser being solemnly sworn, or pledged, to confine his practice to his own district, and to keep the secret of the methods.

A major portion of this book's criticism was directed at Alexander Brinkerhoff (CR8 and CR19). Further editions were published in 1889 and 1892.

CR16. **WILLIAM JEFFERSON GUERNSEY** (?–?). *The homoeopathic therapeutics of hemorrhoids*. 142pp. Philadelphia: Boericke & Tafel, 1882.

Guernsey was a homeopathic physician who practiced in Philadelphia. This work contains neither a table of contents nor an index, which makes it difficult to read. It was interleaved with blank pages so notes could be taken. Guernsey notes in the preface to the second edition:

> Pathology is not within the scope of this work: but that method of therapeutics which will produce a cure in the surest and easiest manner, with absolute safety to the patient, shall claim our attention. As Homeopaths we believe that our tenets are based upon a law of nature and that we are the possessors of the only positive system of cure in existence. That it is so true in its action; so universal in its application; that it alone meets all the requirements for general practice; as it should be able to cure all curable ailments and must be the best treatment for the disease in question . . . . And the writer begs to repeat with emphasis . . . that we have proven remedies enough to easily, surely and safely restore to health all patients suffering with uncomplicated piles. And, indeed, the complicated cases should not be too quickly turned over to the surgeon, simply because they are such . . . .

CR17. **LEWIS H. ADLER** (?–?). *Fissure of the anus and fistula in ano.* 78pp. Detroit: G. S. Davis, 1892.

Adler was an instructor in diseases of the rectum at the Philadelphia Polyclinic and College for Graduates in Medicine. This monograph is divided into two parts: "Anal fissure, or irritable ulcer of the rectum" and "Fistula in ano." Chapter 3 in the first part and chapter 4 in the second part give detailed instructions on the operative treatment of these conditions. Adler notes in the preface:

> While the two subjects treated in this volume have been ably written on at various times and by different authorities, it is undeniable that no organ of the body is more neglected by both the laity and the profession than is the rectum . . . . As a result of this unattractiveness, even amounting to repulsiveness, to the general practitioner, most of the affections of the lower bowel are treated by him as "piles," the diagnosis being usually made by the patient, and accepted by the physician without questions or personal examination . . . . A knowledge of these facts has led me to hope that a brochure upon the subjects might excite a deeper professional interest in rectal maladies if issued as a volume of the Physicians' Leisure Library Series, which by its moderate price permits of a wide circulation . . . .

(See also GS151.)

CR18. **JOSEPH MCDOWELL MATHEWS** (1847–1928). *A treatise on diseases of the rectum, anus, and sigmoid flexure.* 537pp. New York: D. Appleton, 1892.

An 1877 graduate of the University of Louisville School of Medicine, Mathews became interested in the specialty of proctology after having studied in London. He spent all his professional life in practice in Louisville. In 1880 he was appointed professor of surgery at the Kentucky School of Medicine, and when the Department of Proctology was established in 1883, he was chosen as its head. He helped organize the American Proctological Society in 1899. Mathews is best remembered for having served as the fifty-first president of the American Medical Association in 1899. He is considered America's first proctologist and the first orthodox physician anywhere in the world to limit his practice to rectal diseases. He took proctology out of the hands of quacks and charlatans and placed it on a firm, scientific basis. Interestingly, Mathews exerted a conservative influence in rectal surgery, opposing most radical operations because of their demonstrated failure to save or prolong life. In 1894, he started *Mathews's medical quarterly*, the first journal on proctology in the United States. The preface provides Mathews's reason for writing the book:

> I have written this book because of a desire to record my individual experience of fifteen years as a rectal specialist, in answer to the demand of my students and friends. During this time I have learned that many things that are taught are not true, and that many true things have not been taught. I have therefore not taken other men's opinions as my guide, but have accepted as truths only those things which could be substantiated by fact, and here recorded them. In differing from others

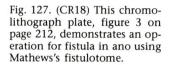

Fig. 127. (CR18) This chromo-lithograph plate, figure 3 on page 212, demonstrates an operation for fistula in ano using Mathews's fistulotome.

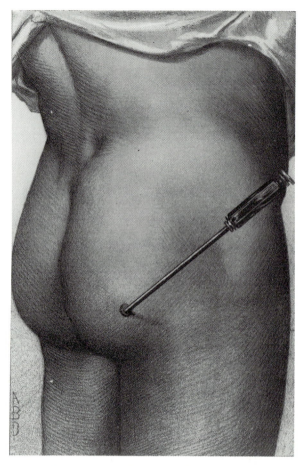

> on any special point I have tried first to state fairly and fully their views, and then my own. The verdict is left to the reader . . . .

The twenty-four chapters cover a wide range of material, including "Antiseptics in rectal surgery" (chapter 4); "The nervous or hysterical rectum" (chapter 10); and "Cancer of the rectum with its operative treatment" (chapters 16–18). There are six chromolithograph plates. Further editions were published in 1896 and 1903. Mathews's other medical book is *How to succeed in the practice of medicine* (Louisville: J. P. Morton, 1902).

CR19. **ALEXANDER W. BRINKERHOFF** (?–1887). *Haemorrhoids (piles), rectal ulcer, fistula in ano, fissure, pruritus, polypus recti, stricture, &c., &c.; a statement of facts sustained by indisputable evidence written for the public.* 80pp. Chicago: Thayer & Jackson, 1895.

An intriguing follow-up to Brinkerhoff's previous work (CR8), *Haemorrhoids* is actually a revision of it by Alexander's son William C. Brinkerhoff. Clearly, it represents the son's attempt to rescue his father's sullied reputation. The elder Brinkerhoff was regarded as a quack who plied his trade of curing piles. Brinkerhoff's son defends his father in the preface:

> To the memory of my honorable, able and beloved father . . . . His life was marred by repeated reverses both in health and fortune, but the

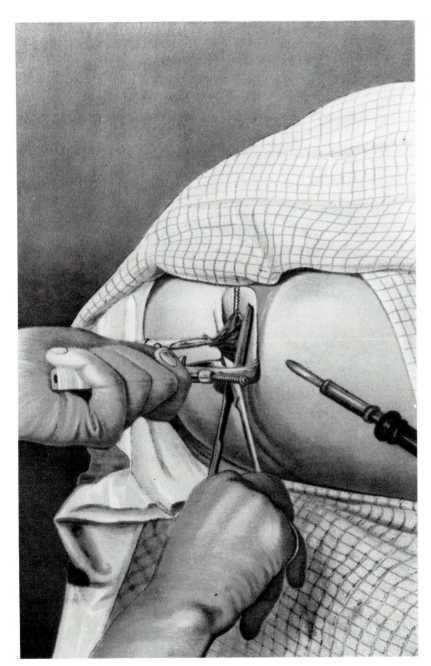

Fig. 128. (CR20) Gant's chromolithographic plates were quite graphic. Here (number 15, page 216) he demonstrates his clamp and position of the scissors just prior to excision of the hemorrhoids. Burk and McFetridge of Philadelphia were the lithographers.

indomitable will, perseverance and high sense of honor with which he was imbued surmounted all obstacles in his way. It is to his learning, ability and wisdom that suffering humanity owe a debt of gratitude for a system of rectal treatment that is humane, successful and wonderful in its workings. That the treatment may be honorably, creditably and successfully perpetuated is the wish and will be the effort of his son.

The title page contains the gist of the entire text:

Part 1st. diseases of the rectum and their reflex results—surgical operations for the cure of piles, absolutely unnecessary—Dr. Alexander W. Brinkerhoff's system of rectal treatment; and, Part 2d. medical code of ethics—the protection it affords to the medical professor's advertising

trust and a curiosity that exists under its provisions whereby the owner-
ship of a hospital (be it ever so small) forever saves a man from being
called a quack.

It is worth noting that the younger Brinkerhoff is careful to report that
he matriculated at the Regular Graduate College of Physicians and Surgeons in Chicago. Among the more fascinating contents in the first part
are "A history of the Brinkerhoff system" (pages 7–8); "The medical
profession and its interaction with the Brinkerhoff system" (page 43);
"Medical opinions of the system" (page 45); and a lengthy set of endor-
sements of the system by prominent citizens (pages 45–68). The second
part includes "What is a medical quack" (page 75); "In defense of advertising doctors" (page 76); and "Statistics, operations and surgeons'
opinions" (pages 78–80). This second part is particularly important because it provides a detailed look at how medicine reacted to advertising
at a time when American surgery was undergoing profound changes.
The book was available for $1.00.

CR20. **SAMUEL GOODWIN GANT** (1869–1944). *Diagnosis and treatment
of diseases of the rectum, anus, and contiguous textures.* 399pp.
Philadelphia: F. A. Davis, 1896.

This work is an amazing effort since Gant wrote it when he was
only twenty-seven years old. He had recently been appointed professor
of diseases of the rectum and anus at the University and Woman's Medical Colleges and lecturer on intestinal diseases at the Scarritt Training-
School for Nurses in Kansas City. Gant later moved to New York, where
he became professor of diseases of the rectum and anus at New York
Post-Graduate Medical School and Hospital and attending surgeon for
rectal diseases at St. Mary's Hospital and the German Polyclinic Dispensary. The *Diagnosis* is dedicated to his father, Jackson D. Gant, and contains thirty-two chapters. Among the more interesting are "Relation of
pulmonary tuberculosis to fistula" (pages 99ff.); "Auto-infection from
the intestinal canal" (pages 268ff.); and "Railroading as an etiological
factor in rectal diseases" (pages 379ff.). Herbert William Allingham
provided two chapters on cancer and colotomy. There are sixteen full-
page chromolithographic plates and 115 wood engravings in the text.
Gant notes in the preface that "this treatise is the result of an effort to
give to the practitioners and students of medicine a concise, yet practical, work. I have not attempted to give a detailed discussion of theories
and antiquated views of unrecognized value . . . . " A second edition was
published in 1902 and a third edition in 1905. Among Gant's other
books is *Constipation and intestinal obstruction (obstipation)* (Philadelphia:
W. B. Saunders, 1909).

CR21. **CHARLES BOYD KELSEY** (1850–1917). *Surgery of the rectum and
pelvis.* 573pp. New York: Richard Kettles, 1897.

This work is a complete revision of Kelsey's previous books (CR9
and CR12), and is actually the fifth edition of the original treatise. For
reasons unknown it was published by Richard Kettles instead of William

Wood. In 1902, a sixth and final edition was published, again by Wood. Kelsey notes in the preface:

> A comparison of this work with those on diseases of the rectum by the same author which have preceded it will show at a glance its increased scope . . . . In enlarging this work, to include surgical procedures necessary for the cure of allied affections, the author has simply followed what experience has proved to be the natural course of his own practice. He can only hope that in its new form the book will meet with the same favor that has attended former editions.

There are twenty-seven chapters, including "Pelvis abscess in women" and "Kraske's excision of the rectum." The final seven chapters discuss pelvic surgery, including "Salpingectomy and oophorectomy"; "Vagina, uterus and the round ligaments"; "Hernia"; "Male genito-urinary organs"; "Ureters"; and "Appendicitis." There are a few halftone plates and 281 additional illustrations. (See also CR14 and CR22.)

CR22. **CHARLES BOYD KELSEY** (1850–1917). *The office treatment of hemorrhoids, fistula, etc. without operation.* 68pp. New York: E. R. Pelton, 1898.

Kelsey, who had recently resigned as professor of surgery at New York Post-Graduate Medical School and Hospital, writes in the preface:

> Of the three lectures contained in the following pages one only has previously appeared in print, and that the last. In presenting them in this form the author has done what is in his power to counteract the far too prevalent idea in the medical profession, that the only radical treatment of these affections is by operations; as well as to call attention to what he considers the far too frequent misuse of one of the most important of all the operations.

The contents are "The cure of hemorrhoids, fistula, fissure and other affections of the rectum by office treatment without operation"; "On the relation between diseases of the rectum and other diseases in both sexes, but especially in women"; and "On the abuse of the operation of colostomy, or the formation of an artificial anus." There are no plates. (See also CR9, CR12, CR14, and CR21.)

VIII. NEUROLOGICAL SURGERY

NS1. **JOHN BINGHAM ROBERTS** (1852–1924). *The field and limitation of the operative surgery of the human brain.* 80pp. Philadelphia: P. Blakiston & Son, 1885.

Although initially presented as a paper at the 1885 meeting of the American Surgical Association, Roberts's paper was later revised and expanded to be published in book form. At the time of its publication Roberts was professor of anatomy and surgery at the Philadelphia Polyclinic. According to the *Transactions of the American Surgical Association*, Roberts had been asked to prepare a paper on cerebral surgery for the meeting. Nine theses were presented, most of which remain scientifically sound. Roberts strongly espoused immediate operation for all depressed skull fractures, an opinion which was considered quite radical. However, in his first thesis, he proposed that infection and not pressure displacement was the cause of symptoms and death in depressed fractures. Subsequent discussion of the paper occupied thirty-eight pages of text in the *Transactions*. There are three chapters in the monograph: "Principles of cerebral surgery"; "Cerebral localization"; and "Operative treatment of cerebral lesions." The chapter on localization cites cases of Rickman John Godlee (1849–1925), William Macewen (1848–1924), and others, and gives a detailed description of the localizing significance of the various neurological signs. This was the only edition. (See also GS99, GS102, GS143, OR53, and OR60.)

NS2. **SHOBAL VAIL CLEVENGER** (1843–1920). *Spinal concussion: surgically considered as a cause of spinal injury, and neurologically restricted to a certain symptom group, for which is suggested the designation Erichsen's disease, as one form of the traumatic neuroses.* 359pp. Philadelphia: F. A. Davis, 1889.

One of the more intriguing of nineteenth-century American physicians, Clevenger was born in Florence, Italy, although his parents were citizens of the United States. He graduated from Chicago Medical School in 1879 and became interested in neuropathological studies. This work led to his criticism of abuses in the treatment of patients in asylums. Clevenger soon became a target of the politicians who ran the mental health system and was eventually blacklisted. His subsequent professional career was filled with turmoil, and he was unable to remain for long in one position. He remained a prolific writer, however. This volume was published when Clevenger was consulting physician to the

Fig. 129. (NS5) A photograph of a sarcoma removed from the frontal lobe of a forty-year-old farmer (figure 58 on page 235). Starr localized the tumor, and Charles McBurney performed the surgery.

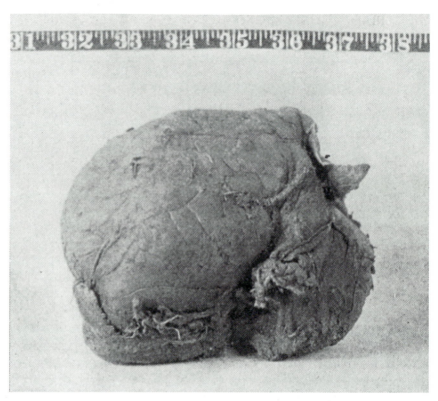

Reese and Alexian Brothers hospitals in Chicago. It is illustrated with twelve plates and thirty wood engravings. He writes in the preface:

> A class of injuries that is frequently caused by railway accidents can be studied to advantage in any large metropolis . . . . The need of a new work on spinal concussion is apparent in the scattered condition of the essays on the subject . . . . The recent Franco-German contest concerning the pathology of the disorder has ended in an advance of our knowledge, but the change from a spinal to a cerebral explanation of the symptoms, and their inclusion with other widely different phenomena, resulting from wounds in general, under the title traumatic neuroses, appears to be unjustified. An attempt has therefore been made in this work to carefully review the entire subject, with reference to anatomical derangements that will best explain the symptoms . . . . The author regrets the unavoidable polemics of parts of the book, though it is by controversy that the truth is often evolved from error; and his strong feeling against the political corruption in our country is explained by its opposition to all progress through the mediocrity and ignorance in most of our public institutions, scientific and medical, placed there by men of like character. A spring cannot rise higher than its source . . . .

Among the chapter headings are "Spinal concussion"; "Injuries of the spine and spinal cord"; "Traumatic neuroses"; "Traumatic insanity"; "Electro-diagnosis"; and "Medico-legal considerations." Clevenger's other books are the two-volume *Medical jurisprudence of insanity; or, forensic psychiatry* (Rochester: Lawyers' Cooperative, 1898) and *Therapeutics, materia medica and the practice of medicine* (Atlantic City: Evolution, 1905).

NS3. **BERIAH ANDRE WATSON** (1836–92). *An experimental study of lesions arising from severe concussions.* 76pp. Philadelphia: P. Blakiston & Son, 1890.

Watson was surgeon to the Jersey City and Christ hospitals in New Jersey. A fellow of the American Surgical Association, he held no academic position but obviously had a scientific mind. In 1895 Watson helped persuade the New Jersey legislature to legalize the dissection of human cadavers. He was reputed to have one of the largest medical libraries in New Jersey, but its disbursement remains unknown. This small brochure contains eight chapters: "Description of apparatus"; "Study of cases"; "Post-mortem examinations"; "Experiments—first series"; "Second series"; "Results of the experiments"; "Classification of injuries"; and "Conclusions." It is one of the earliest examples of basic science research in neurosurgery to be conducted by an American surgeon. (See also OR44.)

NS4. **PHILLIP COOMBS KNAPP** (1858–1920). *The pathology, diagnosis, and treatment of intracranial growths. Fiske Fund Prize Essay.* 165pp. Boston: Rockwell & Churchill, 1891.

Knapp was one of America's earliest neurologists, and at the time this essay was published was clinical instructor in diseases of the nervous system at Harvard Medical School. He served as president of the American Neurological Association in 1895. He notes in the introduction:

> Since this essay was presented for the Fiske prize, in May, 1890, I have been enabled, by the kindness of the Trustees of the Fiske Fund, to make a thorough revision of it . . . . The essay is based on the records of forty cases with autopsies . . . . In the chapter on treatment I have . . . given a tolerably complete list of the cases operated upon . . . .

Surgical treatment and an extensive group of tables of operations are found on pages 135–62. Chapter 5 ("Special symptomatology") is especially significant for its in-depth discussion of various tumors by anatomical site.

NS5. **MOSES ALLEN STARR** (1854–1932). *Brain surgery.* 295pp. New York: William Wood, 1893.

Starr was not a surgeon but professor of diseases of the mind and nervous system at the College of Physicians and Surgeons of Columbia University in New York. He writes in the preface to this book, which was the first full-length American treatise to deal with neurosurgery:

> Brain surgery is at present a subject both novel and interesting. It is within the past five years only that operations for the relief of epilepsy and of imbecility, for the removal of clots from the brain, for the opening of abscesses, for the excision of tumors, and for the relief of intra-cranial pressure have been generally attempted . . . . Brain surgery has as its essential basis the accurate diagnosis of cerebral lesions, which was impossible until the localization of cerebral functions had been determined. And this diagnosis must be made by the physician before the surgeon is called in to remove the disease. It is the object of this book to state clearly those facts regarding the essential features of brain disease which will enable the reader to determine in any case both the nature and the

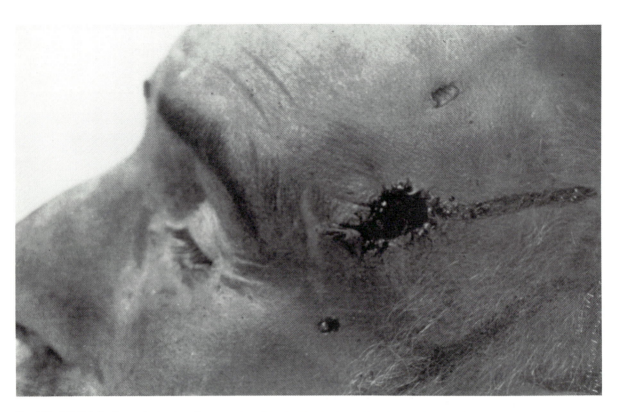

Fig. 130. (NS6) A fatal gunshot injury from a 0.44 caliber bullet. Brain matter is noted on the skin surface in this photograph which Phelps had taken in the Coroner's Office of New York City (figure 15 page 268).

situation of the pathological process in progress, to settle the question whether the disease can be removed by surgical interference, and to estimate the safety and probability of success by operation. The facts have been reached by a careful study of the literature of the subject and by a considerable personal experience . . . . While in no way disregarding the work of foreign observers, I have endeavored to utilize American observations and to cite American cases in preference to others. And this has in no way hampered me, for it is to the industry and genius of American surgeons that much of the great advance in this department of surgery is due. To this collection of facts I am able to contribute a considerable number of cases of cerebral disease, operated upon under my direction . . . . It is my hope that this work may aid the physician to diagnosticate brain diseases with more accuracy, and to select such cases as are properly open to surgical treatment by trephining; and also that it may enable the surgeon to perform his delicate task with more precision and with a fuller knowledge of those principles of local diagnosis which should form his constant guide.

The ten chapters are "Diagnosis of cerebral disease"; "Trephining for epilepsy"; "Imbecility due to microcephalus"; "Cerebral hemorrhage"; "Abscess of the brain"; "Tumor of the brain"; "Hydrocephalus and the relief of intracranial pressure"; "Insanity"; "Headache and other conditions"; and "The operation of trephining." There are fifty-nine illustrations, five of which are photographs. Most of the surgical operations cited were performed by Charles McBurney (1845–1913). Starr's other books include *Familiar forms of nervous disease* (New York: William Wood,

1890), *Atlas of nerve cells* (New York: Macmillan for the Columbia University Press, 1896), and *Organic nervous diseases* (New York: Lea Brothers, 1903).

NS6. **CHARLES PHELPS** (1834–1913). *Traumatic injuries of the brain and its membranes, with a special study of pistol-shot wounds of the head in their medico-legal and surgical relations.* 582pp. New York: D. Appleton, 1897.

Phelps was a graduate of Brown College and received his M.D. from the College of Physicians and Surgeons in New York in 1858. Following active military service during the Civil War, he settled in New York where he practiced until his death. Phelps never held an academic post, but was surgeon at Bellevue and St. Vincent's hospitals. In his later years he became especially interested in the study of injuries of the brain following fractures of the skull and of pistol-shot wounds of the head. This work is

> ... designed to be a concise and systematic exposition of the injuries which the brain suffers from external violence, a division of brain surgery which has the greatest practical importance and has received the least careful attention. It is believed that it will not only be of interest to surgeons, but will meet the requirements of general practitioners in whose experience such injuries are infrequent, and who in exceptional instances have urgent need of the aid to be derived from a wider clinical observation than their own opportunities have permitted. It has been based essentially, if not exclusively, upon an observation of five hundred consecutive cases of recent occurrence ....

The book is divided into two parts: "General traumatic lesions" and "Pistol-shot wounds of the head." The chapter headings include "Preliminary consideration of cranial fracture"; "Pathology"; "Symptomatology"; "Diagnosis"; "Prognosis"; "Principles of treatment"; "Medico-legal relations"; and "Surgical relations." The most fascinating section of the work appears on pages 395–581, which detail the condensed histories of 300 intracranial traumatisms, most of which were verified by necropsy. The vast majority of the forty-nine illustrations are clinical photographs of cadavers who suffered gunshot wounds to the head. A second edition was published in 1902.

Short Title List

GENERAL SURGERY

GS1. **JONES, J.** *Plain concise practical remarks on the treatment of wounds and fractures . . . .* New York, 1775.

GS2. **SEAMAN, V.** *Pharmacoepia [sic] chirurgica in usum Nosocomii Novi Eboracencis.* New York, 1811.

GS3. **DORSEY, J. S.** *Elements of surgery . . . .* Philadelphia, 1813.

GS4. **MANN, J.** *Medical sketches of the campaigns of 1812, 13, 14.* Dedham, MA, 1816.

GS5. **ANDERSON, W.** *System of surgical anatomy.* New York, 1822.

GS6. **THACHER, J.** *A military journal during the American Revolutionary War, from 1775 to 1783.* Boston, 1823.

GS7. **GIBSON, W.** *The institutes and practice of surgery; being the outlines of a course of lectures.* Philadelphia, 1824.

GS8. **SMITH, N. R.** *Surgical anatomy of the arteries.* Baltimore, 1830.

GS9. **BEAUMONT, W.** *Experiments and observations on the gastric juice, and the physiology of digestion.* Plattsburgh, 1833.

GS10. **ATKINS, D.** *Medical and surgical cases and observations.* New York, 1834.

GS11. **CHASE, H.** *A treatise on the radical cure of hernia by instruments; . . .* Philadelphia, 1836.

GS12. **DOANE, A. S.** *Surgery illustrated, compiled from the works of Cutler, Hind, Velpeau and Blasius.* New York, 1836.

GS13. **PARRISH, J.** *Practical observations on strangulated hernia, and some of the diseases of the urinary organs.* Philadelphia, 1836.

GS14. **CHASE, H.** *The final report of the committee of the Philadelphia Medical Society on the construction of instruments, and their mode of action, in the radical cure of hernia . . . .* Philadelphia, 1837.

GS15. **WARREN, J. C.** *Surgical observations on tumours, with cases and operations.* Boston, 1837.

GS16. **GROSS, S. D.** *Elements of pathological anatomy.* Boston, 1839.

GS17. **PARSONS, U.** *Boylston prize dissertations on: (1) inflammation of the periosteum; (2) eneuresis irritata; (3) cutaneous diseases; (4) cancer of the breast; also remarks on malaria.* Boston, 1839.

GS18. CHAPMAN, N. *Essays on practical medicine and surgery.* Philadelphia, 1841.

GS19. GROSS, S. D. *Experimental and critical inquiry into the nature and treatment of wounds of the intestines.* Louisville, 1843.

GS20. MÜTTER, T. D. *Syllabus of the course of lectures on the principles and practice of surgery.* Philadelphia, 1843.

GS21. SMITH, H. H. *Minor surgery; or, hints on the every-day duties of the surgeon.* Philadelphia, 1843.

GS22. PANCOAST, J. *A treatise on operative surgery; . . .* Philadelphia, 1844.

GS22.1. SMITH, H. H. *Anatomical atlas, illustrative of the structure of the human body.* Philadelphia, 1844.

GS23. McCLELLAN, G. *Principles and practice of surgery.* Philadelphia, 1848.

GS24. NEILL, J. and SMITH, F. G. *A handbook of surgery, being a portion of an analytical compend of the various branches of medicine.* Philadelphia, 1848.

GS25. SARGENT, F. *On bandaging and other operations of minor surgery.* Philadelphia, 1848.

GS26. WARREN J. C. *Etherization with surgical remarks.* Boston, 1848.

GS27. ROGERS, D. L. *Surgical essays and cases in surgery.* Newark, 1849.

GS27.1. WARREN, J. C. *Effects of chloroform and of strong chloric ether, as narcotic agents.* Boston, 1849.

GS28. HILL, B. L. *Lectures on the American eclectic system of surgery.* Cincinnati, 1850.

GS29. BRYANT, H. *The radical cure of inguinal hernia; . . .* Boston, 1851.

GS29.1. FLAGG, J. F. *Ether and chloroform; . . .* Philadelphia, 1851.

GS30. PIPER, R. U. *Operative surgery.* Boston, 1852.

GS31. SMITH , H. H. *A system of operative surgery: . . .* Philadelphia, 1852.

GS32. BOWDITCH, H. I. *A treatise on diaphragmatic hernia.* Buffalo, 1853.

GS33. GLOVER, R. *A treatise on orthopedic surgery and hernia; . . .* New York, 1853.

GS34. GROSS, S. D. *A practical treatise on foreign bodies in the air-passages.* Philadelphia, 1854.

GS35. HAYWARD, G. *Surgical reports and miscellaneous papers on medical subjects.* Boston, 1855.

GS36. HELMUTH, W. T. *Surgery and its adaptation to homoeopathic practice.* Philadelphia, 1855.

GS37. HILL, B. L. and HUNT, J. G. The homoeopathic practice of surgery, together with operative surgery. Cleveland, 1855.

GS38. SMITH, H. H. *Syllabus of the lectures on the principles and practice of surgery.* Philadelphia, 1855.

GS39. SMITH, H. H. *A treatise on the practice of surgery.* Philadelphia, 1856.

GS40. CARNOCHAN, J. M. *Contributions to operative surgery, and surgical pathology.* Philadelphia, 1857.

GS41. EVE, P. F. *A collection of remarkable cases in surgery.* Philadelphia, 1857.

GS42. COOK, W. H. *A treatise on the principles and practice of physio- medical surgery.* Cincinnati, 1858.

GS43. HODGES, R. M. *Practical dissections.* Cambridge, 1858.

GS44. SIMS, J. M. *Silver sutures in surgery.* New York, 1858.

GS45. GEDDINGS, E. *Outlines of a course of lectures on the principles and practice of surgery delivered by E. Geddings, . . .* Charleston, 1858.

GS46. GROSS, S. D. *A system of surgery; . . .* Philadelphia, 1859.

GS47. FRANCIS, S. W. *Report of Professor Valentine Mott's surgical cliniques in the University of New York, session 1859–60.* New York, 1860.

GS48. CHISOLM, J. J. *A manual of military surgery, for the use of surgeons in the Confederate States army; . . .* Richmond, 1861.

GS49. GROSS, S. D. *A manual of military surgery; . . .* Philadelphia, 1861.

GS50. HAMILTON, F. H. *A practical treatise on military surgery.* New York, 1861.

GS50.1. JACKSON, C. T. *A manual of etherization: . . .* Boston, 1861.

GS51. TRIPLER, C. S. and BLACKMAN, G. C. *Handbook for the military surgeon: . . .* Cincinnati, 1861.

GS52. BUCHANAN, J. *The eclectic practice of medicine and surgery.* Philadelphia, 1867.

GS53. SMITH, S. *Hand-book of surgical operations.* New York, 1862.

GS53.1. HELMUTH, W. T. *A treatise on diphtheria; . . .* St. Louis, 1862.

GS54. PACKARD, J. H. *A manual of minor surgery.* Philadelphia, 1863.

GS55. SMITH, H. H. *The principles and practice of surgery, embracing minor and operative surgery; . . .* Philadelphia, 1863.

GS56. WARREN, E. *An epitome of practical surgery for field and hospital.* Richmond, 1863.

GS56.1. SURGEON-GENERAL OF THE CONFEDERATE STATES. *A manual of military surgery, prepared for the use of the Confederate States Army.* Richmond, 1863.

GS57. HAMMOND, W. A. *Military medical and surgical essays, prepared for the United States Sanitary Commission.* Philadelphia, 1864.

GS58. MITCHELL, S. W., MOREHOUSE G. R., and KEEN, W. W. *Gunshot wounds and other injuries of nerves.* Philadelphia, 1864.

GS59. PACKARD, J. H. *Lectures on inflammation.* Philadelphia, 1865.

GS60. VAN BUREN, W. H. *Contributions to practical surgery.* Philadelphia, 1865.

GS61. CANNIFF, W. *A manual of the principles of surgery, based on pathology.* Philadelphia, 1866.

GS62. OTIS, G. A. *Histories of two hundred and ninety-six surgical photographs, prepared at the Army Medical Museum.* Washington, 1865–72?

GS63. OTIS, G. A. *Photographs of surgical cases and specimens: taken at the Army Medical Museum.* Washington, 1865–72?

GS64. WOODHULL, A. A. *Catalogue of the Surgical Section of the United States Army Museum.* Washington, 1866.

GS65. FRANKLIN, E. C. *The science and art of surgery, embracing minor and operative surgery; . . .* St. Louis, 1867–73.

GS66. WALTER, A. G. *Conservative surgery in its general and successful adaptation in cases of severe traumatic injuries of the limbs; . . .* Pittsburgh, 1867.

GS67. WARREN, J. M. *Surgical observations, with cases and operations.* Boston, 1867.

GS68. BARNES, J. K. *The medical and surgical history of the war of the rebellion, 1861–65.* Washington, 1870–88.

GS69. CHEEVER, D. W. *First medical and surgical report of the Boston City Hospital.* Boston, 1870.

GS70. HAMILTON, F. H. *Surgical memoirs of the war of the rebellion; . . .* New York, 1870–71.

GS71. PACKARD, J. H. *A handbook of operative surgery.* Philadelphia, 1870.

GS72. ASHURST, J. *The principles and practice of surgery.* Philadelphia, 1871.

GS73. HOWE, J. W. *Emergencies and how to treat them; . . .* New York, 1871.

GS74. OTIS, G. A. *A report of surgical cases treated in the army of the United States from 1865 to 1871.* Washington, 1871.

GS75. HAMILTON, F. H. *The principles and practice of surgery.* New York, 1872.

GS76. HEWSEN, A. *Earth as a topical application in surgery, . . .* Philadelphia, 1872.

GS77. WARREN, J. C. *The anatomy and development of rodent ulcer; . . .* Boston, 1872.

GS78. GILCHRIST, J. G. *The homoeopathic treatment of surgical diseases.* Chicago, 1873.

GS79. NORRIS, G. W. *Contributions to practical surgery.* Philadelphia, 1873.

GS80. WYETH, J. A. *A handbook of medical and surgical reference.* New York, 1873.

GS81. PEUGNET, E. *The nature of gunshot wounds of the abdomen, and their treatment;* . . . New York, 1874.

GS82. BRIGHAM, C. B. *Surgical cases.* Cambridge, 1876.

GS83. BUCK, G. *Contributions to reparative surgery;* . . . New York, 1876.

GS84. HOWE, A. J. *The art and science of surgery.* Cincinnati, 1879.

GS85. DOWELL, G. *A treatise on hernia:* . . . Philadelphia, 1876.

GS86. OSTROM, H. I. *A treatise on the breast and its surgical diseases.* Philadelphia, 1877.

GS87. TOLAND, H. H. *Lectures on practical surgery.* Philadelphia, 1877.

GS88. AGNEW, D. H. *Principles and practice of surgery, being a treatise on surgical diseases and injuries.* Philadelphia, 1878–83.

GS89. MEARS, J. E. *Practical surgery:* . . . Philadelphia, 1878.

GS90. NAPHEYS, G. H. *Modern surgical therapeutics:* . . . Philadelphia, 1878.

GS91. STIMSON, L. A. *A manual of operative surgery.* Philadelphia, 1878.

GS92. STONE, J. O. *Clinical cases, medical and surgical.* New York, 1878.

GS93. TURNBULL, L. *The advantages and accidents of artificial anaesthesia.* Philadelphia, 1878.

GS94. RANNEY, A. L. *A practical treatise on surgical diagnosis.* New York, 1879.

GS95. SMITH, S. *Manual of the principles and practice of operative surgery.* Boston, 1879.

GS96. WYETH, J. A. *Essays in surgical anatomy and surgery.* New York, 1879.

GS97. GROSS, S. W. *A practical treatise on tumors of the mammary glands, embracing their histology, pathology, diagnosis, and treatment.* New York, 1880.

GS98. MORTON, T. G. and HUNT, W. *Surgery in the Pennsylvania Hospital, being an epitome of the practice of the hospital since 1756;* . . . Philadelphia, 1880.

GS99. ROBERTS, J. B. *Paracentesis of the pericardium, a consideration of the surgical treatment of pericardial effusions.* Philadelphia, 1880.

GS100. ASHURST, J. *The international encyclopedia of surgery;* . . . New York, 1881–86.

GS101. GILCHRIST, J. G. *Surgical principles and minor surgery.* Chicago, 1881.

GS101.1. LYMAN, H. M. *Artificial anaesthesia and anaesthetics.* New York, 1881.

GS102. ROBERTS, J. B. *The compend of anatomy, for use in the dissecting room, and in preparing for examinations.* Philadelphia, 1881.

GS103. VON TAGEN, C. H. *Biliary calculi; perineorrhaphy; hospital gangrene and its kindred diseases, with their respective treatments.* New York, 1881.

GS104. **WARREN, J. H.** *Hernia, strangulated and reducible, with cure by sub-cutaneous injections, together with suggested and improved methods for kelotomy;* . . . Boston, 1881.

GS105. **BERMINGHAM, E. J.** *An encyclopaedic index of medicine and surgery.* New York, 1882.

GS106. **BUTLER, J.** *Electricity in surgery.* New York, 1882.

GS107. **FRANKLIN, E. C.** *A complete minor surgery.* Chicago, 1882.

GS108. **FRANKLIN, E. C.** *The practitioner's and student's manual of the science of surgery.* Ann Arbor, 1882.

GS109. **RANNEY, A. L.** *Practical medical anatomy;* . . . New York, 1882.

GS110. **GILLIAM, D. T.** *The essentials of pathology.* Philadelphia, 1883.

GS111. **DULLES, C. W.** *What to do first in accidents and emergencies;* . . . Philadelphia, 1883.

GS112. **HOPKINS, W. B.** *The roller bandage.* Philadelphia, 1883.

GS113. **HORWITZ, O.** *A compend of surgery.* Philadelphia, 1883.

GS114. **PILCHER, L. S.** *The treatment of wounds;* . . . New York, 1883.

GS115. **SALTER, S. F.** *Principles and practice of American medicine and surgery.* Atlanta, 1883.

GS116. **BRYANT, J. D.** *Manual of operative surgery.* New York, 1884.

GS117. **GILCHRIST, J. G.** *Surgical emergencies and accidents.* Chicago, 1884.

GS118. **KNIGHT, C. H.** *A year-book of surgery for 1883.* New York, 1884.

GS119. **VAN BUREN, W. H.** *Lectures on the principles of surgery.* New York, 1884.

GS120. **WARREN, J. H.** *A plea for the cure of rupture;* . . . Boston, 1884.

GS121. **CORNING, J. L.** *Local anesthesia in general medicine and surgery, being the practical application of the author's recent discoveries.* New York, 1885.

GS122. **PARKER, W.** *Cancer: a study of three hundred and ninety-seven cases of cancer of the female breast, with clinical observations.* New York, 1885

GS123. **TAYLOR, G. H.** *Pelvic and hernial therapeutics.* New York, 1885.

GS124. **TURNBULL, L.** *The new local anaesthetic;* . . . Philadelphia, 1885.

GS125. **MORRIS, R. T.** *How we treat wounds today;* . . . New York, 1886.

GS126. DE **NANCREDE, C. B. G.** *Essentials of anatomy including the anatomy of the viscera.* Philadelphia, 1887.

GS127. **WARREN, J. C.** *The healing of arteries after ligature in man and animals.* New York, 1886.

GS128. **FOWLER, G. R.** *Syllabus of a course of lectures on first aids to the injured, arranged for the medical officers of the second brigade, National Guard of the State of New York.* New York, 1887.

GS129. GARMANY, J. J. *Operative surgery on the cadaver.* New York, 1887.

GS130. HOMANS, J. *Three hundred and eighty-four laparotomies for various diseases, with tables showing the results of the operations and the subsequent history of the patients . . . .* Boston, 1887.

GS131. PRATT, E. H. *Orificial surgery and its application to the treatment of chronic diseases.* Chicago, 1887.

GS132. WYETH, J. A. *A text-book on surgery, general, operative, and mechanical.* New York, 1887.

GS133. GERSTER, A. G. *The rules of aseptic and antiseptic surgery.* New York, 1888.

GS134. MARTIN, E. *Questions and answers of the essentials of surgery: . . .* Philadelphia, 1888.

GS135. NEWELL, O. K. *The best surgical dressing; . . .* Boston, 1888.

GS136. WYMAN, H. C. *Abdominal surgery.* Detroit, 1888.

GS137. MARCY, H. O. *A treatise on hernia, the radical cure by the use of the buried antiseptic animal suture.* Detroit, 1889.

GS138. SENN, N. *Experimental surgery.* Chicago, 1889.

GS139. SENN, N. *Intestinal surgery.* Chicago, 1889.

GS140. SENN, N. *Surgical bacteriology.* Philadelphia, 1889.

GS141. YOUNG, J. K. *Synopsis of human anatomy; . . .* Philadelphia, 1889.

GS142. MARTIN, E. *Essentials of minor surgery and bandaging, with an appendix on venereal diseases.* Philadelphia, 1890.

GS143. ROBERTS, J. B. *A manual of modern surgery; . . .* Philadelphia, 1890.

GS144. SENN, N. *Principles of surgery.* Philadelphia, 1890.

GS145. STEMEN, C. B. *Railway surgery, a practical work on the special department of railway surgery; . . .* St. Louis, 1890.

GS146. HAMILTON, J. B. *Lectures on tumors from a clinical standpoint.* Detroit, 1891.

GS147. MARTIN, E. *The surgical treatment of wounds and obstruction of the intestines.* Philadelphia, 1891.

GS148. McCLELLAN, G. *Regional anatomy in its relation to medicine and surgery.* Philadelphia, 1891–92.

GS149. ROBINSON, F. B. *Practical intestinal surgery.* Detroit, 1891.

GS150. WHARTON, H. R. *Minor surgery and bandaging, including the treatment of fractures and dislocations, . . .* Philadelphia, 1891.

GS151. WILLARD, D. and ADLER, L. H. *Artificial anaesthesia and anaesthetics.* Detroit, 1891.

GS152. **BROCKWAY, F. J.** and **O'MALLEY, A.** *Anatomy; a manual for students and practitioners.* Philadelphia, 1892.

GS153. **PARK, R.** *The Mütter lectures on surgical pathology.* St. Louis, 1892.

GS154. **KEEN, W. W.** and **WHITE, J. W.** *An American text-book of surgery.* Philadelphia, 1892.

GS155. **MARCY, H.O.** *The anatomy and surgical treatment of hernia.* New York, 1892.

GS156. **GALLAUDET, B. B.** and **DIXON-JONES, C. N.** *Surgery, a manual for students and practitioners.* Philadelphia, 1893.

GS157. **MANLEY, T. H.** *Hernia; . . .* Philadelphia, 1893.

GS158. **CHEEVER, D. W.** *Lectures on surgery.* Boston, 1894.

GS159. **DaCOSTA, J. C.** *A manual of modern surgery, general and operative.* Philadelphia, 1894.

GS160. **FOWLER, G. R.** *A treatise on appendicitis.* Philadelphia, 1894.

GS161. **ROBB, H.** *Aseptic surgical technique; . . .* Philadelphia, 1894.

GS162. **SENN, N.** *Syllabus of lectures on the practice of surgery, arranged in conformity with the American text-book of surgery.* Philadelphia, 1894.

GS163. **BECK, C.** *A manual of the modern theory and technique of surgical asepsis.* Philadelphia, 1895.

GS164. **BUCHANAN, C. M.** *Antisepsis and antiseptics.* Newark, 1895.

GS165. **DENNIS, F. S.** *System of surgery.* Philadelphia, 1895–96.

GS166. **GILCHRIST, J. G.** *The elements of surgical pathology with therapeutic hints.* Minneapolis, 1895.

GS167. **MORRIS, R. T.** *Lectures on appendicitis and notes on other subjects.* New York, 1895.

GS168. **SENN, N.** *The pathology and surgical treatment of tumors.* Philadelphia, 1895.

GS169. **WARREN, J. C.** *Surgical pathology and therapeutics.* Philadelphia, 1895.

GS170. **DEAVER, J. B.** *A treatise on appendicitis.* Philadelphia, 1896.

GS171. **FISHER, C. E.** and **MacDONALD, T. L.** *A homeopathic text-book of surgery.* Chicago, 1896.

GS172. **MORTON, W. J.** and **HAMMER, E. W.** *The X ray or photography of the invisible and its value in surgery.* New York, 1896.

GS173. **PARK, R.** *A treatise on surgery by American authors.* Philadelphia, 1896.

GS174. **PARKES, C. T.** *Clinical lectures on abdominal surgery and other subjects.* Chicago, 1896.

GS175. **MYNTER, H.** *Appendicitis and its surgical treatment, with a report of seventy-five operated cases.* Philadelphia, 1897.

GS176. CRUTCHER, H. *A practical treatise on appendicitis.* Chicago, 1897.

GS177. HILLSMAN, B. L. *Notes on principles of surgery from lectures by Stuart McGuire.* Richmond, 1897.

GS178. KEEN, W. W. *The surgical complications and sequels of typhoid fever.* Philadelphia, 1898.

GS179. MacDONALD, J. W. *A clinical textbook of surgical diagnosis and treatment for practitioners and students of surgery and medicine.* Philadelphia, 1898.

GS180. WHARTON, H. R. and CURTIS, B. F. *The practice of surgery; a treatise on surgery for the use of practitioners and students.* Philadelphia, 1898.

GS181. WINANS, W. W. *Quiz-compend on surgery.* Philadelphia, 1898.

GS182. CRILE, G. W. *An experimental research into surgical shock.* Philadelphia, 1899.

GS183. CRILE, G. W. *Experimental research into the surgery of the respiratory system.* Philadelphia, 1899.

GS184. DEAVER, J. B. *Surgical anatomy; . . .* Philadelphia, 1899–1903.

GS185. DE NANCREDE, C. B. G. *Lectures upon the principles of surgery.* Philadelphia, 1899.

GS186. HERRICK, C. B. *Railway surgery, a handbook of the management of injuries.* New York, 1899.

GS187. SKENE, A. J. C. *Electro-haemostasis in operative surgery.* New York, 1899.

GS188. SUMMERS, J. E. *The modern treatment of wounds.* Omaha, 1899.

GS189. TRUAX, C. *The mechanics of surgery, . . .* Chicago, 1899.

GS190. PILCHER, L. S. *The treatment of wounds, its principles and practice, general and special.* New York, 1899.

OPHTHALMOLOGY

OP1. FRICK, G. *A treatise on the diseases of the eye; . . .* Baltimore, 1823.

OP2. GIBSON, J. M. *A condensation of matter upon the anatomy, surgical operations and treatment of diseases of the eye.* Baltimore, 1832.

OP3. WALLACE, W. C. *The structure of the eye with reference to natural theology.* New York, 1836.

OP4. LITTELL, S. *A manual of the diseases of the eye.* Philadelphia, 1837.

OP5. DIX, J. H. *Treatise on strabismus, or squinting and the new mode of treatment.* Boston, 1841.

OP6. POST, A. C. *Observations on the cure of strabismus; . . .* New York, 1841.

OP7. BOLTON, J. *A treatise on strabismus, with a description of new instruments designed to improve the operation for its cure, . . .* Richmond, 1842.

OP8. HAMILTON, F. H. *Monograph on strabismus, with cases.* Buffalo, 1845.

OP9. POWELL, J. W. *The eye: its imperfections and their prevention; . . .* New York, 1847.

OP10. DIX, J. H. *Treatise upon the nature and treatment of morbid sensibility of the retina, or weakness of sight . . .* Boston, 1849.

OP11. CADWELL, F. A. *Treatise on the eye and ear: . . .* Chicago, 1853.

OP12. CLARK, J. H. *Sight and hearing, how preserved, and how lost.* New York, 1856.

OP13. WILLIAMS, H. W. *A practical guide to the study of the diseases of the eye; . . .* Boston, 1862.

OP14. KEYSER, P. D. *Glaucoma, its symptoms, diagnosis, and treatment.* Philadelphia, 1864.

OP15. WILLIAMS, H. W. *Recent advances in ophthalmic science.* Boston, 1866.

OP15.1. ALDEN, W. *The human eye; its use and abuse: . . .* Cincinnati, 1866.

OP16. METZ, A. *The anatomy and histology of the human eye.* Philadelphia, 1868.

OP17. KNAPP, J. H. *A treatise on intraocular tumors, from original observations and anatomical investigations.* New York, 1869.

OP18. PHILLIPS, J. *Ophthalmic surgery and treatment: with advice on the use and abuse of spectacles.* Chicago, 1869.

OP19. ANGELL, H. C. *A treatise on diseases of the eye; . . .* Boston, 1870.

OP20. JEFFRIES, B. J. *The eye in health and disease: . . .* Boston, 1871.

OP21. WILLIAMS, H. W. *Our eyes and how to take care of them.* Boston, 1871.

OP22. HOWE, A. J. *Manual of eye surgery.* Cincinnati, 1874.

OP23. FENNER, C. S. *Vision; its optical defects, and the adaptation of spectacles.* Philadelphia, 1875.

OP24. ALLEN, T. F. and NORTON, G. S. *Ophthalmic therapeutics.* New York, 1876.

OP25. LORING, E. G. *Determination of the refraction of the eye by means of the ophthalmoscope.* New York, 1876.

OP26. ROOSA, D. B. ST. J. and ELY, E. T. *Ophthalmic and optic memoranda.* New York, 1876.

OP27. HART, C. P. *Homeopathic ophthalmic practice: . . .* Detroit, 1877.

OP28. JEFFRIES, B. J. *Color-blindness: its dangers and its detection.* Boston, 1879.

OP29. HARLAN, G. C. *Eyesight, and how to care for it.* Philadelphia, 1880.

OP30. LeCONTE, J. *Sight; an exposition of the principles of monocular and binocular vision.* New York, 1881.

OP31. **MITTENDORF, W. F.** *A manual on diseases of the eye and ear, for the use of students and practitioners.* New York, 1881.

OP32. **NOYES, H. D.** *A treatise on diseases of the eye.* New York, 1881.

OP33. **VILAS, C. H.** *Spectacles; . . .* Chicago, 1881.

OP34. **WILLIAMS, H. W.** *The diagnosis and treatment of the diseases of the eye.* Boston, 1882.

OP35. **VILAS, C. H.** *The ophthalmoscope; . . .* Chicago, 1882.

OP36. **BUFFUM, J. H.** *The diseases of the eye: their medical and surgical treatment.* Chicago, 1884.

OP37. **VILAS, C. H.** *Therapeutics of the eye and ear.* Chicago, 1883.

OP38. **ALT, A.** *A treatise on ophthalmology for the general practitioner.* Chicago, 1884.

OP39. **LORING, E. G.** *Textbook of ophthalmoscopy.* New York, 1886–91.

OP40. **MITTENDORF, W. F.** *Granular lids and contagious diseases of the eye.* Detroit, 1886.

OP41. **BURNETT, S. M.** *A theoretical and practical treatise on astigmatism.* St. Louis, 1887.

OP42. **FOX, L. W.** and **GOULD, G. M.** *A compend of the diseases of the eye, including refraction and surgical operations.* Philadelphia, 1887.

OP43. **ROOSA, D. B. St. J.** *The determination of the necessity for wearing glasses.* Detroit, 1887.

OP44. **CLAIBORNE, J. H.** *The theory and practice of the ophthalmoscope; . . .* Detroit, 1888.

OP45. **PRENTICE, C. F.** *Dioptric formulae for combined cylindrical lenses applicable for all angular deviation of their axes.* New York, 1888.

OP46. **VALK, F.** *Lectures on the errors of refraction and their correction with glasses.* New York, 1889.

OP47. **JACKSON, E.** and **GLEASON, E. B.** *Essentials of refraction and the diseases of the eye, and essentials of diseases of the nose and throat.* Philadelphia, 1890.

OP48. **NOYES, H. D.** *A textbook on diseases of the eye.* New York, 1890.

OP49. **VILAS, C. H.** *Diseases of the eye and ear.* Chicago, 1890.

OP50. **WOOD, C. A.** *Lessons in the diagnosis and treatment of eye diseases.* Detroit, 1891.

OP51. **SKINNER, D. N.** *The care of the eyes in health and disease.* Boston, 1891.

OP52. **DE SCHWEINITZ, G. E.** *Diseases of the eye; . . .* Philadelphia, 1892.

OP53. **HANSELL, H. F.** and **BELL, J. H.** *A manual of clinical ophthalmology.* Philadelphia, 1892.

OP54. JOHNSTON, J. M. *Eye studies, a series of lessons on vision and visual tests.* Chicago, 1892.

OP55. NORTON, A. B. *Ophthalmic diseases and therapeutics.* Philadelphia, 1892.

OP56. PHILLIPS, R. J. *Spectacles and eyeglasses, their forms, mounting, and proper adjustment.* Philadelphia, 1892.

OP57. NORRIS, W. F. and OLIVER, C. A. *A textbook of ophthalmology.* Philadelphia, 1893.

OP58. SAVAGE, G. C. *New truths in ophthalmology.* Nashville, 1893.

OP59. BUFFUM, J. H. *Diseases of the eye and ear in children.* Chicago, 1894.

OP60. ROOSA, D. B. ST. J. *A clinical manual of diseases of the eye, including a sketch of its anatomy.* New York, 1894.

OP61. TIFFANY, F. B. *Anomalies of refraction and of the muscles of the eye.* Kansas City, 1894.

OP62. CLAIBORNE, J. H. *The functional examination of the eye.* Philadelphia, 1895.

OP63. JACKSON, E. *Skiascopy and its practical application to the study of refraction.* Philadelphia, 1895.

OP64. McCORMICK, C. N. *Practical optics for beginners.* Chicago, 1895.

OP65. PRENTICE, C. *The eye in its relation to health.* Chicago, 1895.

OP66. WALKER, G. A. *Students' aid in ophthalmology.* Philadelphia, 1895.

OP67. DE SCHWEINITZ, G. E. *The toxic amblyopias:* . . . Philadelphia, 1896.

OP68. JENNINGS, J. E. *Color-vision and color-blindness;* . . . Philadelphia, 1896.

OP69. VEASEY, C. A. *Ophthalmic operations as practiced on animal's eyes.* Philadelphia, 1896.

OP70. WRIGHT C. D'A. *A handbook of the refraction of the eye, its anomalies and their correction.* Ann Arbor, 1896.

OP71. WRIGHT, J. W. *A textbook of ophthalmology.* Columbus, 1896.

OP72. DUANE, A. *A new classification of the motor anomalies of the eye based upon physiological principles,* . . . New York, 1897.

OP73. NORRIS, W. F. and OLIVER, C. A. *System of diseases of the eye;* . . . Philadelphia, 1897–1900.

OP74. HENDERSON, F. L. *Notes on the eye, for the use of students.* St. Louis, 1897.

OP74.1. LINNELL, E.H. *The eye as an aid in general diagnosis.* Philadelphia, 1897.

OP75. MacBRIDE, N. L. *Diseases of the eye.* New York, 1897.

OP76. RANNEY, A. L. *Eye-strain in health and disease; . . .* Philadelphia, 1897.

OP77. THORINGTON, J. *Retinoscopy (or shadow test) in the determination of refraction at one meter distance, with the plane mirror.* Philadelphia, 1897.

OP78. BOYLE, C. C. *Therapeutics of the eye.* New York, 1898.

OP79. DAILEY, L. J. *Refractive and ophthalmic catechism, . . .* Gloversville, NY, 1898.

OP80. McCORMICK, C. N. *Optical truths, illustrated.* Chicago, 1898.

OP81. STIRLING, A. W. *Glaucoma; . . .* St. Louis, 1898.

OP82. HANSELL, H. F. and REBER, W. *A practical handbook on the muscular anomalies of the eye.* Philadelphia, 1899.

OP83. HENRY, C. E. *A manual of osteopathic treatment of diseases of the eye.* Minneapolis, 1899.

OP84. ROOSA, D. B. ST. J. *Defective eyesight; . . .* New York, 1899.

OTORHINOLARYNGOLOGY

OT1. GREEN, H. *A treatise on diseases of the air passages: . . .* New York, 1846.

OT2. GREEN, H. *Observations on the pathology of croup: . . .* New York, 1849.

OT3. BRYAN, J. *A treatise on the anatomy, physiology and diseases of the human ear.* Philadelphia, 1851.

OT4. GREEN, H. *On the surgical treatment of polypi of the larynx, and oedema of the glottis.* New York, 1852.

OT5. GREEN, H. *A practical treatise on pulmonary tuberculosis, . . .* New York, 1864.

OT6. ELSBERG, L. *Laryngoscopal surgery illustrated in the treatment of morbid growths within the larynx, . . .* Philadelphia, 1866.

OT7. CLARKE, E. H. *Observations on the nature and treatment of polypus of the ear.* Boston, 1867.

OT8. SOLIS COHEN, J. D. *Inhalation: its therapeutics and practice; . . .* Philadelphia, 1867.

OT9. RUPPANER, A. *The principles and practice of laryngoscopy and rhinoscopy in diseases of the throat and nasal passages.* New York, 1868.

OT10. KNAPP, J. H. *A clinical analysis of the inflammatory affections of the inner ear.* New York, 1871.

OT11. SOLIS COHEN, J. D. *Diseases of the throat: . . .* New York, 1872.

OT12. TURNBULL, L. *A clinical manual of the diseases of the ear.* Philadelphia, 1872.

OT13. WILLIAMS, A. D. *Diseases of the ear including the necessary anatomy of the different parts of the organ . . . .* Cincinnati, 1873.

OT14. ROOSA, D. B. ST. J. *A practical treatise on the diseases of the ear, . . .* New York, 1873.

OT15. SOLIS COHEN, J. D. *Croup, in its relation to tracheotomy.* Philadelphia, 1874.

OT16. MORSE, L. D. *On nasal catarrh; . . .* Memphis, 1876.

OT17. BURNETT, C. H. *The ear; its anatomy, physiology, and diseases.* Philadelphia, 1877.

OT18. BOSWORTH, F. H. *Handbook upon diseases of the throat for the use of students.* New York, 1879.

OT19. BURNETT, C. H. *Hearing, and how to keep it.* Philadelphia, 1879.

OT20. SOLIS COHEN, J. D. *The throat and the voice.* Philadelphia, 1879.

OT21. SEILER, C. *Handbook of diagnosis and treatment of diseases of the throat and nasal cavities.* Philadelphia, 1879.

OT22. SHOEMAKER, C. E. *The ear: its diseases and injuries and their treatment.* Reading, PA, 1879.

OT23. BUCK, A. H. *Diagnosis and treatment of ear diseases.* New York, 1880.

OT24. ROBINSON, B. *A practical treatise on nasal catarrh.* New York, 1880.

OT25. RUMBOLD, T. F. *Hygiene and treatment of catarrh; . . .* St. Louis, 1880.

OT26. BOSWORTH, F. H. *A manual of diseases of the throat and nose.* New York, 1881.

OT27. BRIGHAM, G. N. *Catarrhal diseases of the nasal and respiratory organs.* New York, 1881.

OT28. INGALS, E. F. *Lectures on the diagnosis and treatment of diseases of the chest, throat, and nasal cavities.* New York, 1881.

OT29. RUMBOLD, T. F. *The hygiene and treatment of catarrh.* St. Louis, 1881.

OT30. TURNBULL, L. *Imperfect hearing and the hygiene of the ear; . . .* Philadelphia, 1881.

OT31. WAGNER, C. *Habitual mouth-breathing; . . .* New York, 1881.

OT32. BRIGHAM, G. N. *Phthisis pulmonalis; or, tubercular consumption.* New York, 1882.

OT33. LEFFERTS, G. M. *A pharmacopoeia for the treatment of diseases of the larynx, pharynx, and nasal passages, . . .* New York, 1882.

OT34. WINSLOW, W. H. *The human ear and its diseases; . . .* New York, 1882.

OT35. KITCHEN, J. M. W. *Student's manual of diseases of the nose and throat; . . .* New York, 1883.

OT36. KITCHEN, J. M. W. *Catarrh, sore-throat and hoarseness; . . .* New York, 1884.

OT37. **POMEROY, O. D.** *The diagnosis and treatment of diseases of the ear.* New York, 1883.

OT38. **WAGNER, C.** *Diseases of the nose.* New York, 1884.

OT39. **HOUGHTON, H. C.** *Lectures on clinical otology.* Boston, 1885.

OT40. **NICHOL, T.** *Diseases of the nares, larynx and trachea in childhood.* New York, 1885.

OT41. **OSTROM, H. I.** *Epithelioma of the mouth.* New York, 1885.

OT42. **RUMBOLD, T. F.** *Pruritic rhinitis (hay-fever, autumnal catarrh, etc.) . . .* St. Louis, 1885.

OT43. **SAJOUS, C. E. D. M.** *Lectures on the diseases of the nose and throat.* Philadelphia, 1885.

OT44. **SAJOUS, C. E. D. M.** *Hay fever and its successful treatment by superficial organic alteration of the nasal mucous membrane.* Philadelphia, 1885.

OT45. **STERLING, C. F.** *The disease of the ear and their homoeopathic treatment, . . .* New York, 1885.

OT46. **ROBINSON, B.** *A manual on inhalers, inhalations, and inhalants, . . .* Detroit, 1886.

OT47. **SEXTON, S.** *The classification and treatment of over two thousand consecutive cases of ear diseases at Dr. Sexton's aural clinic, New York Eye and Ear Infirmary.* Detroit, 1886.

OT48. **RUMBOLD, T. F.** *A practical treatise on the medical, surgical and hygienic treatment of catarrhal diseases of the nose, throat, and ears; . . .* St. Louis, 1887.

OT49. **SEXTON, S.** *The ear and its diseases; . . .* New York, 1888.

OT49.1. **WAXHAM, F. E.** *Intubation of the larynx.* Chicago, 1888.

OT50. **BOSWORTH, F. H.** *A treatise on diseases of the nose and throat.* New York, 1889–92.

OT51. **BUCK, A. H.** *A manual of diseases of the ear.* New York, 1889.

OT52. **BURNETT, C. H.** *Diseases and injuries of the ear: their prevention and cure.* Philadelphia, 1889.

OT52.1. **BILLINGTON, C.E.** and **O'DWYER, J.** *Diphtheria, its nature and treatment; . . .* New York, 1889.

OT53. **SEXTON, S.** *Deafness and discharge from the ear; . . .* New York, 1891.

OT54. **ALLEN, S. E.** *The mastoid operation, including its history, anatomy, and pathology.* Cincinnati, 1892.

OT55. **MILLER, F. E., McEVOY, J. P.,** and **WEEKS, J. E.** *Diseases of the eye, ear, throat, and nose.* Philadelphia, 1892.

OT56. **TUTTLE, A. H.** *The surgical anatomy and surgery of the ear.* Detroit, 1892.

OT57. BURNETT, C. H. *System of diseases of the ear, nose, and throat.* Philadelphia, 1893.

OT58. IVINS, H. F. *Diseases of the nose and throat.* Philadelphia, 1893.

OT59. DENCH, E. B. *Diseases of the ear.* New York, 1894.

OT60. GLEASON, E. B. *Essentials of the diseases of the ear.* Philadelphia, 1894.

OT61. BOSWORTH, F. H. *A text-book of diseases of the nose and throat.* New York, 1896.

OT62. BUFFUM, J. H. *Manual of the essentials of diseases of the eye and ear.* Chicago, 1896.

OT63. LANE, L. C. *The surgery of the head and neck.* San Francisco, 1896.

OT64. BISHOP, S. S. *Diseases of the ear, nose, and throat and their accessory cavities.* Philadelphia, 1897.

OT64.1. QUAY, G. H. *A monograph of diseases of the nose and throat.* Philadelphia, 1897.

OT65. BACON, G. *A manual of otology.* New York, 1898.

OT66. RUMBOLD, T. F. *The hygiene of the voice.* St. Louis, 1898.

OT67. SCHEPPEGRELL, W. *Electricity in the diagnosis and treatment of diseases of the nose, throat and ear.* New York, 1898.

OT68. BUCK, A. H. *First principles of otology.* New York, 1899.

OT69. COAKLEY, C. G. *A manual of diseases of the nose and throat.* Philadelphia, 1899.

OT70. DE SCHWEINITZ, G. E. and RANDALL, B. A. *An American text-book of diseases of the eye, ear, nose and throat.* Philadelphia, 1899.

OT71. KYLE, D. B. *A textbook of diseases of the nose and throat.* Philadelphia, 1899.

OT72. NAULTEUS, F. *Medical compendium on all acute and chronic, all female and children, eye, ear, nose and throat diseases.* Hastings, NE, 1899.

ORTHOPEDIC SURGERY

OR1. WARREN, J. C. *A letter to the Honorable Isaac Parker, Chief Justice of the Supreme Court of the State of Massachusetts, containing remarks on the dislocation of the hip joint.* Cambridge, 1824.

OR2. GROSS, S. D. *The anatomy, physiology, and diseases of the bones and joints.* Philadelphia, 1830.

OR3. MÜTTER, T. D. *A lecture on loxarthrus or club-foot,* Philadelphia, 1839.

OR4. BIGELOW, H. J. *Manual of orthopedic surgery, . . .* Boston, 1845.

OR5. JARVIS, G. O. *Lectures on fractures and dislocations, explaining new modes of treatment, . . .* Derby, CT, 1846.

OR6. CARNOCHAN, J. M. *A treatise on the etiology, pathology and treatment of congenital dislocations of the head of the femur.* New York, 1850.

OR7. HAMILTON, F. H. *A practical treatise on fractures and dislocations.* Philadelphia, 1860.

OR8. HODGES, R. M. *The excision of joints.* Cambridge, 1861.

OR9. TAYLOR, C. F. *Theory and practice of the movement-cure; . . .* Philadelphia, 1861.

OR10. CLEAVELAND, C. H. *Causes and cure of diseases of the feet; with practical suggestions as to their clothing.* Cincinnati, 1862.

OR11. BAUER, L. *Lectures on orthopedic surgery.* Philadelphia, 1864.

OR12. TAYLOR, C. F. *Infantile paralysis, and its attendant deformities.* Philadelphia, 1864.

OR13. NOTT, J. C. *Contributions to bone and nerve injury.* Philadelphia, 1866.

OR14. PRINCE, D. *Orthopedics; . . .* Philadelphia, 1866.

OR15. ASHHURST, J. *Injuries of the spine; . . .* Philadelphia, 1867.

OR16. DAVIS, H. G. *Conservative surgery, as exhibited in remedying some of the mechanical causes that operate injuriously both in health and disease.* New York, 1867.

OR17. LEE, B. *Contributions to the pathology, diagnosis, and treatment of angular curvature of the spine.* Philadelphia, 1867.

OR18. OTIS, G. A. *A report on amputations at the hip-joint in military surgery.* Washington, 1867.

OR19. SMITH, N. R. *Treatment of fractures of the lower extremity by the use of the anterior suspensory apparatus.* Baltimore, 1867.

OR20. WALES, P. S. *Mechanical therapeutics, a practical treatise on surgical apparatus, . . .* Philadelphia, 1867.

OR21. BAUER, L. *Lectures on causes, pathology, and treatment of joint diseases.* New York, 1868.

OR22. BIGELOW, H. J. *The mechanism of dislocation and fracture of the hip with the reduction of the dislocation by the flexion method.* Philadelphia, 1869.

OR23. OTIS, G. A. *A report on excisions of the head of the femur for gunshot injury.* Washington, 1869.

OR24. SAYRE, L. A. *A practical manual of the treatment of club foot.* New York, 1869.

OR25. HOWE, A. J. *A practical and systematic treatise on fractures and dislocations.* Cincinnati, 1870.

OR26. PRINCE, D. *Plastics and orthopedics.* Philadelphia, 1871.

OR27. LEE, B. *The correct principles of treatment for angular curvature of the spine.* Philadelphia, 1872.

OR28. MARKOE, T. M. *A treatise on diseases of the bones.* New York, 1872.

OR29. ELA, W. *Fractures of the elbow joint.* Cambridge, 1873.

OR30. TAYLOR, C. F. *On the mechanical treatment of disease of the hip-joint.* New York, 1873.

OR31. TAYLOR, R. W. *Syphilitic lesions of the osseous system in infants and young children.* New York, 1875.

OR32. CULBERTSON, H. *Excision of the larger joints of the extremities.* Philadelphia, 1876.

OR33. SAYRE, L. A. *Lectures on orthopedic surgery and diseases of the joint.* New York, 1876.

OR34. SAYRE, L. A. *Spinal disease and spinal curvature, their treatment by suspension and the use of the plaster of Paris bandage.* Philadelphia, 1877.

OR35. FRANKLIN, E. C. *The homoeopathic treatment of spinal curvatures according to the new principle.* St. Louis, 1878.

OR36. SHAFFER, N. M. *Pott's disease, its pathology and mechanical treatment, with remarks on rotary lateral curvature.* New York, 1879.

OR37. HAMILTON, F. H. *Fracture of the patella: . . .* New York, 1880.

OR38. HUTCHISON, J. C. *Contributions to orthopedic surgery; . . .* New York, 1880.

OR39. SHAFFER, N. M. *The hysterical element in orthopaedic surgery.* New York, 1880.

OR40. STIMSON, L. A. *A treatise on fractures.* Philadelphia, 1883.

OR41. GIBNEY, V. P. *The hip and its diseases.* New York, 1884.

OR42. KNIGHT, J. *Orthopaedia or a practical treatise on the aberrations of the human form.* New York, 1874.

OR43. POORE, C. T. *Osteotomy and osteoclasis for deformities of the lower extremities.* New York, 1884.

OR44. WATSON, B. A. *A treatise on amputations of the extremities and their complications.* Philadelphia, 1882.

OR45. STIMSON, L. A. *A treatise on dislocations.* Philadelphia, 1888.

OR46. BRADFORD, E. H. and LOVETT, R. W. *A treatise on orthopedic surgery.* New York, 1890.

OR47. LOVETT, R. W. *The etiology, pathology, and treatment of diseases of the hip joint.* Boston, 1891.

OR48. STILLMAN, C. F. *A practical resumé of modern methods employed in the treatment of chronic articular ostitis of the hip.* Detroit, 1891.

OR49. SENN, N. *Tuberculosis of bones and joints.* Philadelphia, 1892.

OR50. RIDLON, J. and JONES, R. *Chronic joint disease; some preliminary papers.* Chicago, 1894.

OR51. YOUNG, J. K. *A practical treatise on orthopedic surgery.* Philadelphia, 1894.

OR52. ALLIS, O. H. *An inquiry into the difficulties encountered in the reduction of dislocations of the hip.* Philadelphia, 1896.

OR53. ROBERTS, J. B. *A clinical, pathological, and experimental study of fracture of the lower end of the radius, . . .* Philadelphia, 1897.

OR54. FARNUM, E. J. *Deformities; a textbook on orthopedic surgery.* Chicago, 1898.

OR55. MOORE, J. E. *Orthopedic surgery.* Philadelphia, 1898.

OR56. McCURDY, S. L. *Manual of orthopedic surgery.* Pittsburgh, 1898.

OR57. ROBERTS, A. S. *Contributions to orthopedic surgery; . . .* Philadelphia, 1898.

OR58. SHAFFER, N. M. *Brief essays on orthopedic surgery, . . .* New York, 1898.

OR59. RIDLON, J. and JONES, R. *Lectures on orthopedic surgery.* Philadelphia, 1899.

OR60. ROBERTS, J. B. *Notes on the modern treatment of fractures.* New York, 1899.

OR61. STIMSON, L. A. *A practical treatise on fractures and dislocations.* New York, 1899.

GYNECOLOGY

GY1. DEWEES, W. P. *A treatise on the diseases of females.* Philadelphia, 1826.

GY2. DIXON, E. H. *Woman, and her diseases, from the cradle to the grave:* . . . New York, 1847.

GY3. MEIGS, C. D. *Females and their diseases; . . .* Philadelphia, 1848.

GY4. LYMAN, G. H. *Non-malignant diseases of the uterus; . . .* Boston, 1854.

GY5. MEIGS, C. D. *A treatise on acute and chronic diseases of the neck of the uterus.* Philadelphia, 1854.

GY6. BEDFORD, G. S. *Clinical lectures on the diseases of women and children.* New York, 1855.

GY7. LYMAN, G. H. *The history and statistics of ovariotomy and the circumstances under which the operation may be regarded as safe and expedient.* Boston, 1856.

GY8. SCUDDER, J. M. *A practical treatise on the diseases of women; . . .* Cincinnati, 1857.

GY9. HODGE, H. L. *On diseases peculiar to women, including displacements of the uterus.* Philadelphia, 1860.

GY10. BYFORD, W. H. *A treatise on the chronic inflammation and displacement of the unimpregnated uterus.* Philadelphia, 1864.

GY11. BYFORD, W. H. *The practice of medicine and surgery, applied to the diseases and accidents incident to women.* Philadelphia, 1865.

GY12. SIMS, J. M. *Clinical notes on uterine surgery; . . .* New York, 1866.

GY13. EMMET, T. A. *Vesico-vaginal fistula from parturition and other causes: with cases of recto-vaginal fistula.* New York, 1868.

GY14. THOMAS, T. G. *A practical treatise on the diseases of women.* Philadelphia, 1868.

GY15. LUDLAM, R. *Lectures, clinical and didactic, on the diseases of women.* Chicago, 1870.

GY16. TAYLOR, G. H. *Diseases of women: . . .* Philadelphia, 1871.

GY17. CHAPMAN, E. N. *Hysterology: . . .* New York, 1872.

GY18. PEASLEE, E. R. *Ovarian tumors; . . .* New York, 1872.

GY19. AGNEW, D. H. *Lacerations of the female perineum; and vesico-vaginal fistula; . . .* Philadelphia, 1873.

GY20. ATLEE, W. L. *General and differential diagnosis of ovarian tumors, with specific references to the operation of ovariotomy; . . .* Philadelphia, 1873.

GY21. SKENE, A. J. C. *Diseases of the bladder and urethra in women.* New York, 1878.

GY22. CLARK, A. L. *A treatise on the medical and surgical diseases of women.* Chicago, 1879.

GY23. EMMET, T. A. *The principles and practice of gynaecology.* Philadelphia, 1879.

GY24. GOODELL, W. *Lessons in gynecology.* Philadelphia, 1879.

GY25. ATKINSON, W. B. *The therapeutics of gynecology and obstetrics, . . .* Philadelphia, 1880.

GY26. EATON, M. M. *A treatise on the medical and surgical diseases of women, with their homeopathic treatment.* New York, 1880.

GY27. MUNDE, P. F. *Minor surgical gynecology: . . .* New York, 1880.

GY28. DONALDSON, S. J. *Contributions to practical gynecology.* New York, 1882.

GY29. GARRIGUES, H. J. *Diagnosis of ovarian cysts by means of the examination of their contents.* New York, 1882.

GY30. MAY, C. H. *Manual of the diseases of women, . . .* Philadelphia, 1885.

GY31. MANN, M. D. *A system of gynecology by American authors.* Philadelphia, 1887–1888.

GY32. COWPERTHWAITE, A. C. *A textbook of gynecology.* Chicago, 1888.

GY33. SKENE, A. J. C. *Treatise on the diseases of women.* New York, 1888.

GY34. SOUTHWICK, G. R. *A practical manual of gynaecology.* Boston 1888.

GY35. DAVENPORT, F. H. *Diseases of women: . . .* Philadelphia, 1889.

GY35.1. WEAVER, B. F. *Woman's guide to health: . . .* Bucyrus, OH, 1889.

GY36. CRAGIN, E. B. *Essentials of gynaecology.* Philadelphia, 1890.

GY37. HOWE, A. J. *Operative gynaecology.* Cincinnati, 1890.

GY38. GRANDIN, E. H. and GUNNING, J. H. *Practical treatise on electricity in gynaecology.* New York, 1891.

GY38.1. MORRIS. H. *A compend of gynaecology.* Philadelphia, 1891.

GY39. BRATENAHL, G. W. and TOUSEY, S. *Gynecology.* Philadelphia, 1892.

GY40. GOELET, A. H. *The electro-therapeutics of gynaecology.* Detroit, 1892.

GY41. BUSHONG, C. H. *Modern gynecology: . . .* New York, 1893.

GY42. MARTIN, F. H. *Electricity in diseases of women and obstetrics.* Chicago, 1893.

GY43. BALDY, J. M. *An American text-book of gynecology, medical and surgical.* Philadelphia, 1894.

GY44. MUNDE, P. F. *A report of the gynecological service of Mount Sinai Hospital, New York, for the twelve years from January 1st, 1883, to December 31st, 1894.* New York, 1894.

GY45. WOOD, J. C. *A textbook of gynecology.* Philadelphia, 1894.

GY46. GARRIGUES, H. J. *A text-book of the diseases of women.* Philadelphia, 1894.

GY47. ROBINSON, F. B. *Landmarks in gynecology.* Detroit, 1894.

GY48. BYFORD, H. T. *Manual of gynecology.* Philadelphia, 1895.

GY49. KEATING, J. M and COE, H. C. *Clinical gynaecology, medical and surgical by eminent American teachers.* Philadelphia, 1895.

GY50. LONG, J. W. *Syllabus of gynecology based on the American text-book of gynecology.* Philadelphia, 1895.

GY51. SKENE, A. J. C. *Medical gynecology, a treatise on the diseases of women from the standpoint of the physician.* New York, 1895.

GY52. PENROSE, C. B. *Syllabus of the lectures on gynecology.* Philadelphia, 1896.

GY53. WELLS, W. H. *A compend of gynecology.* Philadelphia, 1896.

GY54. PENROSE, C. B. *A textbook of diseases of women.* Philadelphia, 1897.

GY55. DUDLEY, E. C. *Diseases of women; . . .* Philadelphia, 1898.

GY56. KELLY, H. A. *Operative gynecology.* New York, 1898.

UROLOGY

GU1. STEVENS, A. H. *Lectures on lithotomy.* New York, 1838.

GU2. DIXON, E. H. *A treatise on diseases of the sexual organs; . . .* New York, 1846.

GU3. BOSTWICK, H. *A treatise on the nature and treatment of seminal diseases, impotency, and other kindred affections: . . .* New York, 1847.

GU4. BOSTWICK, H. *A complete practical work on the nature and treatment of venereal diseases, and other affections of the genito-urinary organs of the male and female.* New York, 1848.

GU5. GROSS, S. D. *A practical treatise on the disease and injuries of the urinary bladder, the prostate gland, and the urethra.* Philadelphia, 1851.

GU6. GOLDSMITH, A. G. *Diseases of the genito-urinary organs.* New York, 1857.

GU6.1. MORLAND, W. W. *Diseases of the urinary organs; . . .* Philadelphia, 1858.

GU7. BUMSTEAD, F. J. *The pathology and treatment of venereal diseases: . . .* Philadelphia, 1861.

GU8. GOULEY, J. W. S. *Diseases of the urinary organs: . . .* New York, 1873.

GU9. VAN BUREN, W. H. and KEYES, E. L. *A practical treatise on the surgical diseases of the genito-urinary organs, including syphilis.* New York, 1874.

GU10. KING, J. *Urological dictionary: containing an explanation of numerous technical terms; . . .* Cincinnati, 1878.

GU11. OTIS, F. N. *Stricture of the male urethra, its radical cure.* New York, 1878.

GU12. KEYES, E. L. *The venereal diseases, including strictures of the male urethra.* New York, 1880.

GU13. GROSS, S. W. *A practical treatise on impotence, sterility, and allied disorders of the male sexual organs.* Philadelphia, 1881.

GU14. STEIN, A. W. *A study of tumors of the bladder, with original contributions and drawings.* New York, 1881.

GU15. HELMUTH, W. T. *Suprapubic lithotomy; . . .* New York, 1882.

GU16. FRANKLIN, E. C. *A manual of venereal diseases; . . .* Chicago, 1883.

GU17. OTIS, F. N. *Practical clinical lessons on syphilis and the genitourinary diseases.* New York, 1883.

GU18. BELFIELD, W. T. *Diseases of the urinary and male sexual organs.* New York, 1884.

GU19. WALKER, H. O. *The treatment of diseases of the bladder, prostate, and urethra.* Detroit, 1887.

GU20. KEYES, E.L. *The surgical diseases of the genito-urinary organs.* New York, 1888.

GU21. OTIS, F. N. *The male urethra, its diseases and reflexes.* Detroit, 1888.

GU22. WATSON, F. S. *The operative treatment of the hypertrophied prostate.* Boston, 1888.

GU23. WYMAN, H. C. *Diseases of the bladder and prostate.* Detroit, 1891.

GU24. CHETWOOD, C. H. *Genito-urinary and venereal diseases.* Philadelphia, 1892.

GU25. GOULEY, J. W. S. *Diseases of the urinary apparatus; phlegmasic affections.* New York, 1892.

GU26. LYDSTON, G. F. *Varicocele and its treatment.* Chicago, 1892.

GU27. LYDSTON, G. F. *Gonorrhoea and urethritis.* Detroit, 1892.

GU28. LYDSTON, G. F. *Stricture of the urethra.* Chicago, 1893.

GU29. MORROW, P. A. *A system of genito-urinary diseases, syphilology and dermatology.* New York, 1893–94.

GU30. CARLETON, B. G. *A manual of genito-urinary and venereal diseases.* New York, 1895.

GU31. MARTIN, E. *Impotence and sexual weakness in the male and female.* Detroit, 1895.

GU32. FULLER, E. *Disorders of the male sexual organs.* Philadelphia, 1895.

GU33. TAYLOR, R. W. *The pathology and treatment of venereal diseases.* Philadelphia, 1895.

GU34. STEWART, R. W. *The diseases of the male urethra.* New York, 1896.

GU35. DOUGHTY, F. E. *A practical working handbook in the diagnosis and treatment of diseases of the genito-urinary system and syphilis.* Philadelphia, 1897.

GU36. SENN, N. *Tuberculosis of the genito-urinary organs, male and female.* Philadelphia, 1897.

GU37. TAYLOR, R. W. *A practical treatise on sexual disorders of the male and female.* Philadelphia, 1897.

GU38. WHITE, J. W. and MARTIN, E. *Genito-urinary surgery and venereal diseases.* Philadelphia, 1897.

GU39. BANGS, L. B. and HARDAWAY, W. A. *An American textbook of genito-urinary diseases, syphilis and diseases of the skin.* Philadelphia, 1898.

GU40. CARLETON, B. G. *Medical and surgical diseases of the kidneys and ureters.* New York, 1898.

GU41. CARLETON, B. G. *A practical treatise on the sexual disorders of men.* New York, 1898.

GU42. PHILLIPS, G. M. *A handbook of genito-urinary surgery and venereal diseases.* St. Louis, 1898.

GU43. WAITE, K. B. *A textbook of genito-urinary surgery.* Cleveland, 1898.

GU44. KIRBY, E. R. *Manual of genito-urinary diseases.* Philadelphia, 1899.

GU45. LYDSTON, G. F. *The surgical diseases of the genito-urinary tract, venereal and sexual diseases.* Philadelphia, 1899.

GU46. MORGAN, A. R. *Repertory of the urinary organs and prostate gland, including condylomata.* Philadelphia, 1899.

COLON AND RECTAL SURGERY

CR1. BUSHE, G. M. *A treatise on the malformations, injuries, and diseases of the rectum and anus (plus atlas).* New York, 1837.

CR2. BODENHAMER, W. *Practical observations on some of the diseases of the rectum, anus, and contiguous textures; . . .* Cincinnati, 1847.

CR3. BODENHAMER, W. *A practical treatise on the etiology, pathology, and treatment of the congenital malformations of the rectum and anus.* New York, 1860.

CR4. BODENHAMER, W. *Practical observations on the etiology, pathology, diagnosis, and treatment of anal fissure.* New York, 1868.

CR5. BODENHAMER, W. *The physical exploration of the rectum; with an appendix on the ligation of haemorrhoidal tumours.* New York, 1870.

CR6. VAN BUREN, W. H. *Lectures upon diseases of the rectum.* New York, 1870.

CR7. BODENHAMER, W. *An essay on rectal medication.* New York, 1878.

CR8. BRINKERHOFF, A. W. *Diseases of the rectum and new method of rectal treatment.* Columbus, 1881.

CR9. KELSEY, C. B. *Diseases of the rectum and anus.* New York, 1882.

CR10. AYRES, M. *Some of the diseases of the rectum and their homeopathic and surgical treatment.* Chicago, 1884.

CR11. BODENHAMER, W. *A theoretical and practical treatise on the hemorrhoidal disease, . . .* New York, 1884.

CR12. KELSEY, C. B. *The pathology, diagnosis, and treatment of diseases of the rectum and anus.* New York, 1884.

CR13. WRIGHT, J. W. *Lectures on diseases of the rectum.* New York, 1884.

CR14. KELSEY, C. B. *The diagnosis and treatment of haemorrhoids; . . .* Detroit, 1887.

CR15. ANDREWS, E. and ANDREWS, E. W. *Rectal and anal surgery, with a description of the secret methods of the itinerants.* Chicago, 1888.

CR16. GUERNSEY, W. J. *The homoeopathic therapeutics of hemorrhoids.* Philadelphia, 1882.

CR17. **ADLER, L. H.** *Fissure of the anus and fistula in ano.* Detroit, 1892.

CR18. **MATHEWS, J. M.** *A treatise on diseases of the rectum, anus, and sigmoid flexure.* New York, 1892.

CR19. **BRINKERHOFF, A. W.** *Haemorrhoids (piles), rectal ulcer, fistula in ano, fissure, pruritus, polypus recti, stricture, &c., &c; . . .* Chicago, 1895.

CR20. **GANT, S. G.** *Diagnosis and treatment of diseases of the rectum, anus, and contiguous textures.* Philadelphia, 1896.

CR21. **KELSEY, C. B.** *Surgery of the rectum and pelvis.* New York, 1897.

CR22. **KELSEY, C. B.** *The office treatment of hemorrhoids, fistula, etc. without operation.* New York, 1898.

NEUROLOGICAL SURGERY

NS1. **ROBERTS, J. B.** *The field and limitation of the operative surgery of the human brain.* Philadelphia, 1885.

NS2. **CLEVENGER, S. V.** *Spinal concussion: . . .* Philadelphia, 1889.

NS3. **WATSON, B. A.** *An experimental study of lesions arising from severe concussions.* Philadelphia, 1890.

NS4. **KNAPP, P. C.** *The pathology, diagnosis, and treatment of intracranial growths.* Boston, 1891.

NS5. **STARR, M. A.** *Brain surgery.* New York, 1893.

NS6. **PHELPS, C.** *Traumatic injuries of the brain and its membranes, with a special study of pistol-shot wounds of the head in their medico-legal and surgical relations.* New York, 1897.

References

I. BIBLIOGRAPHIES:

American College of Surgeons. *A catalogue of the H. Winnett Orr historical collection.* Chicago: American College of Surgeons, 1960.

Austin, Robert B. *Early American medical imprints: a guide to works printed in the United States, 1668–1820.* Washington, DC: U.S. Department of Health, Education, and Welfare, 1961.

Cordasco, Francesco. *American medical imprints, 1820–1910.* Totowa, NJ: Rowan & Littlefield, 1985.

Fulton, John F. and Stanton, Madeline E. *The centennial of surgical anesthesia: an annotated catalogue of books and pamphlets bearing on the early history of surgical anesthesia.* New York: Henry Schuman, 1946.

Guerra, Francisco. *American medical bibliography, 1639–1783.* New York: Lathrop C. Harper, 1962.

Index catalogue of the library of the Surgeon-General's Office, 1st series. 16 vols. Washington, DC: U.S. Government Printing Office, 1880–95.

Index catalogue of the library of the Surgeon-General's Office, 2d series. 21 vols. Washington, DC: U.S. Government Printing Office, 1896–1916.

Index catalogue of the library of the Surgeon-General's Office, 3d series. 5 vols. Washington, DC: U.S. Government Printing Office, 1918–25.

Morton, Leslie T. *A medical bibliography (Garrison and Morton): an annotated check-list of texts illustrating the history of medicine.* Hampshire, Great Britain: Gower, 1983.

II. BIOGRAPHICAL COMPILATIONS:

Anonymous. *Biographies of physicians and surgeons.* Chicago: J. H. Beers, 1904.

Atkinson, William B. *The physicians and surgeons of the United States.* Philadelphia: Charles Robson, 1878.

—. *A biographical dictionary of contemporary American physicians and surgeons.* Philadelphia: D. G. Brinton, 1880.

Cleave, E. *Biographical cyclopaedia of homoeopathic physicians and surgeons.* Philadelphia: Galaxy, 1873.

Francis, Samuel W. *Biographical sketches of distinguished living New York surgeons.* New York: John Bradburn, 1866.

Gross, Samuel. *Lives of eminent American physicians and surgeons of the nineteenth century.* Philadelphia: Lindsay & Blakiston, 1861.

Holloway, Lisabeth M. *Medical obituaries, American physicians' biographical notices in selected medical journals before 1907.* New York: Garland, 1981.

Kaufman, Marvin; Galishoff, Stuart; and Savitt, Todd L. *Dictionary of American medical biography.* Westport, CT: Greenwood Press, 1984.

Kelly, Howard A. *A cyclopedia of American medical biography comprising the lives of eminent deceased physicians and surgeons from 1610 to 1910.* Philadelphia: W. B. Saunders, 1912.

Kelly, Howard A. and Burrage, Walter L. *American medical biographies.* Baltimore: Norman & Remington, 1920.

—. *Dictionary of American medical biography; lives of eminent physicians of the United States and Canada, from the earliest times.* New York: D. Appleton, 1928.

Leonardo, Richard. *Lives of master surgeons.* New York: Froben Press, 1948.

Stone, Richard F. *Biography of eminent American physicians and surgeons.* Indianapolis: Carlon & Hollenbeck, 1894.

—. *Biography of eminent American physicians and surgeons.* Indianapolis: C. E. Hollenbeck, 1898.

Surgery, gynecology, and obstetrics. From 1922 through 1939, this monthly journal ran a series entitled "Master Surgeons of America," which included more than 150 biographies of American surgeons.

Thacher, James. *American medical biography: or memoirs of eminent physicians who have flourished in America.* Boston: Richardson & Lord and Cottons & Barnard, 1828.

Watson, Irving A. *Physicians and surgeons of America: a collection of biographical sketches of the regular medical profession.* Concord, MA: Republican Press Association, 1896.

Willard, Sylvester D. *Annals of the Medical Society of the County of Albany, 1806–1851; with biographical sketches of deceased members.* Albany, NY: J. Munsell, 1864.

Williams, Stephen. *American medical biography: or, memoirs of eminent physicians, embracing principally those who have died since the publication of Dr. Thacher's work on the same subject.* Greenfield, MA: L. Merriam, 1845.

III. DIRECTORIES:

American Medical Association. *Directory of American physicians, 1906.* Subsequent editions appeared every two, three, or four years.

Butler, Samuel W. *The medical register and directory of the United States.* Philadelphia: Office of the Medical and Surgical Reporter, 1874. A second, updated edition appeared in 1877.

Flint, J. B. *Medical and surgical directory of the United States.* New York: J. B. Flint, 1897.

Polk, R. L. *Medical and surgical register of the United States.* Detroit: R. L. Polk, 1886. Later editions appeared in 1890, 1893, 1896, 1898, 1900, 1902, 1904, and 1906.

IV. NECROLOGICAL LISTINGS:

Biographical cyclopedia of homeopathic physicians and surgeons. Chicago: American Homeopathic Biographical Association, 1893.

Transactions of the American Institute of Homeopathy, 1895. Pages 1092–1101.

Transactions of the American Institute of Homeopathy, 1906. Pages 879–95.

Transactions of the American Medical Association. Beginning in 1850 with volume 3, *Transactions* published obituaries together with a yearly index.

V. HISTORIES OF SURGERY (BOOKS AND BOOK CHAPTERS):

American Association of Genito-urinary Surgeons. *A brief history of the organization and transactions of the American Association of Genito-urinary surgeons; October 16th, 1886 to October 16th, 1911.* New York: private printing, 1911.

American Otological Society. *History of the American Otological Society, Inc.* New York: American Otological Society, 1968.

American Urological Association. "Early history of urology in the United States." In *History of urology,* vol. 1, pp. 1–120. Baltimore: Williams & Wilkins, 1933.

Berman, Jacob K. *The Western Surgical Association, 1891–1900; impressions and selected transactions.* Indianapolis: Hackett, 1976.

Billings, John S. "The history and literature of surgery." In *The system of surgery,* edited by Frederic Dennis, vol. 1, pp. 17–144. Philadelphia: Lea Brothers, 1895.

Blaisdell, Frank. *One hundred years of New Hampshire surgery, 1800–1900.* Goffstown, NH: private printing, 1907.

Conway, H. and Stark R. B. *Plastic surgery at the New York Hospital one hundred years ago with biographical notes on Gurdon Buck.* New York: Paul B. Hoeber, 1953.

Earle, A. Scott. *Surgery in America: from the colonial era to the twentieth century, selected writings.* Philadelphia: W. B. Saunders, 1965.

—. *Surgery in America: from the colonial era to the twentieth century.* New York: Praeger, 1983.

Franklin, Edward Carroll. "Surgery in the United States." In *The science and art of surgery, embracing minor and operative surgery; compiled from standard allopathic authorities, and adapted to homoeopathic therapeutics, with a general history of surgery from the earliest periods to the present time,* pp. 25–41. St. Louis: Missouri Democrat Book and Job Print, 1867–73.

Garrison, Fielding H. "American surgery." In *An introduction to the history of medicine with medical chronology, suggestions for study, and bibliographic data,* pp. 498–512, 598–601, and 730–34. Philadelphia: W. B. Saunders, 1929.

Gross, Samuel D. *Report on Kentucky surgery.* Louisville: Webb and Levering, 1853.

Hubbell, Alvin A. *The development of ophthalmology in America, 1800 to 1870.* Chicago: W. T. Keener, 1908.

Kelly, Howard A. "Medicine in America." In *A cyclopedia of American medical biography comprising the lives of eminent deceased physicians and surgeons from 1610 to 1910,* pp. 11–85. Philadelphia: W. B. Saunders, 1912.

Leonardo, Richard A. "American Surgery." In *History of surgery,* pp. 297–331. New York: Froben Press, 1948.

Marr, James Pratt. *Pioneer surgeons of the Woman's Hospital; the lives of Sims, Emmet, Peaslee, and Thomas.* Philadelphia: F. A. Davis, 1957.

Moore, Francis D. "American surgery, progress over two centuries." In *Advances in American medicine: essays at the bicentennial,* edited by John Z. Bowers and Elizabeth F. Purcell, vol. 2, pp. 614–84. New York: Josiah Macy, 1976.

Mumford, James G. "American surgery." In *Surgical memoirs and other essays,* pp. 72–93. New York: Moffat & Yard, 1908.

Organ, Claude and Kosiba, Margaret. *A century of black surgeons: the U.S.A. experience.* Norman, OK: Transcript Press, 1987.

Pool, Eugene H. and McGowan, Frank J. *Surgery at the New York Hospital one hundred years ago.* New York: Paul B. Hoeber, 1929.

Ravitch, Mark M. *A century of surgery, the history of the American Surgical Association.* Philadelphia: J. B. Lippincott, 1981.

Ricci, James V. "The rise of American gynaecology." In *One hundred years of gynaecology, 1800–1900,* pp. 38–47. Philadelphia: Blakiston, 1945.

Shands, Alfred Rives. *The early orthopaedic surgeons of America.* St. Louis: C. V. Mosby, 1970.

Smith, Henry H. "Historical record of American surgery." In *A system of operative surgery: based upon the practice of surgeons in the United States*, pp. 17–111. Philadelphia: Lippincott & Grambo, 1852.

—. "A bibliographical index of American surgical writers from the year 1783 to 1860." In *The principles and practice of surgery*, pp. 33–61. Philadelphia: J. B. Lippincott, 1863.

Smith, Stephen. "The evolution of American surgery." In *American practice of surgery*, edited by Joseph D. Bryant and Albert Buck, vol. 1, pp. 3–67. New York: William Wood, 1906–11.

Sparkman, Robert S. and Shires, G. Tom. *Minutes of the American Surgical Association, 1880–1968*. Dallas: Taylor Publishing, 1972.

Speert, Harold. *Obstetrics and gynecology in America: a history*. Chicago: American College of Obstetricians and Gynecologists, 1980.

Stevens, Audrey. *American pioneers in abdominal surgery*. Melrose, MA: American Society of Abdominal Surgeons, 1968.

Thacher, James. "History of medicine in America." In *American medical biography: or memoirs of eminent physicians who have flourished in America*, pp. 9–85. Boston: Richardson & Lord and Cottons & Barnard, 1828.

Thoms, Herbert. *Chapters in American obstetrics*. Springfield, MA: Charles C Thomas, 1933.

Whipple, Allen O. *The evolution of surgery in the United States*. Springfield, MA: Charles C Thomas, 1963.

VI. HISTORIES OF SURGERY (PERIODICAL LITERATURE):

Brieger, Gert H. A portrait of surgery: surgery in America, 1875–1889. *Surgical clinics of North America* 67 1987: 1181–1216.

—. American surgery and the germ theory of disease. *Bulletin of the history of medicine* 40 1966: 135-45.

Dennis, Frederic. The achievements of American surgery. *Medical record* (NY) 42 1892: 637–48.

Gross, Samuel D. A century of American surgery. *American journal of the medical sciences* 71 1876: 431–84.

Hall, Courtney. The rise of professional surgery in the United States: 1800–1865. *Bulletin of the history of medicine* 26 1952: 231–62.

Rutkow, Ira M. American surgical biographies. *Surgical clinics of North America* 67 1987: 1153–180.

—. I. Reference works related to United States surgical history. II. A chronologic bibliography of American textbooks, monographs, and treatises relating to the surgical sciences, 1775–1900. *Surgical clinics of North America* 67 1987: 1127–152.

Shrady, George. American achievements in surgery. *The forum* 17 1894: 167–78.

Souchon, Edmund. Original contributions of America to medical sciences. *Transactions of the American Surgical Association* 35 1917: 65–171.

Tinker, Martin B. America's contributions to surgery. *Johns Hopkins Hospital bulletin* 13 1902: 209–13.

VII. GENERAL HISTORIES OF MEDICINE:

Bordley, James and Harvey, A. McGehee. *Two centuries of American medicine, 1776–1976.* Philadelphia: W. B. Saunders, 1976.

Brieger, Gert. *Medical America in the nineteenth century.* Baltimore: Johns Hopkins Press, 1972.

Clarke, Edward H. *A century of American medicine, 1776–1876.* Philadelphia: H. C. Lea, 1876.

Fishbein, Morris. *A history of the American Medical Association, 1847 to 1947.* Philadelphia: W. B. Saunders, 1947.

Gross, Samuel D. *History of American medical literature from 1776 to the present time.* Philadelphia: Collins, 1876.

Haller, John. *American medicine in transition, 1840–1910.* Urbana, IL: University of Illinois, 1981.

King, W. H. *History of homeopathy and its institutions in America.* New York: Lewis, 1905.

Ludmerer, Kenneth. *Learning to heal: the development of American medical education.* New York: Basic Books, 1985.

Mumford, James. *A narrative of medicine in America.* Philadelphia: J. B. Lippincott, 1903.

Packard, Francis R. *History of medicine in the United States.* New York: P. B. Hoeber, 1931.

Rosenberg, Charles E. *The care of strangers: the rise of America's hospital system.* New York: Basic Books, 1987.

Rothstein, William. *American physicians in the nineteenth century.* Baltimore: Johns Hopkins Press, 1972.

Shafer, Henry B. *The American medical profession, 1783 to 1850.* New York: Columbia University, 1936.

Shryock, Richard H. *American medical research, past and present.* New York: Commonwealth Fund, 1947.

—. *Medicine in America: historical essays.* Baltimore: Johns Hopkins Press, 1966.

Sigerist, Henry E. *Amerika und die Medizin.* Leipzig: G. Thieme, 1933.

Starr, Paul. *The social transformation of American medicine.* New York: Basic Books, 1982.

Toner, Joseph M. *Contributions to the annals of medical progress and medical education in the United States before and during the War of Independence.* Washington, DC: U.S. Government Printing Office, 1874.

VIII. BIOGRAPHICAL DICTIONARIES:

Appleton's Cyclopedia of American Biography. 16 vols. New York: D. Appleton, 1887–89.

Dictionary of American Biography. 21 vols. plus supplements. New York: Scribner, 1943–.

National Cyclopedia of American Biography. 21 vols. New York: J. T. White, 1893–1927.

Index

A

Abdomen
affections of, GS39
kneading, GY16
relaxed, OR42
surgery on, GS118, GS136, GS170; GY56
"belly rippers" criticized, GS136
Deaver incision, GS170
observations about, GS67
lectures on, GS174
resume of experiences with, GS130
surgical anatomy of, GS184
surgical diagnosis of, GS94
tumors of, GS15
unusual problems of, GS41
wounds to, GS51
arrow, GS74
gunshot, GS81, GS147
healing of by first intention, GS169
penetrating, GS1
treatment of, GS190
The abdominal brain and automatic visceral ganglia
(Robinson), GS149
Abdominal surgery (Wyman), GS136
Abdominal tumors, GS15
Abdominal viscera, diseases of, GS18
Abdominal wall, surgical anatomy of, GS184
Abdominotomy, GY37
Ablation of the tonsils, in diphtheria, GS53.1
Abnormalities, encyclopedic collection of, OP42. *See also*
Deformities
Abortion
as gynecology landmark, GY47
Keating disclaimer on, GY49
Abortion and its treatment . . . (Thomas), GY14
Abscess, GS7, GS23
anal-rectal, CR6
brain, NS5, OT65
genitourinary, GU4
in kidney of rabbit, GS173
milk abscess of breast, GY1
rectal, CR9, CR13
homeopathic treatment of, CR10
retro-pharyngeal, homeopathic view of, OT64.1
tubercular, OR36
Accidental injuries. *See* Injuries
Accommodation, OP75, OP79
errors of, OP23, OP38, OP48, OP60
correction of, OP33, OP57
osteopathic treatment of, OP83
therapeutics for, OP37

homeopathic view of, OP75
Acetabulum, accessory Y ligament of, hip dislocation
and, OR22
Acoustic nerve, diseases of, OT37
Actinomycosis, GS144
Adams, J. Howe, on Agnew, GS88
Addresses and essays (Lydston), GU26
Addresses and other papers (Keen), GS154
Adler, Lewis H.
on anal fistula and fissure, CR17
on anesthesia, GS151
Adolescents, diseases of heart and circulation in, GY49
The advantages and accidents of artifical anaesthesia
(Turnbull), GS93
Advertising, reactions to, CR19
Agassiz, Louis, LeConte and, OP30
Agnew, Cornelius Rea, Loring and, OP25
Agnew, David Hayes
biography of, GS88
Martin and, GS134
in multiauthor text, GS100
on perineal lacerations and vesico-vaginal fistula, GY19
surgical treatise by, GS88
Young book dedicated to, OR51
Air-passages
See also Respiratory tract
acute and chronic inflammation of, OT26
catarrhal inflammation of, OT26
foreign bodies in, GS34
malignant follicular disease of, OT1
Air pressure variations, experimental research on, GS183
Albany Medical college, Herrick at, GS186
Albertype, as frontispiece, OP45
Albion College, Walker degree from, GU19
Albumen photography, early use of, GS69
Albuminuria, ophthalmoscopy and, OP18
Alcohol
diphtheria and, GY17
in preparation of medicines, GS26
toxic amblyopia and, OP67
Alden, Walter, OP15.1
Alexander, Samuel, GU29
Alexian Brothers Hospital (Chicago)
Clevenger at, NS2
Wood at, OP50
Alimentary system
anatomy of, GS141
physiology of digestion, GS9
Alimentation, rectal, CR9
Allen, Dudley P., GY49
Allen, Harrison, OT70
Allen, Samuel Ellsworth, OT54

Fractures of the elbow joint (Ela), OR29
Fractures of the lower extremity or base of the nadius
    (Pilcher), GS114
Francis, Samuel Ward, GS47
Franklin, Edward Carroll
    on homeopathic treatment of spinal curvature, OR35
    lectures on surgery by, GS108
    on minor surgery, GS107
    on science and art of surgery, GS65
    on venereal diseases, GU16
Fraud, Buchanan involvement in, GS52
French Hospital (San Francisco), Brigham at, GS82
French authors, in multiauthor texts, GS100; OP73
French orthopedic surgery, OR4
French urology, errors of, GU11
Fresh air, with Swedish movement therapy, OR12
Frick, George, OP1
Frost-bite, GS158
Fuller, Eugene
    on genitourinary disease, GU32, GU39
    on male sexual disorders, GU32
    on urine testing significance, GU29
The functional examination of the eye (Jackson), OP62
The fundus oculi of birds . . . (Wood), OP50
Fundus-reflex test, OP57
Furunculus, GS23

G

Galactocele, homeopathic view of, GU35
Gallaudet, Bern Budd, GS156
Gallstones, solvents on, GS167. *See also* Biliary calculi
Galvanic current, use of, OR10; GY40, GY42
Galvanism (Cleaveland), OR10
Ganglionectomy, for trigeminal neuralgia, GS89
Gangrene
    of foot, GS82
    hospital, GS50, GS70, GS113
        homeopathic view of, GS103
Gant, Jackson D., Samuel Gant work dedicated to, CR20
Gant, Samuel Goodwin, CR20
Garfield, President James, Agnew and, GS88
Garfield Hospital and Central Dispensary and Emergency
    Hospital (Washington, D.C.), Burnett at, OP41
Gargles, OT33
Garmany, Jasper Jewett, GS129
Garrigues, Henry Jacques
    on diseases of women, GY46
    on genital malformations, GY31
    on ovarian cysts, GY29
Gasserian ganglionectomy, GS89
Gastralgia, OR17
Gastrectomy, first in U.S., GY43
Gastro-elytrotomy, as cesarean section substitute, GY14
Gastroenterostomy, GS149
Gastrointestinal anastomosis, GS138
Gastrointestinal system
    anatomy of, GS141
    disturbances in, eyestrain as cause of, OP76
    injury to, testing for, GS139
Geddings, Eli, GS45
General and differential diagnosis of ovarian tumors . . .
    (Atlee), GY20

General health
    exercise and, GS123
    eye as aid to diagnosis in, OP74.1
    eye problems and, OP65
    eyestrain and, OP76
    home medical guides to, GU10, GU18
    preservation of, GS26
    for women, GS123
        education and, GY21
General Medical Board, Martin on, GY42
General medicine
    See also General practitioners; Medicine
    as applied to dentistry, OR56
    essays on, GS18
    Gould works on, OP42
    theory and practice of, GS18
General practitioners
    anatomy manual for, GS152
    electricity in surgery for, GS106
    gynecology for, GY48
    nasal catarrh treatments by, GS105
    nose and throat question-compends for, OP47
    ophthalmology for, OP31, OP34, OP38, OP42, OP47,
        OP50, OP52, OP53
        as aid to general diagnosis, OP74.1
        astigmatism text, OP41
        homeopathic view of, OP19, OP27, OP55, OP75
        on need for spectacles, OP43
        ophthalmoscopy and, OP68, OP74
        principles of spectacle correction, OP84
        outline of, OP26
        refraction guide, OP79
    orthopedic treatise for, OR14
    otology for, OP31
    rectal diseases and, CR15, CR17
    surgery for, GS72, GS138, GS156, GS180
        diagnosis and treatment, GS179
        for traumatic brain injuries, NS6
    tumor text for, GS168
    urology for, GU24
        genitourinary diseases, GU24, GU45
        homeopathic view of, GU16
        sexual disorders, GU13, GU37, GU45
        sterility, GU13
        venereal diseases, GU16, GU24, GU45
    venereal disease guide for, GU12, GU16
General surgery, GS12, GS22, GS27, GS118
    See also Anesthesia; Antiseptic surgery; Aseptic surgery;
        Operative surgery; Surgery; *specific types of surgery*
    blood pressure in, GS182
    complications of. See Postoperative complications
    essays on, GS18
    experimentation in, GS182
    exposure techniques, GS8
    first American works on, GS1, GS3
    first operation using anesthesia, GS26
    history of. *See* History of medicine and surgery
    lectures on, GS45, GS158, GS162, GS177, GS185
        syllabus of, GS38
    manual of, GU44
    minor. *See* Minor surgery
    orthopedic surgery and, OR58

Massage, pelvic, GY55
Mastication, in digestive process, GS9
The mastodon giganteus of North America (Warren), GS26
Mastoid
 affections of, OT37
 diseases of, OT23, OT30, OT51, OT64
 surgery on, OT54, OT56, OT64
  first U.S., OT12
The mastoid operation . . . (Allen), OT54
Masturbation, GU37
 excessive, GS73
 surgical treatment of, GU2
Materia medica, NS2
 See also Formularies; Medications; Therapeutics
 American eclectic, GY8
 Cook on, GS42
 cyclopedia of, OP42
 elementary text of, GY32
 handbook on, GS24
 homeopathic, OP24, OP27, OP55; GU30
 index of, GY30
 ophthalmologic, OP78
 therapeutics and, GS18
 urological, GU30
Maternity Hospital. *See* New York Maternity Hospital
Mathews, Joseph McDowell, CR18
Mathews's medical quarterly, CR18
Mütter lectures
 on inflammation, GS59
 on surgical pathology, GS153
Maxillary nerve, superior, first excision of, GS40
Mayall, J. R., early photos by, OR34
May, Charles Henry, GY30
The meaning and method of life . . . (Gould), OP42
Mears, James Ewing, GS89
Mechanical aids in the treatment of chronic . . . disease (Taylor), GS123
Mechanical appliances. *See* Equipment; Mechanical therapeutics
Mechanical causes of disease, OR16
Mechanical or conservative surgery, OR16
Mechanical photography, GS76, GS82. *See also* Woodburytypes
Mechanical therapeutics, OR20
 See also Movement therapy
 for bony lesions of hip, OR41
 for dislocations, GS25
 for fractures, GS25
 for hip disease, OR30
 Lee and, OR17
 for Pott's disease, OR36
 for spinal curvatures, OR35
 for spinal diseases and deformities, OR17
 Taylor as advocate of, GS123
Mechanical therapeutics . . . (Wales), OR20
On the mechanical treatment of disease of the hip-joint (Taylor), OR30
The mechanics of surgery . . . (Truax), GS189
The mechanism of dislocation and fracture of the hip . . . (Bigelow), OR22
A mechanistic view of war and peace (Crile), GS182
Mechano-movement cure. *See* Movement therapy
Medical anomalies and curiosities, OP42

Medical bulletin, Morris book reviewed in, GS125
Medical and Chirurgical Faculty of Maryland, Gibson as member of, OP2
Medical College of Georgia, Eve at, GS41
Medical College of Ohio
 See also Ohio Medical University
 Blackman at, GS51
 Byford degree from, GY10
 Conner at, GS185
 Gilliam degree from, GS110
 Goldsmith at, GU6
 Prince at, OR14
 Tripler lectures at, GS51
Medical College of South Carolina
 Chisolm at, GS48
 Geddings at, GS45
 Scheppegrell degree from, OT67
 Thomas degree from, GY14
Medical College of Toledo, Robinson at, GS149
Medical College of Virginia, Long at, GY50
Medical compendium on all . . . female and children, eye, ear, nose and throat diseases (Naulteus), OT72
Medical dictionaries. *See* Dictionaries
Medical education, diatribe against, GU2
Medical electricity . . . (Tousey), GY39
Medical ethics, conversations on, GS50
Medical Gazette, Wright lectures in, CR13
Medical gynecology, GY35, GY35.1, GY51, GY56
Medical gynecology . . . (Skene), GY51
Medical illustration, Broedel and, GY56
The medical investigator, Gilchrist as editor of, GS78
Medical jurisprudence. *See* Legal aspects of medicine
Medical jurisprudence of insanity . . . (Clevenger), NS2
The medical men of New Jersey (Clark), OP12
Medical news, Gould as editor of, OP41
Medical record of New York, Hutchison papers in, OR38
Medical research and human welfare . . . (Keen), GS154
Medical sketches of the campaigns of 1812, 13, 14 (Mann), GS4
Medical Society of Norway, Emmet in, GY13
The medical student's guide . . . (Chase), GS14
Medical and surgical cases and observations (Atkins), GS10
Medical and surgical diseases of the kidneys and ureters (Carleton), GU40
Medical and surgical history of the War of the Rebellion (Barnes), GS68
 catalogue descriptions and, GS64
 reconstructive surgery case in, GS83
Medical and surgical reporter, on perineal lacerations, GY19
The medical and surgical uses of electricity (Rockwell), GY38
Medical terminology, Cleaveland on, OR10. *See also* Dictionaries
Medications
 See also Formularies; Materia medica; Therapeutics
 alcohol in, GS26
 amblyopias induced by, OP67, OP73
 American medical botanists, GY56
 botanic, GS28, GS52
 dietetic and remedial, GS90
 for ear problems, OP37; OT60
 earth, GS76
 in eclectic medicine, GS28; GY8; GU10
 electric diffusion of, GS172

for eye problems, OP15, OP37, OP38
    spectacles vs., OP3
homeopathic. *See* Homeopathic medicine; Materia
    medica
hypodermic injection of, for neuralgia, rheumatism,
    and gout, OT9
inhalation of, OT8, OT46; GY8
King introduction of, GU10
medical therapeutics, GS90
morphine, GS81
for nose and throat diseases, OT33, OT35, OT69
physiomedical, GS42
popular medicine handbook, GS90
practical therapeutics, GS105
rectal, CR7
skin eruptions from, GU29
surgical use of, GS90
tonics, OR42
Medicine
    See also General medicine
    anomalies and curiosities of, OP42
    cyclopedia of, OP42
    history of. *See* History of medicine and surgery
    mature, system of, OP64
    practice of. *See* Practice of medicine
Medico-Chirurgical College (Philadelphia)
    Gleason at, OT60
    Keyser at, OP14
    Kirby at, GU44
    Roberts at, GS102
Medico-legal problems. *See* Legal aspects of medicine
Medico-Legal Society of New York City, Peugnet address
    to, GS81
Medico-surgical aspects of the Spanish American War (Senn),
    GS138
Meigs, Arthur Vincent, GY5
Meigs, Charles Delucena, GY3, GY5
    Hodge text dedicated to, GY9
Meigs, John Forsyth, GY5
    Robinson book dedicated to, OT24
Meisenbach process, in Gerster book, GS133
Membrana tympani. *See* Eardrum (tympanum);
    Tympanic membrane
Membranous sore throat, OT26
Membranous textures, tumors of, GS15
A Memoir of Henry Jacob Bigelow (William Bigelow), OR4
Memoir of Jonathan Mason Warren, M.D., GS67
Memoirs of military surgery (Larrey), GS4
Memoir of Thomas Addis and Robert Emmet (Emmet), GY13
Memoir of Valentine Mott (Gross), GS16
Memorial oration in honor of Ephraim McDowell . . .
    (Gross), GS16
Men
    genitourinary disorders in, GU21
    See also Genitourinary system; *specific organs*
    surgery for, CR21
    surgical diagnosis of, GS94
    tuberculosis, GU36
    mammary gland tumors in, GS97
    sexual disorders in, GU36, GU41
    hygiene concerns, GS90
    medical counseling for, GS90
Meningitis, surgical treatment of, OT56

Menopause, GY51
Menstruation
    disorders of, GY25, GY30, GY35, GY46
        eclectic view of, GY37
    dysmenorrhoea, GY13
    as gynecology landmark, GY47
    menorrhagia, GY35
    uterine health shown by, GY12
Mental health profession, Clevenger blacklisted by, NS2
Mental affections, homeopathic view of, GS78; OP27. *See
    also* Hysteria; Insanity; Nervous affections
Merchant vessels
    passenger problems on, GS17
    color-blindness danger for, OP28, OP68
Mercury
    iritis treatment without, OP13
    for syphilis, GU9
Mercy Hospital (Chicago), Edward Andrews at, CR15
Mercy Hospital (Pittsburgh), Stewart at, GU34
Metatarsalgia, anterior, first complete description of, GS98
Methodist Episcopal Hospital (New York), Pilcher at,
    GS190
Metritis, GY22
Metropolitan Hospital (New York), Carleton at, GU30,
    GU40
Metropolitan Throat Hospital (New York), Kitchen at,
    OT35
Metrorrhagia, GY35, GY46
Metz, Abram, OP16
Meyer, Willy, GU29
Miami Medical College, Williams at, OT13
Michigan College of Medicine and Surgery, Wyman at,
    GS136, GU23
Michigan Homeopathic Medical Society, Wood and, GY45
Michigan, University of. *See* University of Michigan
Microcephalus, imbecility due to, NS5
Microorganisms, wound treatment and, GS190
The microscopist's companion . . . (King), GU10
Microscopy
    of breast tumors, GS97
    early textbook examples of, GS39
    of ear polyps, OT7
    guide to, OT21; GU10
    histological, GS22.1
        early preparations, GS110
    of kidney abscess in rabbit, GS173
    ophthalmic, OP32
    of urine, GU10
Micturition. *See* Urination
Middle age, vision problems in, OP12. *See also* Presbyopia
Midwifery, GS28
    See also Childbirth; Obstetrics
    antiseptic, GY29
    domestic handbook of, GY34
    eclectic view of, GS28
    essays on, GY1
    evolution to obstetrics from, GY1
    Philadelphia practice of, GY3
    texts on, GS2, GY9
The midwives monitor . . . (Seaman), GS2
Military hospitals, GS1
Military medical concerns, GS50, GS51
    See also Military surgery

eye problems and, OP65, OP76
familiar forms of, NS5
hearing and, OT30
homeopathic view of, GS7; OP27
movement therapy for, OR9
organic, NS5
orthopedic implications of, OR46
paralysis, GS123
in women, GY16, GY48
Nervous diseases. *See* Nervous affections
Nervous or hysterical rectum, CR18
Nervous prostration, eye-treatment of, OP76
Nervous supply, uterine diseases and, GY34
Nervous system
anatomy of, GS94, GS141
ocular, OP58
syphilis of, GU29
Neuralgia
of anus, CR2, CR6
in eye, OP4
eyestrain as cause of, OP76
facial, excision of superior maxillary nerve for, GS40
homeopathic view of, OP27
hypodermic injections for, OT9
of rectum, CR1, CR6, CR9
treatise on, GS121
Neurological disorders, electro-diagnosis of, NS2
Neurological signs, cerebral localization and, NS1
Neurological surgery
on brain, NS1, NS5
cerebral localization for, GS94; NS1, NS5
earliest American basic science research on, NS3
electrocoagulation in, GS106
first full-length American treatise on, NS5
intracranial growths, NS4
Neurology, anatomy for, GS152
Neuroses
functional, ocular muscle changes with, OP73
nose and throat diseases and, OT71
sexual, GU35
traumatic, NS2
first detailed study of, GS58
spinal concussion vs., NS2
Neurosurgery. *See* Neurological surgery
Nevus of face, congenital, GS82
New Aid Series, nose and throat text from, OT71
Newberry Library (Chicago), Senn library bequest to, GS138
A new classification of the motor anomalies of the eye . . . (Duane), OP72
Newcomb, James Edward, Burnett and, OT17
Newell, Otis Kimball, GS135
New England Hospital for Women and Children, Jeffries at, OP28
New England journal of medicine, predecessor of, GU6.1
The new local anaesthetic . . . (Turnbull), GS124
A new medical dictionary (Gould), OP42
A new pronouncing dictionary of medicine . . . (Keating), GY49
Newton, Robert S., GY8
New truths in ophthalmology (Savage), OP58
New York Academy of Medicine
Bedford and, GY6

Claiborne papers to, OP44
Grandin and, GY38
Ranney and, OP76
Roosa and, OP60
Simms address to, GS44
Taylor library donated to, GU37
unpublished Green autobiography at, OT1
New York Botanical Gardens, Allen and, OP24
New York, University of the City of. *See* University of the City of New York
New York City, day-to-day surgical practice in, GU2
New York City Commissioners of Health
Bryant as, GS116
Smith as, GS53
New York College of Dentistry, Stein at, GU14
New York College of Veterinary Surgery, Stein at, GU14
New York County Medical Society, Wagner paper to, OT31
New York Dispensary, Robert William Taylor at, OR31
New York Ear Dispensary, *See also* New York Eye and Ear Infirmary
New York Eye and Ear Infirmary
Buck at, OT23, OT68
Loring at, OP25
Mittendorf at, OP31, OP40
Noyes and, OP32, OP48
Post at, OP6
Sexton and, OT47, OT49
Weeks at, OT55
Wood at, OP50
New York Foundling Hospital, O'Dwyer at, OT52.1
New York gynecological and obstetrical journal, Skene as editor of, GY21
New York Homeopathic Medical College
Allen at, OP24; OT39
Buffum degree from, OP36
Carleton at, GU30
Doughty at, GU35
Helmuth at, GS36; GU15
Houghton at, OT39
Sterling at, OT45
New York Hospital
Buck at, GS83
Cornell University Medical School and, GS91
Jones and, GS1
Markoe at, OR28
Post at, OP6
Seaman at, GS2
Stevens at, GU1
Stimson at, GS91, OR45
surgical formulary for, GS2
New York Infirmary, Woman's Medical School of, Curtis at, GS180
New York Institution for the Blind, Wallace at, OP3
New York journal of homeopathy, Allen and, OP24
New York Laryngological Society
Bosworth and, OT18
Coakley and, OT69
Wagner and, OT38
New York Maternity Hospital
Garrigues at, GY29
Grandin at, GY38
New York Medical College

Ophthalmia, OP1
  sympathetic, OP32
Ophthalmic and Aural Institute of New York
  Duane at, OP72
  Knapp and, OP17; OT10
Ophthalmic Hospital (Heidelberg, Germany)
  Cole at, OP17
  Knapp at, OP17
Ophthalmic lenses. *See* Spectacle lenses
Ophthalmic lenses . . . (Prentice), OP45
Ophthalmic myology (Savage), OP58
Ophthalmic neuro-myology . . . (Savage), OP58
Ophthalmic operations as practiced on animal's eyes
  (Veasey), OP69
Ophthalmic and optic memoranda (Roosa and Ely), OP26
Ophthalmic record
  Savage as founder of, OP58
  Wood as editor of, OP50
Ophthalmic surgery, GS71; OP2, OP18, OP20, OP26,
    OP38, OP52, OP53, OP58, OP60
  brief description of, OP66
  common operations, OP73
  compend of, OP42
  eclectic manual on, OP22
  on eyelids, OP73
  first female eye surgeon, OP66
  homeopathic view of, OP19, OP36, OP75
  international authors on, OP73
  on ocular muscles, OP69, OP76, OP82
  surgical anatomy for, GS184
  system of, OP50
  text on, OP53
Ophthalmic surgery and treatment . . . (Phillips), OP18
Ophthalmic therapeutics, OP24, OP50
Ophthalmic therapeutics (Field and Norton), OP24
Ophthalmologists, diatribe against, OP80
Ophthalmology
  See also Eye; Ophthalmic surgery; *specific parts of eye*
  advances in, OP15
  Alt and, OP38
  clinical, OP53
  de Schweinitz and, OP52
  dictionary of, OP50
  encyclopedia of, OP50
  first American book on, OP1
  first American specialist in, OP1
  first female eye surgeon, OP66
  first non-allopathic text on, OP19
  for general practitioners. *See* General practitioners,
    ophthalmology for
  glossary of, OP79
  Gould and, OP42
  handbook on, OP52, OP74
  homeopathic view of. *See* Homeopathic medicine,
    ophthalmology
  international compendium on, OP73
  Knapp and, OT10
  new truths in, OP58
  Noyes and, OP32
  practical treatise on, OP42
  principles and practice of, OP52, OP53
  students' aid in, OP66
  text on, OP16, OP52, OP57, OP71

  homeopathic, OP19
  multiauthor, OT70
  Williams and, OP13
Ophthalmometry, OP71, OP79
  skiascopy vs., OP63
Ophthalmoscope, OP20, OP29, OP48, OP61, OP70, OP73
  discounting of, OP22, OP74
  early discussions of, OP13, OP15, OP18, OP27
  Hewsen as champion of, GS76
  history of, OP43
  homeopathic use of, OP19, OP35
  lectures on, OP46
  skiascopy vs., OP63
  text on, OP39
  theory of, OP39, OP44, OP52
  use of, OP44, OP47, OP52, OP57, OP77, OP79
    manual of, OP68
    for refraction, OP25
The ophthalmoscope (Loring), OP25
The ophthalmoscope . . . (Vilas), OP35
The ophthalmoscope and how to use it (Thorington), OP77
Opium, toxic amblyopia and, OP67
Optical instruments, OP66
Optical terms, glossary of, OP80
Optical truths (McCormick), OP80
Optician, OP54
Opticians, refraction guide for, OP79
Optic nerve, OP53, OP66
  atropy of, OP65
  diseases of, OP32, OP38, OP39
    homeopathic view of, OP36
    osteopathic view of, OP83
Optico-ciliary neurectomy, OP32
Optics, OP9, OP57, OP77
  practical, OP64
Optometry, OP54
  ophthalmoscopic, OP35
  Prentice as father of, OP45
Oral surgery (McCurdy), OR56
Orbit, OP53, OP66
  diseases of, OP4, OP32, OP38, OP60, OP73
    homeopathic view of, OP36
  surgical anatomy of, GS184
Orchidectomy, for hypertrophy of the prostate, GU38
Organic nervous diseases (Starr), NS5
Orgasm, first sexual therapy discussion on, GY46
Orificial surgery . . . (Pratt), GS131
The origin and nature of the emotions (Crile), GS182
Orphan Asylum (New York), Wallace at, OP3
Orr, Hiram Winnett, on Ridlon-Jones relationship, OR50
Orthopaedia . . . (Knight), OR42
Orthopaedic surgery (Lovett and Jones), OR47
Orthopedic Dispensary (Brooklyn), Hutchison at, OR38
Orthopedic pathology, OR51
Orthopedics . . . (Prince), OR14
Orthopedic surgery, OR46, OR51, OR54, OR55, OR56,
    OR57
  See also specific orthopedic problems
  on children, GS151
  conservative or expectant, OR42
  conservative or mechanical, OR16
  contributions to, OR50, OR57
  first chair in, OR24

Bushe at, CR1

S

Sachs, Bernard, GU29
Sacrum, artificial, OR35
Safety, color-blindness and, OP28, OP68
Sailor's physician (Parsons), GS17
St. Bartholomew's Hospital (London), hip dislocation
    specimen in, OR1
St. Elizabeth's Hospital (New York), Munde at, GY44
St. Francis Hospital (Jersey City, New Jersey), Watson at,
    OR44
St. Joseph's Hospital (New York), Miller at, OT55
St. Joseph's Hospital (Philadelphia), Keating at, GY49
St. Louis College of Homeopathic Physicians and
    Surgeons, Helmuth at, GS36
St. Louis University, Pope at, GS31
St. Luke's Hospital (New York)
    Bangs at, GU39
    Bumstead at, GU7
St. Mark's Hospital, Beck at, GS163
St. Martin, Alexis, as Beaumont's patient, GS9
St. Mary's Free Hospital for Children (New York), Poore
    at, OR43
St. Mary's Hospital (New York), Gant at, CR20
St. Mary's Infirmary (St. Louis), Henderson at, OP74
St. Paul's Infirmary (New York), Kelsey at, CR9
St. Vincent's Hospital (New York), Phelps at, NS6
St. Vitus's dance, eye-treatment of, OP76
Sajous, Charles Euchariste de Médicis
    on diseases of nose and throat, OT43
    on hay fever, OT44
    on nose and throat diseases, OT70
Salaries of military physicians, GS50
Salicylic acid, toxic amblyopia and, OP67
Saline, for circulatory collapse, GS182
Salivary fistula, GS60
Salpingectomy, CR21
Salter, Seaborn Freeman, GS115
Samuel D. Gross Prize essay, by Allis, OR52
Sands, Henry B., GS105
San Francisco City and County Hospital, Toland at, GS87
Sanitary Commission, essays for, GS57
Sanitary reform, Smith as pioneer in, GS53
Sapremia, GS185
Saratoga mineral waters, GS2
Sarcoma
    in breast, GS97
    of left upper jaw, Grover Cleveland's "secret"
        operation, GS116
    osteosarcoma, GS27
Sargent, Fitzwilliam, GS25
Sargent, John Singer, GS25
Saunders, W.B. & Co., multiauthor surgical text
    published by, GS154
Saunders's American Text-Book Series
    on eye, ear, nose, and throat diseases, OT70
    on genitourinary diseases, syphilis, and diseases of the
        skin, GU39
    on gynecology, GY43
        syllabus based on, GY50
    volumes listed, GY43, OT70

Saunders's New Aid Series
    on nose and throat diseases, OT71
    purpose of, GS159
    Question Compends Series and, GS159
    surgery manual in, GS159
Saunders's pocket medical lexicon . . . (Keating), GY49
Saunders's Question Compends Series
    on anatomy, GS126
    on ear diseases, OT60
    on essentials of surgery and bandaging, GS134
    format of, GS134
    on gynecology, GY36
    on minor surgery and bandaging, GS142
    New Aid Series and, GS159
    on nose and throat diseases, OP47
    popularity of, GS134
    on refraction errors and eye diseases, OP47
Savage, Giles Christopher, OP58
Sayre, Lewis Albert
    on chronic articular ostitis of the hip, OR48
    on clubfoot, OR24
    mention of, by Bradford and Lovett, OR46
    on orthopedic surgery and joint diseases, OR33
    Shaffer criticism of, OR36
    on spinal disease and spinal curvature, OR34
Scalds, GS23, GS145
Scalp
    surgical anatomy of, GS184
    wounds of, silver sutures for, GS44
The scalpel, Dixon as publisher of, GU2
Scalping, GS6
Scarification, GS21
Scarlatinal croup, OT40
Scarritt Training-School for Nurses (Kansas City), Gant at,
    CR20
Scenes in the practice of a New York surgeon (Dixon), GY2
Scheppegrell, William, OT67
Schirrus, GS3
School hygiene, OP73; OT19; OR38
School and industrial hygiene (Lincoln), OT19
Schwartz, Professor, OT54
Science and art of surgery (Franklin), GS107
A scientific man and the Bible (Kelly), GY56
Sclera, OP53, OP66
    diseases of, OP4, OP32, OP38, OP50, OP73
        homeopathic view of, OP36, OP75
        osteopathic view of, OP83
    surgery on, OP69
Sclerotic. *See* Sclera
Scoliosis, OR34
    plaster-of-paris support for, OR24
    Swedish movement therapy for, OR9
Scratches of a surgeon (Helmuth), GS36
Scribner's handbook series, on sight and hearing, OP12
Scrofula, surgical therapeutics, GS90
Scrotum
    diseases of, GU44
    elephantiasis of, GU35
    tumors in, GU42
Scudder, John Milton, GY8
    Hill work revised by, GS28
Sea-air and sea-bathing (Packard), GS54; OT19
Sea-bathing, problems from, GS54; OT19, OT49

478

V

Vermont Medical College, Brigham degree from, OT27
Vertigo, OT53
    aural, OT30
Vesical calculus, GU30, GU39
    treatment of, GU6.1
Vesical fistula, GU6.1
Vesical specula, GY56
Vesico-vaginal fistula, GY13, GY19, GY20, GY23, GS35
    operation for, GY20
    Sims and, GS44
A vest-pocket medical dictionary . . . (Buck), OT23
A vest-pocket medical lexicon . . . (Roosa), OT14
Victoria University (Toronto), Canniff at, GS61
Virginia, Medical College of, Long at, GY50
Virginia, University of, Claiborne degree from, OP44
Vilas, Charles Harrison
    on ear therapeutics, OP37
    on eye and ear diseases, OP49
    on eye therapeutics, OP37
    on ophthalmoscopy, OP35
    on spectacles, OP33
Visceral syphilis, GU29
Vision; its optical defects, and the adaptation of spectacles
        (Fenner), OP23
Vision, OP23, OP54, OP62, OP63
    See also Eye(s); Vision problems; Vision testing
    accommodation, OP15. *See also* Accommodation
    American Health Primer on, OT19
    binocular, OP30, OP48
    care of, OP29
    homeopathic view of, OP75
    monocular, OP30
    normal. *See* Emmetropia
    physical optics, OP23
    physiology of, OP29, OP30, OP51, OP53
    practical optics, OP64
    preservation and loss of, OP12
    preservation and restoration of, OP11
    principles of, OP52, OP75
    routine in eye-work, OP58
    school life and, OP29
Vision aids, OP33
    See also Spectacle lenses; Spectacles
    homeopathic view of, OP27
    proper use of, OP15.1
Vision problems, OP4, OP15.1, OP23, OP29, OP51,
        OP60, OP84
    accommodation errors. *See* Accommodation, errors of
    aemetropia (abnormal sight), OP54
    amaurosis, partial or incipient, OP10
    amblyopia, OP10
        toxic, OP67, OP73
    artificial light and, OP9, OP12
    asthenopia. *See* Asthenopia
    astigmatism. *See* Astigmatism
    blindness
        one-sided simulated, detection of, OP38
        statistics on, OP73
        from worms in eye, GS41
    color-blindness, OP28, OP54, OP68
        bibliography on, OP28
        dangers of, OP28, OP68
        detection of, OP38, OP68, OP73

    tests for compared, OP80
    diet and, OP9
    in elderly, OP12
    exercise and, OP9
    eye paralysis, OP50
    eyestrain as cause of, OP76
    farsightedness. *See* Hypermetropia; Hyperopia
    in middle age, OP12
    nearsightedness. *See* Myopia
    presbyopia. *See* Presbyopia
    prevention of, OP9
    refraction errors. *See* Refraction, errors of
    spectacles for. *See* Spectacles lenses; Spectacles
    squint, OP20, OP50
    strabismus. *See* Strabismus
    testing for. *See* Vision testing
    tobacco and, OP9
Visions: a study of false sight (pseudopia) (Clarke), OT7
Vision testing, OP54, OP76, OP80, OP84
    charts for, OP34, OP84. *See also* Vision testing,
        test-types
    for color-blindness, OP68, OP80
    concave mirror in, OP63
    description of, OP62
    diagrams for, OP34
    dioptrics, OP73, OP80
    homeopathic view of, OP27
    instruments for, OP15
    measurement of visual power, OP84
    methods compared, OP80
    mirrors in, OP63, OP77
    perimetery, OP71, OP79
    test-types, OP20, OP57, OP62
        history of, OP43
        Jaeger, OP23, OP62
        Snellen, OP23, OP36, OP54, OP62
Visual acuity, OP70
Visual field testing, OP71, OP79
Vitreous, OP53, OP66
    diseases of, OP32, OP38
        homeopathic view of, OP36
Vitreous humor, diseases of, OP4
Vitry, Benjamin A., plates by, GS5
Vocal cords
    removal of polyps from, OT8
    voice problems and, OT66
Voice
    American Health Primer on, OT19, OT20
    anatomy of vocal system, GS141
    care of, OT66
    causes of vocal disability, OT66
    hoarseness, OT36
    physiology of, OT21
The voice in speaking (Seiler), OT21
Vomiting, with spinal irritation, GY15
Von Graefe, Professor A., Keyser as follower of, OP14
von Mikulicz-Radecki, Johann, Newell as translator of,
        GS135
Von Tagen, Charles H., GS103
Vulva
    affections of, GY30, GY35
    diseases of, GY46
    traumatic lesions of, GY49

Norman Publishing is a division of Jeremy Norman & Company, Inc., leading international dealers in rare books and manuscripts in the history of medicine and science.

The following people have collaborated on the production of
The History of Surgery in the United States, 1775-1900, Vol. 1:

Steven Hiatt, Copy Editor
Diana Hook, Associate Editor
Peter Rutledge Koch, Designer
Elinor Lindheimer, Indexer
Jill Rotenberg, Project Manager

The layout was done by Donna Kelley at Zetatype Desktop Publishers of San Francisco, using Ventura Publisher.™ The type is Stone Serif, a Postscript® font from Adobe Systems.

Linotronic output by: Pinnacle Type, San Francisco

Printed and bound by: Braun-Brumfield, Ann Arbor